Workbook to accompany
Saunders Textbook of
MEDICAL ASSISTING

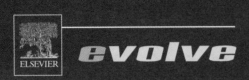

ELSEVIER

evolve

To access your Student Resources, visit the web address below:

http://evolve.elsevier.com/klieger/medicalassisting

- **Content updates**
  Updated with the most current information for medical assisting practice

- **Scored chapter quizzes**
  With answers and rationales for review of concepts

- **Internet research activities**
  To challenge and intrigue while broadening comprehension

- **WebLinks**
  Links to hundreds of websites carefully chosen to supplement the content of each chapter of the textbook; regularly updated, with new links added as they develop

Workbook to accompany
Saunders Textbook of
MEDICAL
ASSISTING

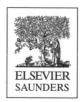

ELSEVIER
SAUNDERS

ELSEVIER
SAUNDERS

11830 Westline Industrial Drive
St. Louis, Missouri 63146

WORKBOOK TO ACCOMPANY
SAUNDERS TEXTBOOK OF MEDICAL ASSISTING   ISBN 0-7216-9575-2
Copyright © 2005 by Elsevier Inc.

NOTICE

International Standard Book Number 0-7216-9575-2

Publisher: Michael S. Ledbetter
Developmental Editor: Celeste Clingan
Publishing Services Manager: Patricia Tannian
Project Manager: Sarah Wunderly
Designer: Kathi Gosche

Printed in United States

Last digit is the print number: 9 8 7 6 5 4 3 2 1

To the Student

This workbook is designed to help you apply and master key concepts and skills presented in *Saunders Textbook of Medical Assisting*. Completing the variety of exercises in each chapter in this workbook will help reinforce the material you have studied in the textbook and learned in class.

You'll find exercises specially tailored to help you master objectives in both the theory and practice of medical assisting:

- A **vocabulary review** begins each chapter. This includes a comprehensive list of important words in each chapter and tests your knowledge of their definitions.

- **Skills application exercises** encourage you to put concepts into practice.

- A variety of questions test your knowledge of concepts in the book, including **matching**, **true-false**, and **multiple choice** questions.

- **Short answer** response questions apply what you've learned to a variety of situations.

- **Critical thinking exercises** take information presented in the textbook to the next level and prepare you for the real world through patient case scenarios.

- **Internet exercises** guide you in finding answers to current, important patient care and health issues facing the medical community today. You'll gain valuable knowledge and hone your skills in finding high quality medical information using the Internet.

- **Chapter quizzes** help reinforce what you learned from the textbook.

- **Skills competency checklists** help you monitor your progress and can be used by your instructor to evaluate your competency. These are designed to accompany the skills presented in the textbook.

Best wishes as you begin your journey to becoming a medical assistant.

Contents

SECTION VI • **Employment and Beyond**

Procedure Checklists

Workbook to accompany
Saunders Textbook of
MEDICAL ASSISTING

CHAPTER ONE

Becoming a Successful Student

VOCABULARY REVIEW

Matching: Match each term with the correct definition.

A. attitude

B. concept map

C. day planner

D. goals

E. habit

F. mnemonic device

G. prioritize

H. short-term memory

I. time management

J. Venn diagram

_____ 1. Diagram using circles to represent concepts; overlapping areas of the circles represent similarities between concepts, whereas the other areas represent differences.

_____ 2. Memory that holds a small amount of information for a short time

_____ 3. Set of beliefs one holds about something

_____ 4. Organizational system for planning and recording deadlines, tasks to be completed, events, and other activities

_____ 5. Established pattern of thinking or behaving

_____ 6. To decide which situation requires the most attention; to organize tasks or activities according to their level of importance

_____ 7. Drawing that uses words to describe and define a main idea. Relationships between items are shown by connecting them with lines or arrows.

_____ 8. Organization of time to accomplish your goals; the choices that are made about how time is used

_____ 9. Plans that are developed to reach one's mission in life; includes long-term plans and short-term plans

_____ 10. Creative device used to aid memory

1

THEORY RECALL

True/False

Indicate whether the sentence or statement is true or false.

_____ 1. Information stored in long-term memory can be recalled throughout your lifetime.

_____ 2. If you manage your time efficiently, you will not need to delegate tasks to others.

_____ 3. Planning one's time to meet established goals is a skill. It takes patience and practice.

_____ 4. Being organized is often an accident.

_____ 5. It is recommended that a 20-minute break after 3 hours of study is most effective and will prepare your mind to retain more information.

Multiple Choice

Identify the letter of the choice that best completes the statement or answers the question.

1. One way to start setting your goals is to develop a(n) _____.
   A. mind map
   B. personal mission statement
   C. anticipation guide
   D. learning log

2. SQ3R is a method used to increase reading comprehension. The second R stands for _____.
   A. recite
   B. read
   C. review
   D. recover

3. To determine your background knowledge of a subject, do all of the following EXCEPT _____.
   A. use an anticipation guide
   B. take a pretest
   C. surf the Internet
   D. read the chapter objectives and see how many you know or are able to do

4. Answering questions such as "What do I want to know about a subject?" and "What have I learned about the subject?" is an example of
   A. SQ3R
   B. KWL
   C. LAB RAT
   D. matrixing

5. _____ is (are) a simplified method of outlining that help(s) you make connections between the concepts presented in lecture and/or reading material.
   A. KWL
   B. SQ3R
   C. Venn diagram
   D. Power notes

6. _____ is (are) another way to create variety and interest as you write and helps you plug concepts into long-term memory.
   A. KWL
   B. RAFTs
   C. Learning logs
   D. SQ3R

7. One of the most common methods of _____ learning is simply asking questions.
   A. actively
   B. memorizational
   C. inadequate
   D. repetitive

8. The use of _____ can help you learn and can prove to be beneficial discussion time.
   A. partnered reading
   B. prediction questions
   C. learning logs
   D. concept maps

9. Step 1 of preparing effectively for a test is to _____.
   A. get adequate sleep and rest the night before the examination
   B. take a deep breath and relax
   C. start early
   D. review how you did on your last exam

10. _____ is most essential to a well-functioning brain.
    A. Breakfast
    B. Protein
    C. Water
    D. Sugar

11. Feedback comes from your instructor in several ways, including all of the following EXCEPT _____.
    A. homework assignments
    B. grades
    C. written/oral communication
    D. facial expressions

12. To change or break a habit, the habit must be replaced and consistently repeated for _____.
    A. 10 to 15 days
    B. 21 to 28 days
    C. 1 to 2 weeks
    D. 6 to 8 weeks

13. One method for choosing goals is by being _____.
    A. SMART
    B. BUFF
    C. YOUNG
    D. GOOD

14. Which of the following is NOT a reason some students may find it hard to say "No"? _____
    A. I do not want to be selfish.
    B. I want to be liked.
    C. I do not want to look like I cannot handle a challenge.
    D. All of the above reasons may make it difficult to say "No."

15. When answering multiple-choice questions, the word _____ requires the question to be studied a little more carefully, as the question may be confusing.
    A. "challenge"
    B. "option"
    C. "not"
    D. "topic"

Sentence Completion

Complete each sentence or statement.

1. _____ represents a note-taking strategy in which main concepts and subconcepts are

   identified and recorded in a simple format.

2. When we first encounter a new concept or piece of information, it goes into our _____

   memory.

3. There are several ways to learn: through _____, through _____, and through

   _____, _____, and _____.

4. _____ are the tools you use to put knowledge into your long-term memory.

5. The most beneficial feedback to you as a student is _____ feedback.

Short Answers

1. Describe the four phases of preparing for a test.

   _____

   _____

   _____

   _____

2. Describe three negative and three positive effects of stress.

_____

_____

_____

_____

3. List three values of good study habits.

_____

_____

4. List nine tips for successful test taking.

_____

_____

_____

_____

_____

_____

_____

_____

_____

CRITICAL THINKING

1. Susan has recently enrolled in a medical assistant program at her local community college. She really wants to do well in school so she can graduate and get a good job, but she is starting to wonder if she is going to be able to make it. Susan is a single parent with a 4-year-old daughter and a 6-month-old son, and she does not have a very solid support system. Susan took her first exam on Monday morning. She tried to study the night before the exam, but the baby is teething and was fussy most of the night. Her daughter does not like the idea that mom is suddenly busy with homework and does everything she can to get Susan's attention. Susan did not have time to make flash cards, and when she tried to read the chapter and review the information prior to the exam, it just would not stick. She looked at her class notes a day or so before the exam, but they did not make a lot of sense to her when she tried to create an outline. She is really worried that she did not pass.

    A. What suggestions do you have for Susan?

_____

_____

    B. How can she schedule her time more efficiently?

_____

_____

    C. What should Susan do in the future regarding her class notes?

_____

_____

2. What suggestions would you give Susan specifically regarding how to prepare for exams?

_____

_____

_____

3. Explain to Susan two mnemonic devices that might help her when studying.

    A. _____

_____

    B. _____

_____

4. Describe the SQ3R method to Susan to help build her reading comprehension.

_____

_____

_____

_____

INTERNET RESEARCH

Keyword: Study Skills. Research and discover two study skills that are different than what is presented in the chapter. Write a short paragraph about the two techniques, quote the source, and list the Web site address. Your instructor may ask you to give an oral presentation to the class.

_____

_____

_____

_____

_____

_____

_____

_____

_____

WHAT WOULD YOU DO?

If you have accomplished the objectives in this chapter, you will be able to make better choices as a medical assistant. Take a look at this situation and decide what you would do.

Alex is a student enrolled in a medical assisting class at her local vocational school. The program provides the opportunity to complete the program of study, then take the credentialing examination within 2 weeks.
   Alex likes to study with others but has experienced situations in which the others in her study group wanted to play rather than study. She wants to be well prepared to take the examination without having to do a lot of cramming. She notices two other students, Jake and Mary Lou, studying together and approaches them to see if she can join them. They welcome her, and a new study group is formed. As she talks with them, she quickly learns that their study methods are to memorize, pass the test, and move on to the next assignment.
   Because they seem to be serious students, Alex decides to stay with them and will try to teach them some new tricks. She also decides that she will schedule some study time to be on her own.

Do you think this arrangement will be helpful to Alex? What would you do in this situation?

1. **What are some advantages to Alex trying to stay with a study group whose skills are not as refined as hers?**

_____

_____

_____

2. **What are three study skills you would suggest that Alex teach Mary Lou and Jake?**

_____

_____

_____

3. **How will these suggested study skills help to take the fear out of taking the exam?**

_____

_____

_____

4. **Alex, Mary Lou, and Jake will need to set priorities as they determine how to use their time. What steps would you suggest they follow?**

_____

_____

5. **What are some advantages for Alex to have study time alone, away from her new friends?**

_____

_____

_____

6. **How will working on a study team help Alex to be better prepared to work on a medical team?**

_____

_____

_____

APPLICATION OF SKILLS

1. List three short-term goals for this week. At the end of the week, evaluate how well the goals were met.

_____

_____

_____

2. List three long-term goals—one to be accomplished in the next 6 months, one to be achieved within 1 year, and one you wish to achieve within the next 5 years.

_____

_____

_____

3. On the first 5-day planner provided, outline your schedule for the upcoming week, using the guidelines described in the chapter. At the end of the week, evaluate where your schedule changed and where your schedule can be adjusted for more efficient use of time. After evaluation of the first week, using the second 5-day planner provided, outline your schedule for a second week, making adjustments as necessary. At the end of the second week, evaluate your use of time.

OCTOBER 17–23 20XX

17 Monday

6:00 a.m.	11:30	5:00	10:30
6:30	12:00 p.m.	5:30	11:00
7:00	12:30	6:00	Notes
7:30	1:00	6:30	
8:00	1:30	7:00	
8:30	2:00	7:30	
9:00	2:30	8:00	
9:30	3:00	8:30	
10:00	3:30	9:00	
10:30	4:00	9:30	
11:00	4:30	10:00	

18 Tuesday

6:00 a.m.	11:30	5:00	10:30
6:30	12:00 p.m.	5:30	11:00
7:00	12:30	6:00	Notes
7:30	1:00	6:30	
8:00	1:30	7:00	
8:30	2:00	7:30	
9:00	2:30	8:00	
9:30	3:00	8:30	
10:00	3:30	9:00	
10:30	4:00	9:30	
11:00	4:30	10:00	

19 Wednesday

6:00 a.m.	11:30	5:00	10:30
6:30	12:00 p.m.	5:30	11:00
7:00	12:30	6:00	Notes
7:30	1:00	6:30	
8:00	1:30	7:00	
8:30	2:00	7:30	
9:00	2:30	8:00	
9:30	3:00	8:30	
10:00	3:30	9:00	
10:30	4:00	9:30	
11:00	4:30	10:00	

OCTOBER 20XX 17–23

20 Thursday

6:00 a.m.	11:30	5:00	10:30
6:30	12:00 p.m.	5:30	11:00
7:00	12:30	6:00	Notes
7:30	1:00	6:30	
8:00	1:30	7:00	
8:30	2:00	7:30	
9:00	2:30	8:00	
9:30	3:00	8:30	
10:00	3:30	9:00	
10:30	4:00	9:30	
11:00	4:30	10:00	

21 Friday

6:00 a.m.	11:30	5:00	10:30
6:30	12:00 p.m.	5:30	11:00
7:00	12:30	6:00	Notes
7:30	1:00	6:30	
8:00	1:30	7:00	
8:30	2:00	7:30	
9:00	2:30	8:00	
9:30	3:00	8:30	
10:00	3:30	9:00	
10:30	4:00	9:30	
11:00	4:30	10:00	

22 Saturday / **23 Sunday**

A.M.	P.M.	A.M.	P.M.
Notes		Notes	

OCTOBER
17–23   20XX

17 Monday

6:00 a.m.	11:30	5:00	10:30
6:30	12:00 p.m.	5:30	11:00
7:00	12:30	6:00	Notes
7:30	1:00	6:30	
8:00	1:30	7:00	
8:30	2:00	7:30	
9:00	2:30	8:00	
9:30	3:00	8:30	
10:00	3:30	9:00	
10:30	4:00	9:30	
11:00	4:30	10:00	

18 Tuesday

6:00 a.m.	11:30	5:00	10:30
6:30	12:00 p.m.	5:30	11:00
7:00	12:30	6:00	Notes
7:30	1:00	6:30	
8:00	1:30	7:00	
8:30	2:00	7:30	
9:00	2:30	8:00	
9:30	3:00	8:30	
10:00	3:30	9:00	
10:30	4:00	9:30	
11:00	4:30	10:00	

19 Wednesday

6:00 a.m.	11:30	5:00	10:30
6:30	12:00 p.m.	5:30	11:00
7:00	12:30	6:00	Notes
7:30	1:00	6:30	
8:00	1:30	7:00	
8:30	2:00	7:30	
9:00	2:30	8:00	
9:30	3:00	8:30	
10:00	3:30	9:00	
10:30	4:00	9:30	
11:00	4:30	10:00	

OCTOBER
20XX   17–23

20 Thursday

6:00 a.m.	11:30	5:00	10:30
6:30	12:00 p.m.	5:30	11:00
7:00	12:30	6:00	Notes
7:30	1:00	6:30	
8:00	1:30	7:00	
8:30	2:00	7:30	
9:00	2:30	8:00	
9:30	3:00	8:30	
10:00	3:30	9:00	
10:30	4:00	9:30	
11:00	4:30	10:00	

21 Friday

6:00 a.m.	11:30	5:00	10:30
6:30	12:00 p.m.	5:30	11:00
7:00	12:30	6:00	Notes
7:30	1:00	6:30	
8:00	1:30	7:00	
8:30	2:00	7:30	
9:00	2:30	8:00	
9:30	3:00	8:30	
10:00	3:30	9:00	
10:30	4:00	9:30	
11:00	4:30	10:00	

22 Saturday / 23 Sunday

A.M.	P.M.	A.M.	P.M.
Notes		Notes	

4. Select one undesirable study habit that you would like to change. On a 3 × 5 card, write the habit at the top of the card. Underneath create a replacement plan using a more effective study habit. Put the plan into place for the next 21 to 28 days. Journal the outcome.

CHAPTER QUIZ

Multiple Choice

Identify the letter of the choice that best completes the statement or answers the question.

1. Consistent study habits will prevent you from feeling the need to cram and will store information in your _____ memory.
   A. short-term
   B. long-term
   C. quick-term
   D. action-term

2. _____ on a test will help you prepare for the next exam, as well as for learning the next block of material.
   A. Cheating
   B. A passing grade
   C. Feedback
   D. Writing in ink

3. Which of the following is NOT a successful test-taking tip?
   A. Answer the easiest questions first.
   B. Arrive early and be prepared.
   C. Never guess at an answer.
   D. Briefly outline essay questions.

4. Who is primarily responsible for a student learning new information?
   A. Parent
   B. Teacher
   C. Administrator
   D. Student

5. A prereading guide that presents questions and statements about what will be presented in the text and what you will be learning is called a(n) _____.
   A. concept map
   B. anticipation guide
   C. road map
   D. day planner

6. _____ is the process of talking with others about a concept or information for the purpose of understanding or clarification.
   A. Partnered reading
   B. Prioritizing
   C. Learning log
   D. Discussion

7. _____ are plans you develop to reach your mission in life.
   A. Mission statements
   B. Goals
   C. To-do lists
   D. Organizational skills

8. A _____ is a drawing that depicts what an individual or a group knows about a subject.
   A. mind map
   B. learning log
   C. partnered reading
   D. habit

9. A _____ is a list of tasks to be completed in a given time period; items are crossed off as they are completed.
   A. learning log
   B. mind map
   C. to-do list
   D. study list

10. RAFT is a _____ study strategy.
    A. writing
    B. verbal
    C. reading
    D. mathematical

11. Developing additional study skills will help you be more efficient with your time.
    A. True
    B. False

12. Good study habits are like riding a bicycle; you will never forget them.
    A. True
    B. False

13. When setting goals, it is important to set goals we do not think we can ever achieve. This is to keep our goals challenging.
    A. True
    B. False

14. _____ is a process in which we decide which situations require the most attention and then list each in descending order of importance.
    A. Goal setting
    B. Prioritizing
    C. Creating to-do lists
    D. Venn diagramming

15. When setting priorities, a "Want to Do" item is also classified as a Priority _____.
    A. "A"
    B. "B"
    C. "C"
    D. "D"

16. During study time, effective breaks could include ALL of the following EXCEPT _____.
    A. exercise
    B. water
    C. fresh air
    D. television programs

17. Short-term memory can hold information for approximately _____.
    A. 15 to 20 seconds
    B. 2 minutes
    C. 15 to 20 minutes
    D. 2 days

18. Short-term memory can typically hold _____ pieces, or "chunks," of information.
    A. 2
    B. 4
    C. 7
    D. 12

19. Paying attention to the format of the textbook can give you important clues about the main points and concepts you need to understand. Which one of the following is NOT something to which you should pay attention?
    A. Text boxes
    B. Objectives
    C. Print that is underlined, boldfaced, or italicized
    D. Page numbers

20. Which one of the following is not a method of actively reading?
    A. Taking notes
    B. Reading aloud
    C. Reading silently
    D. Telling someone else about what you have read

CHAPTER TWO

Diversity in Health Care Delivery

VOCABULARY REVIEW

Matching: Match each term with the correct definition.

A. corporation

B. diversity

C. entity

D. group practice

E. management service organization (MSO)

F. partnership

G. sole proprietorship

H. specialization

_____ 1. Particular type of business

_____ 2. Business owned by one person who is legally responsible for the debts and taxes of the business

_____ 3. Large business entity that has incorporated to avoid personal liability from the company's debts and taxes

_____ 4. Occurs when additional training and educational requirements have been met in a specific area of medicine

_____ 5. Having a variety of skills or types

_____ 6. Organization (e.g., hospital) that handles patient services (e.g., billing and payment services) for a medical practice

_____ 7. Business owned by two people who are held legally responsible for the debts and taxes of the business

_____ 8. Practice that is owned by three or more people who are held legally responsible for the debts and taxes of the business.

THEORY RECALL

True/False

Indicate whether the sentence or statement is true or false.

_____ 1. In corporate practices that are handled by an MSO, the physician is technically an employee of the MSO.

_____ 2. Most medical practices today are sole proprietorships.

_____ 3. Nationally, many physicians are general practitioners.

_____ 4. A specialist is a physician who has completed additional training and educational requirements.

_____ 5. Hippocrates is known as the "Father of Inventions."

Multiple Choice

Identify the letter of the choice that best completes the statement or answers the question.

1. The healthcare team member solely responsible for diagnosing and treating patients is a _____.
   A. certified medical assistant
   B. physician
   C. certified nursing assistant
   D. registered nurse

2. The medical specialty that provides treatment for patients with heart and vascular disease is _____.
   A. internal medicine
   B. emergency medicine
   C. aerospace medicine
   D. cardiology

3. A(n) _____ treats disorders of the female reproductive system.
   A. gynecologist
   B. dermatologist
   C. obstetrician
   D. urologist

4. A(n) _____ treats diseases with the use of radionuclides.
   A. aerospace medical specialist
   B. radiologist
   C. nuclear medicine specialist
   D. nephrologist

5. Holistic treatment that focuses on disease prevention and natural treatments is called _____.
   A. nuclear medicine
   B. naturopathy
   C. naprapathy
   D. neurology

6. The field of _____ involves the treatment of myofascial disorders.
   A. chiropractic medicine
   B. orthopedic medicine
   C. naprapathy
   D. naturopathy

7. A(n) _____ provides inpatient care and treatment for acute conditions.
   A. home health care agency
   B. hospice
   C. hospital
   D. assisted living facility

8. A(n) _____ provides 24-hour-a-day nursing services to those who are unable to function on their own on a long-term basis.
   A. ambulatory surgery center
   B. assisted living center
   C. skilled nursing home
   D. hospice

9. A _____ is a practice owned by one person who is legally responsible for the debts and taxes of the business.
   A. partnership
   B. group practice
   C. sole proprietorship
   D. corporate practice

10. Physicians are considered board certified once they have _____.
    A. completed additional training and examination by the board of their specialty
    B. performed 3 years of additional training and 2 years of board certification training
    C. completed a state registry examination and performed 2 years of board certification training
    D. performed 2 years of board certification training only

Sentence Completion

Complete each sentence or statement.

1. A(n) ——————— is a multiskilled professional who is knowledgeable about both administrative

   and clinical procedures.

2. In a(n) ——————— , the practice is responsible for the debt incurred.

3. A(n) ——————— treats diseases of the skin.

4. A(n) ——————— treats problems of conception and maintaining pregnancy.

5. A(n) ——————— tests vision and prepares lenses to correct refractive problems.

Short Answers

1. Explain the importance of being knowledgeable about the various healthcare delivery settings in your community.

2. List seven healthcare delivery settings other than a medical office.

3. Describe the differences between a long-term care facility and a short-term care facility.

4. Explain the difference between a group practice and a corporation.

CRITICAL THINKING

1. Janet has been studying the different types of medical practices in her medical assistant program. She never realized there were so many different specialties. Janet has seen the same family physician from the time she was born for everything from tonsillitis to her yearly physical exams. She always thought she would work for a general practitioner when she graduated, but now she is not sure. She has enjoyed studying the cardiovascular system and thinks working for a cardiologist might be interesting. But she also has been intrigued with naturopathy and maybe emergency medicine. She could go back to school after she graduates and obtain her RN degree and become a flight nurse.

   A. What suggestions do you have for Janet?

   _____

   _____

   _____

   B. How can she learn more about each specialty?

   _____

   _____

2. What specialties are you considering for employment? (List a minimum of two specialties.)

   _____

3. Describe why you believe you may be suited for the specialties you are considering.

   _____

   _____

   _____

4. If you are unsure of the type of practice you would like to pursue for employment, what steps can you take to narrow your choices?

   _____

   _____

   _____

INTERNET RESEARCH

Keyword: One of the American boards listed in Figure 2-1. Write a one-page typed report (double spaced with 1-inch margins) describing the specialty.

WHAT WOULD YOU DO?

If you have accomplished the objectives in this chapter, you will be able to make better choices as a medical assistant. Take a look at this situation and decide what you would do.

Jade is a recent graduate of a medical assisting program. She is looking for a job that will fit her credentials. She has not taken the credentialing examinations for medical assisting and has not had any experience in the medical field except her externship in a pediatric clinic.

Jade finds two ads in the local paper for a medical assistant. One ad specifically asks for a certified medical assistant for a group practice in a management service organization. The other ad asks for a medical assistant for a solo practice for an internist; no medical assisting credentials are specified, but applicants should have experience appropriate to the internal medicine setting. In the solo practice Jade would be the only clinical employee for the practice. Jade decides to apply for both positions. Jade thinks that the job of a medical assistant is the same in each setting and that she is prepared for both employment opportunities.

While reading the same paper, Jade also sees an ad for a nurse for a physician partnership in obstetrics-gynecology. She decides to apply for this position as well.

What advice would you give Jade if she asked for your input?

1. **Does Jade have the credentials for these employment opportunities? If so, which ones? If not, why are some or all not appropriate?**

   _____

   _____

   _____

2. **What advantages would a new graduate have in a group practice rather than a solo practice where he or she is the only clinical medical assistant? What experiences should Jade expect to find in each setting? What are the advantages and disadvantages of each?**

   _____

   _____

   _____

3. **Should Jade assume that she could take a nursing position? What are the implications of using that title? In what scope of practice does the title "nurse" place Jade?**

   _____

   _____

   _____

4. **What would be the legal implications for the physicians in each setting if Jade is hired?**

_____

_____

_____

5. **What influence could Jade have on the community's perception of the physician's abilities or the scope of practice if she does not understand her own abilities and scope of training? Will her scope of practice have any effect on the physician's office? If so, how?**

_____

_____

_____

6. **Is the physician legally responsible for Jade's actions? Explain why or why not.**

_____

_____

_____

APPLICATION OF SKILLS

1. Contact a healthcare facility in your area. Ask, and then answer, the following questions.

   A. What type of business entity is the facility?

   _____

   B. What types of healthcare providers make up the healthcare team?

   _____

   _____

   C. What is the name, address, and telephone number of the medical practice?

   _____

   D. What are the hours of operation? _____

   E. What is the practice's specialty? _____

   F. How many years has the practice been in operation?

   _____

2. Clip two job listings for medical assistants from your local newspaper, and attach them to a blank piece of paper. Identify the type of practice (e.g., family practice, ob/gyn).

CHAPTER QUIZ

Multiple Choice

Identify the letter of the choice that best completes the statement or answers the question.

1. A _____ can perform certain procedures under the supervision of a physician, examine and treat patients, order and interpret laboratory texts and radiographs, and make diagnoses.
   A. registered nurse
   B. physician assistant
   C. certified medical assistant
   D. licensed practical nurse

2. A(n) _____ provides services and assistance to people who require minimal help, such as cooking, laundry, and help with medications.
   A. hospice
   B. home health agency
   C. ambulatory surgery center
   D. assisted living facility

3. A(n) _____ assists and meets the needs of terminally ill patients and their families.
   A. hospice
   B. home health agency
   C. ambulatory surgery center
   D. assisted living facility

4. A(n) _____ is NOT a type of medical practice setting.
   A. independent contractor
   B. sole proprietorship
   C. partnership
   D. corporate practice

5. _____ treat all patients, from the newborn to the elderly.
   A. Internists
   B. Gerontologists
   C. Family practitioners
   D. Pediatricians

6. A(n) _____ requires a license to work.
   A. certified medical assistant
   B. registered nurse
   C. insurance specialist
   D. phlebotomy technician

7. Advantages of a _____ practice are the greater potential for profit; shared decision making; and shared facilities, equipment, and employees.
   A. private
   B. partnership
   C. group
   D. corporate

8. The liability of a _____ practice includes being responsible for all debts of the practice.
   A. private
   B. partnership
   C. group
   D. corporate

9. A _____ medical practice has more than three practitioners and several employees.
   A. private
   B. partnership
   C. group
   D. corporate

10. During surgery, this practitioner administers and maintains the medications given to the patient to keep him or her unconscious during the procedure.
    A. Immunologist
    B. Hematologist
    C. Anesthesiologist
    D. Oncologist

11. A(n) _____ treats conditions and disorders of the male reproductive system.
    A. urologist
    B. gynecologist
    C. oncologist
    D. neurologist

12. A(n) _____ treats disorders of the eyes.
    A. optician
    B. ophthalmologist
    C. neurologist
    D. optometrist

13. A(n) _____ counsels patients with stress or emotional-related disorders.
    A. neurologist
    B. psychologist
    C. physiologist
    D. psychiatrist

14. A(n) _____ examines tissue samples for signs of disease.
    A. pathologist
    B. oncologist
    C. internist
    D. radiologist

15. A(n) _____ treats diseases and disorders of the teeth and gums.
    A. oral surgeon
    B. orthodontist
    C. dental hygienist
    D. dentist

16. A _____ treats the patient through manipulation of the spine to relieve musculoskeletal disorders.
    A. certified medical assistant
    B. family practitioner
    C. chiropractor
    D. podiatrist

17. Which one of the following does NOT need a 4-year degree to practice their profession? _____
    A. MD
    B. DPM
    C. DO
    D. CMA

18. A _____ is a healthcare professional who works in a laboratory and performs venipunctures.
    A. radiology technician
    B. pharmacy technician
    C. phlebotomy technician
    D. histology technician

19. In a _____, the practice ends when the owner dies or closes the practice.
    A. sole proprietorship
    B. corporate practice
    C. group practice
    D. partnership

20. A(n) _____ treats disorders of the blood.
    A. anesthesiologist
    B. hematologist
    C. cardiologist
    D. internist

CHAPTER THREE

Law and Ethics in Health Care

VOCABULARY REVIEW

Matching: Match each term with the correct definition.

A. age of majority

B. contract

C. damages

D. euthanasia

E. Good Samaritan Act

F. infraction

G. noncompliance

H. reciprocity

I. subpoena

J. vicarious liability

_____ 1. Liability of an employer for the wrong-doing of an employee while on the job

_____ 2. Legislation that provides protection from lawsuits for an individual providing lifesaving or emergency treatment

_____ 3. Occurs when one state accepts another state's licensing requirements

_____ 4. Failure of a patient to comply with the physician's treatment plan; grounds for dismissal of a patient from a practice

_____ 5. Person who is considered by law to have acquired all the rights and responsibilities of an adult (age 18 in most states)

_____ 6. Payment used to compensate for physical injury, damaged property, or a loss of personal freedom or used as a punishment

_____ 7. Violation of a law, resulting in a fine

_____ 8. Legal document that requires a person to appear in court or be available for a deposition

_____ 9. Intentional ending of life for the terminally ill

_____ 10. Agreement between two or more persons resulting in a consideration

THEORY RECALL

True/False

Indicate whether the sentence or statement is true or false.

_____ 1. Certification is the strongest form of professional regulation, as it is a legal document.

_____ 2. Under the "Good Samaritan Act," implied consent applies if no one is available to consent for the patient and if a "reasonable" person would consent under similar circumstances.

_____ 3. Under the Uniform Anatomical Gift Act, incompetent individuals may donate their body or body parts after they die.

_____ 4. Confidentiality breaches occur most often as a result of carelessness in elevators or hallways and over lunches in medical facilities.

_____ 5. It is the medical assistant's responsibility to know the laws and to follow them to the letter.

Multiple Choice

Identify the letter of the choice that best completes the statement or answers the question.

1. The failure to make arrangements for a patient's medical coverage is termed _____.
   A. battery
   B. gross negligence
   C. abandonment
   D. implied contract

2. _____ is a written form of defamation.
   A. libel
   B. felony
   C. slander
   D. misfeasance

3. _____ is the performance of an unlawful act causing harm.
   A. abandonment
   B. malfeasance
   C. misfeasance
   D. *quid pro quo*

4. A branch of law that deals with offenses or crimes against the welfare or safety of the public is _____.
   A. public law
   B. administrative law
   C. criminal law
   D. international law

5. _____ is the science of understanding the complete genetic inheritance of an organism.
   A. fiduciary
   B. naturopathy
   C. naprapathy
   D. genomics

6. The document that was formulated by the American Hospital Association to define the rights of patients is the _____.
   A. Patient Care Partnership
   B. Patient Bill of Rights
   C. Private law
   D. Good Samaritan Act

7. Which one of the following is NOT a means of obtaining licensure?
   A. Examination
   B. On-the-job training
   C. Reciprocity
   D. Endorsement

8. Physicians are required to renew their license every _____ years.
   A. 2
   B. 3
   C. 4
   D. 5

9. The doctrine _____ places the liability on the physician for his or her employee's actions.
   A. *quid pro quo*
   B. *res ipsa loquitur*
   C. *respondeat superior*
   D. *subpoena duces tecum*

10. _____ is a voluntary process that professionals can go through to earn certification and other proof of their knowledge and skills.
    A. Endorsement
    B. Reciprocity
    C. Continuing education
    D. Credentialing

11. _____ deals with the rights and responsibilities of the government to the people and the people to the government.
    A. Administrative law
    B. Public law
    C. Criminal law
    D. Civil law

12. A(n) _____ is one that is specifically stated aloud or written and is understood by all parties.
    A. implied contract
    B. illegal contract
    C. breach of contract
    D. expressed contract

13. A(n) _____ is a negligent, wrongful act committed by a person against another person or property that causes harm.
    A. tort
    B. implied contract
    C. slander
    D. fiduciary

14. A threat or the perceived threat of doing bodily harm by another person is _____.
    A. slander
    B. libel
    C. assault
    D. battery

15. Ordinary _____ is not doing (or doing) something that a reasonable person would do (or would not do).
    A. negligence
    B. malfeasance
    C. misfeasance
    D. nonfeasance

16. _____ is the failure to do what is expected, thereby resulting in harm to the patient.
    A. Negligence
    B. Malfeasance
    C. Misfeasance
    D. Nonfeasance

17. Which one of the following is NOT a component that must be present before an attorney will pursue a case for professional negligence?
    A. Duty
    B. Dereliction of duty
    C. Direct cause or proximate cause
    D. Payment for services rendered

18. The _____ of 1990 requires healthcare institutions to give patients written information about advance directives before life-sustaining measures become necessary.
    A. Patient Bill of Rights
    B. Patient Care Partnership
    C. Patient Self-Determination Act
    D. Uniform Anatomical Act

19. The _____ provides guidelines for collecting money owed.
    A. Bankruptcy Act
    B. Fair Debt Collection Practices Act
    C. Consumer Debt Act
    D. Occupational Safety and Health Act

20. _____ refers to "this for that" or the "something for something" issues that may occur in the workplace.
    A. *quid pro quo*
    B. *res ipsa loquitur*
    C. *respondeat superior*
    D. *subpoena duces tecum*

Sentence Completion

Complete each sentence or statement.

1. A(n) _____ is an agreement between two or more people promising to work toward a
   specific goal for adequate consideration.

2. A(n) _____ is an underage person who has legally separated from parents for various
   reasons and is legally capable of consent to treatment.

3. All states require the reporting of _____, including births, deaths, and communicable
   diseases.

4. Each chemical used on the job must have a(n) _____ from the manufacturer on file.

5. Employers, by law, must carry _____. This plan covers medical care and rehabilitation
   costs and offers temporary or permanent pay for the injured employee.

Short Answers

1. List three bioethical situations and briefly explain the considerations for each.

   _____

   _____

   _____

   _____

   _____

   _____

   _____

2. Compare the differences between law and ethics.

   _____

   _____

   _____

   _____

3. Create a scenario involving a breach of confidentiality that might occur in a medical office.

_____

_____

_____

_____

4. Describe your opinion of the legality and ethics of genetic engineering.

_____

_____

_____

_____

CRITICAL THINKING

1. On externship Terry overheard two employees of the medical clinic discussing the specifics of a patient's case, in the clinic's break room. The comment that caught Terry's attention was that the patient had been physically abused by her spouse. Terry knew this patient personally; the patient was married to Terry's cousin. Terry could not believe what she had overheard and was appalled that the medical assistants would be making such claims.

   A. Did the two employees in the medical clinic breach confidentiality?

   _____

   B. Should Terry say anything to the patient or to her cousin?

   _____

   C. Legally and ethically, did the two employees violate any laws or regulations? If so, what are the violations?

   _____

   _____

   _____

   D. What would you do if you were in Terry's place?

   _____

   _____

INTERNET RESEARCH

Keyword: Medical Practice Acts, your state. Research the medical practice acts for your state. Identify the section(s) that pertain to medical assistants practicing their profession.

WHAT WOULD YOU DO?

If you have accomplished the objectives in this chapter, you will be able to make better choices as a medical assistant. Take a look at this situation and decide what you would do.

Jill is a medical assistant with on-the-job training in a medical office setting. She always strives to be caring, courteous, and respectful of patients and co-workers. Because of her caring attitude, the patients with whom Jill works all appreciate her attitude and her work. One of Jill's favorite patients, Shandra, a 24-year-old mother of two young children, has been diagnosed with cancer and recently was told by the physician that her condition is terminal. Shandra is at the office for an appointment and, feeling very upset about her terminal illness, she pours out her heart and fears to Jill. Wanting to comfort Shandra, Jill tells her, "Don't worry. You'll be just fine. You know the doctor will make you better."

   Shandra is comforted by Jill's words and tells her how much Jill means to her. In fact, she has so much faith in Jill that she believes that she will be fine and tells her family what Jill has said. Sadly, a few months later, Shandra dies. Believing she would be fine, Shandra had not made any plans for her children and family. Her family is upset with the physician and with Jill. The family thinks they have been betrayed because they believed that Shandra would be fine. The family is discussing what to say to the physician about this betrayal and whether to bring a lawsuit, because Shandra did not have a will.

How might this situation been avoided? What are the possible implications for Shandra's family, Jill, the physician, and the practice?

1. **Jill has been trained on the job and is uncredentialed. What are the disadvantages to Jill of not having a formal medical assisting education? Would having credentialing and an education make a difference in what Jill said to Shandra?**

   _____

   _____

   _____

2. **Would credentialing make a difference if Shandra's family decides to bring a lawsuit? If so, what are the benefits to the physician if the medical assistant is credentialed?**

   _____

   _____

   _____

3. **Why was it important for Shandra to have an advance directive?**

   _____

   _____

   _____

4. **What are the legal ramifications of Jill telling Shandra not to worry and that she would be fine? What ethical guidelines should be considered in this situation? Did Jill do something illegal, something unethical, neither, or both? Explain why or why not.**

_____

_____

_____

APPLICATION OF SKILLS

1. Draft a formal letter to a patient, withdrawing the physician from the physician-patient contract. Include the six required steps. Step 1 is drafting the letter in writing.

2. Clip two current newspaper articles pertaining to medical legal or ethical issues. Summarize each article by writing a paragraph describing your impression of the article and the impact it has on the medical community. Cite the specific legal or ethical implications.

CHAPTER QUIZ

Multiple Choice

Identify the letter of the choice that best completes the statement or answers the question.

1. A legal document that requires a person to appear in court and bring the records is (a) _____.
   A. subpoena
   B. _res ipsa loquitur_
   C. _subpoena duces tecum_
   D. Patient Bill of Rights

2. A legal document that allows a person to offer their skills and knowledge to the public for compensation is a(n) _____.
   A. certification
   B. license
   C. MSDS
   D. diploma

3. The intentional act of touching another person in a socially unacceptable manner without their consent is called _____.
   A. libel
   B. breach of duty
   C. battery
   D. assault

4. _____ is legislation that regulates patients' rights and federal regulation that mandates the protection of privacy and holds information to be confidential.
   A. Health Insurance Portability and Accountability Act
   B. Patient Care Partnership Act
   C. Standard of Care Act
   D. Good Samaritan Act

5. A person of trusted responsibility is a(n) _____.
   A. emancipated minor
   B. fiduciary
   C. dependent
   D. custodian

6. Laws, or _____, are general rules and standards designed to regulate conduct.
   A. torts
   B. medical practice acts
   C. rights
   D. statutes

7. _____ regulates business practices.
   A. Private law
   B. Partnership law
   C. Administrative law
   D. Public law

8. Not making arrangements for a substitute physician to take patient calls if the physician is unavailable could be grounds for a lawsuit and termed as _____.
   A. misfeasance
   B. battery
   C. breach of contract
   D. abandonment

9. For there to be a valid physician-patient contract, the patient must meet or perform all of the following EXCEPT _____.
   A. truthfully disclose past and present medical information
   B. having reached the age of 14 years old
   C. take all medications
   D. be responsible with an appropriate reimbursement plan

10. In order for a physician to withdraw from patient care, all of the following must be achieved EXCEPT _____.
    A. notify the patient in writing
    B. give a date when this is to take effect (minimum of 30 days)
    C. provide a personal telephone call from the physician
    D. provide for transfer of medical records

11. A(n) _____ contract is one that is specifically stated aloud or written and is understood by all parties.
    A. expressed
    B. implied
    C. invalid
    D. assumed

12. A _____ is a negligent, wrongful act committed by a person against another person or property that causes harm.
    A. fiduciary
    B. tort
    C. liability
    D. fraud

13. _____ is intentional negligence, or a wrongful act done (or not done) on purpose.
    A. Malfeasance
    B. Minor negligence
    C. Gross negligence
    D. Nonfeasance

14. _____ is defamation of character in writing.
    A. Slander
    B. Battery
    C. Libel
    D. Assault

15. If a patient were to receive a burn during ultrasound therapy, the charge may be _____.
    A. misfeasance
    B. malfeasance
    C. nonfeasance
    D. none of the above

16. _____ occurs when a healthcare professional fails to meet accepted standards of care.
    A. Breach of contract
    B. Dereliction of duty
    C. Fraud
    D. All of the above

17. Each state has laws that limit the length of time a person has to take legal action. This is called the _____.
    A. duration of care
    B. expressed contractual agreement
    C. standard of care requirements
    D. statute of limitations

18. The best way to avoid a lawsuit is to _____.
    A. keep the lines of communication open
    B. listen to patient's concerns or complaints; chart the facts
    C. keep patient information confidential
    D. all of the above

19. Not providing a child with clothing for the weather could be considered _____.
    A. abandonment
    B. neglect
    C. good parenting
    D. false imprisonment

20. An employer must provide every employee with the opportunity to receive a hepatitis B vaccination. The second dose in the series of three should be given _____ after the first dose.
    A. 10 days
    B. 30 days
    C. 90 days
    D. 120 days

Student Name _____ Date _____

PROCEDURE 3-1: LEGAL AND ETHICAL BEHAVIOR

TASK: Demonstrate the correct procedure for creating a fact sheet identifying the elements of legal and ethical boundaries for the professional medical assistant.

CONDITIONS: Given the proper equipment and supplies, create a fact sheet identifying the elements of legal and ethical boundaries for the professional medical assistant.

EQUIPMENT AND SUPPLIES
- Copy of the AMA Code of Ethics
- Copy of the medical practice act for your state
- AAMA Creed
- Copy of an informed consent form
- Computer
- Paper and pen/pencil

STANDARDS: Complete the procedure within _____ minutes and achieve a minimum score of _____%.

Time began _____   **Time ended** _____

Steps	Possible Points	First Attempt	Second Attempt
1. Gather equipment and supplies.	5		
2. Create and submit to instructor an outline describing the legal and ethical boundaries addressing key points as outlined in the procedure sheet.	20		
3. Research topics and write a rough draft. Submit rough draft to instructor.	25		
4. Proofread the rough draft. Submit to instructor.	25		
5. Make corrections and submit a final draft.	25		

Total Points Possible   100

Comments: Total Points Earned _____ Divided by _____ Total Possible Points= _____ % Score

*Instructor's Signature*_____

CHAPTER **FOUR**

Becoming a Professional

VOCABULARY REVIEW

Matching: Match each term with the correct definition.

A. AAMA

B. ABHES

C. AMT

D. CAAHEP

E. clinical

F. competence

G. confidential

H. dexterity

I. diplomacy

J. empathy

K. ethical standards

L. integrity

M. professional

N. revalidation

O. tactful

___O___ 1. Acting with sensitivity when dealing with people

___B___ 2. Accrediting Bureau of Health Education Schools

___J___ 3. Understanding how someone else feels by placing yourself in his or her place

___G___ 4. Private

___A___ 5. American Association of Medical Assistants

___I___ 6. Ability to be tactful

___E___ 7. Having to do with hands-on patient care

___K___ 8. Person who conforms to the technical and ethical standards of a profession

___M___ 9. Proficiency in identified skills

___C___ 10. American Medical Technologists organization

___N___ 11. Recertification

___D___ 12. Commission on Accreditation of Allied Health Education Programs

___H___ 13. Ability to move with skill and ease

___F___ 14. Guidelines for professional decisions and conduct

___L___ 15. Quality of being honest and straightforward

THEORY RECALL

True/False

Indicate whether the sentence or statement is true or false.

___T___ 1. A professional is someone who displays positive characteristics and demonstrates competence when performing tasks.

___F___ 2. First impressions often take a few hours.

___T___ 3. Both the American Association of Medical Assistants and the American Medical Technologists are nationally recognized associations for medical assistant participation and for credentialing opportunities.

___F___ 4. A person who has integrity is dishonest and deceitful.

___T___ 5. Reliability means that you do your job well and that others can rely on you.

Multiple Choice

Identify the letter of the choice that best completes the statement or answers the question.

1. Being a dependable employee includes all of the following characteristics EXCEPT ___A___.
   A. deceitfulness
   B. punctuality
   C. efficiency
   D. reliability

2. Giving that "extra push" to get the job done in any situation exhibits ___A___.
   A. loyalty
   B. punctuality
   C. efficiency
   D. reliability

3. Being capable of looking at the "big picture" demonstrates ___C___.
   A. dependability
   B. empathy
   C. a positive attitude
   D. diplomacy

4. ___B___ helps build good relationships between people through tact and empathy.
   A. Compromise
   B. Diplomacy
   C. Confidentiality
   D. Consensus

5. A person who has ___A___ is honest and straightforward.
   A. integrity
   B. compassion
   C. empathy
   D. consensus

6. _B_ is the ability to get things done on time and correctly.
   A. Compassion
   B. Competence
   C. Dexterity
   D. Loyalty

7. The ability to move with skill and ease is called _D_.
   A. sympathy
   B. discretion
   C. trustworthiness
   D. dexterity

8. _C_ is an appropriate way to greet both patients and co-workers.
   A. Reservedly
   B. Compassionately
   C. Smiling
   D. Tersely

9. Your _C_ can influence people's final opinion of you as a medical assistant.
   A. nonverbal communication skills
   B. personal appearance
   C. confidence
   D. all of the above

10. One advantage of a career in medical assisting is the _D_ in both administrative and clinical skills.
    A. lack of training
    B. cross-training
    C. limited training
    D. superficial training

11. There are many types of training programs for medical assistants and they vary in length. Some training programs have gone through a process of _C_, establishing standards and guidelines for postsecondary education.
    A. counseling
    B. peer review
    C. accreditation
    D. audit

12. Some states require that medical assistants _B_ with their state for a small fee.
    A. register
    B. certify
    C. file an endorsement
    D. declare loyalty

13. The American Medical Technologists credential for medical assistants is _C_.
    A. AAMA
    B. CMA
    C. AMT
    D. RMA

14. All medical assistants practice under a physician's direct supervision nationwide whether or not they have received a(n) _____.
    A. letter of recognition
    B. statement of intent
    C. assignment
    D. credential

15. The CMA exam is given __B__ times a year.
    A. 2
    B. 3
    C. 4
    D. as requested

16. The CMA exam consists of a total of __A__ questions.
    A. 100
    B. 200
    C. 300
    D. varies from test to test

17. The certified medical assistant must revalidate his or her credentials every _____ year(s) by either exam or continuing education.
    A. 1
    B. 3
    C. 5
    D. 7

18. The American Medical Technologists exam consists of _____ questions.
    A. varies from test to test
    B. 50
    C. 100
    D. more than 200

19. The RMA exam is offered all over the United States at testing sites _____.
    A. weekly
    B. monthly
    C. three times
    D. five times

20. The credentialing exams for medical assistants are _____ to work in the profession.
    A. voluntary, not required,
    B. voluntary, required,
    C. mandated, not required,
    D. mandated, required,

Sentence Completion

Complete each sentence or statement.

1. Continuing Education is a term used to describe education once a credential is received.

2. Reliability means that you do your job well and that others can count on you.

3. Professionals are expected to behave according to the _____ of their chosen profession.

4. Many employers will not hire a person who has a reputation for not being _____.

5. Integrity is *ethically* doing the right thing, even when it is difficult. It means choosing to do what is right for all people even though it may not be what you personally want to do.

Short Answers

1. List six characteristics of a professional medical assistant, and briefly describe the importance of each.

   _____

   _____

   _____

   _____

   _____

   _____

   _____

   _____

2. State 10 things you can do to have a professional appearance at work.

   _____

   _____

   _____

   _____

3. Explain the importance of maintaining professional competence through continuing education other than recertification of credentials.

   _____

   _____

   _____

   _____

4. List four administrative duties and four clinical duties of a medical assistant.

_____

_____

_____

_____

CRITICAL THINKING

1. Susan has been working for Dr. Howard as an extern for the past 2 weeks. She is hoping that she will be given the opportunity to work at the clinic on completion of her hours. She enjoys the patients; the staff is incredible and has been so helpful. Dr. Howard has allowed Susan to assist with almost every procedure and always finds her when something "interesting" occurs.

   A. If you were Dr. Howard, what traits would you look for in an employee?

   B. What professional characteristics do you think Susan possesses?

   C. Do you think that Dr. Howard values the job Susan is doing? If so, what gives you that impression?

   D. What would you do if you were in Susan's place?

INTERNET RESEARCH

Keyword: Medical Assistant Continuing Education. Research three Web sites for the continuing education opportunities.

WHAT WOULD YOU DO?

If you have accomplished the objectives in this chapter, you will be able to make better choices as a medical assistant. Take a look at this situation and decide what you would do.

Robert is a medical assistant in a medical office. His responsibility is to draw blood samples at 8:00 AM, but he often does not show up until 8:15 AM or later. The scheduled patients must wait and be late for work or must reschedule their appointment. When Robert does arrive, often his uniform is blood stained and wrinkled and he has not shaved or bathed before coming to work. Even if another staff member has started drawing blood, the daily operation of the office is already behind schedule. Robert also has a habit of taking a break between patients.

As the office slips even further behind with more patients waiting, Robert draws the blood but does not take time to label the tubes with the patient's name or complete the laboratory request forms. When Robert makes mistakes, the office staff must make the corrections, resulting in even more delays and confusion about which tube of blood belongs to which patient.

One day Robert is sick and stays home but does not call the office. By 8:30 AM, patients have filled the waiting room, and patients coming to see the physicians have no place to sit. The office has insufficient staff, and the patients and the office personnel are stressed.

Robert's lack of professionalism is affecting both patients and staff. What would you do differently from Robert?

1. **Medical assistants who are respected for their professionalism have certain personality characteristics. Which of these characteristics is Robert lacking? How is Robert's lack of professionalism affecting patients? Co-workers? The office as a whole?**

2. **If you were a patient in this office, how would you feel if Robert was going to draw your blood?**

3. **How could Robert be liable for mislabeling blood samples?**

4. **What actions have shown that Robert does not meet the ethical standards of a medical assistant?**

5. How does the daily schedule fall behind in a medical office? Who is affected by this? What other potential problems and mistakes can you think of that might occur as a result of Robert being late?

_____

_____

_____

_____

6. If you were Robert's immediate supervisor, what would you say to Robert? How would you help him meet the professional and ethical standards expected of a medical assistant? What are some things he can do to arrive at work on time?

_____

_____

_____

_____

APPLICATION OF SKILLS

1. Fold a sheet of lined paper into half lengthwise. On the top of the left column, write the heading "I AM"; on the top of the right column, write the heading "I WILL." Beneath the heading "I AM," list 10 characteristics of a professional medical assistant that you already have. Beneath the heading "I WILL," list 10 characteristics on which you are going to improve, before you start working as a medical assistant. For example:

"I AM"	"I WILL"
Compassionate	Be punctual
Loyal	Press my uniforms daily

2. Research on the Internet the next available certification exam for both the AAMA (www.aama-ntl.org) and AMT (www.amt1.com) in your area. For each exam, list the location, date, time, what you need to bring to the exam, how you register, and the eligibility criteria.

3. Describe one time when you were treated unprofessionally and one time when you were treated professionally by a service provider. Identify specific behaviors, how you felt as the recipient of such behavior, how you handled the situation, and, in the case of unprofessional behavior, what could have been done to improve the service.

CHAPTER QUIZ

Multiple Choice

Identify the letter of the choice that best completes the statement or answers the question.

1. "_____" describes having to do with general front office and financial activities.
   A. Clinical
   B. Administrative
   C. Ambulatory
   D. Theoretical

2. Proficiency in identified skills is called _____.
   A. empathy
   B. dexterity
   C. competence
   D. integrity

3. The ability to be on time is _____.
   A. punctuality
   B. reliability
   C. revalidation
   D. diplomacy

4. A person who displays certain positive characteristics and demonstrates competence when performing tasks is thought of as (a) _____.
   A. dexterous
   B. diplomatic
   C. professional
   D. good Samaritan

5. You are _____ when you perform your tasks on time and accurately, to the best of your ability.
   A. ethical
   B. punctual
   C. dependable
   D. loyal

6. Supporting team leaders and members by accepting decisions and behaving according to the ethics of the profession demonstrates _____.
   A. empathy
   B. compassion
   C. punctuality
   D. loyalty

7. Over time, as you prove you are dependable, competent, and _____, the employer will become more loyal to you as an employee.
   A. private
   B. likable
   C. trustworthy
   D. outspoken

8. Which one of the following is NOT a quality of a professional with a positive attitude?
   A. Flexible
   B. Goal oriented
   C. Enthusiastic
   D. Fanatical

9. Wearing excessive jewelry to work as a medical assistant is unacceptable because it _____.
   A. can injure patients
   B. distracts coworkers and patients
   C. harbors pathogens
   D. both A and C

10. A(n) _____ is a title that signifies a person has attained certain competency standards.
    A. credential
    B. associate degree
    C. diploma
    D. letter of recommendation

11. When taking a certification exam, select answers that are _____ centered.
    A. medical assistant
    B. nursing
    C. physician
    D. patient

12. The CMA exam consists of 300 questions, with 100 questions in each of the following areas EXCEPT _____.
    A. general
    B. laboratory
    C. administrative
    D. clinical

13. One advantage of a career in medical assisting is _____ in administrative and clinical duties.
    A. ambulatory training
    B. surgical training
    C. cross-training
    D. political training

14. _____ are (is) guideline(s) for professional decisions and conduct.
    A. Diplomatic standards
    B. Recertification
    C. Ethical standards
    D. Consensus standards

15. To make a decision based on mutual agreement is _____.
    A. to compromise
    B. to use tact
    C. to use revalidation
    D. to be efficient

16. A(n) _____ passes a certification exam with an accredited certifying agency.
    A. CAAHEP
    B. AMA
    C. MAT
    D. RMA

17. Formal training is a requirement for employment as a medical assistant.
    A. True
    B. False

18. One way to promote professionalism is by joining your professional organization and becoming credentialed after taking an exam.
    A. True
    B. False

19. All medical assistants practice under a physician's direct supervision nationwide whether or not they have received a credential.
    A. True
    B. False

20. Even though you are a member of a professional organization, you will not always have a voice in public policy concerning the practice of medical assisting.
    A. True
    B. False

CHAPTER FIVE

Understanding Human Behavior

VOCABULARY REVIEW

Matching: Match each term with the correct definition.

A. anger

B. compensation

C. defense mechanism

D. depression

E. empathy

F. homeostasis

G. perception

H. phobias

I. physiological

J. psychiatry

K. psychology

L. self-esteem

M. stress

N. subconscious

O. sympathy

_____ 1. Having to do with the body's responses to its internal and external environment

_____ 2. Filtering tactic used by the unconscious to avoid unpleasant situations

_____ 3. Understanding how someone else feels by placing yourself in his or her place

_____ 4. Body in balance

_____ 5. Reaction due to the feeling of loss of control

_____ 6. Feeling of self-worth

_____ 7. Body's response to any demand put on it, whether it be positive or negative

_____ 8. Individual's view of a situation based on the environment

_____ 9. Having concern for a patient's situation

_____ 10. Overall feeling of helplessness

_____ 11. Irrational fears of objects, activities, or situations

_____ 12. Scientific study of the mind and the behavioral patterns of humans and animals

_____ 13. Defense mechanism in which a strength is emphasized to cover up a weakness in another area

_____ 14. Part of the conscious that is not fully aware

_____ 15. Medical specialty that deals with the treatment and prevention of mental illness

THEORY RECALL

True/False

Indicate whether the sentence or statement is true or false.

_____ 1. The study of human behavior helps us understand how people learn, feel emotions, and establish relationships.

_____ 2. The id is the part of the personality that is aware of reality and of the consequences of different behaviors.

_____ 3. Sigmund Freud, a German psychologist, was interested in the understanding of dreams.

_____ 4. The superego is concerned with the internalization of values and standards designed to promote proper social balance.

_____ 5. Knowing how to manage stress in the short term provides long-term rewards.

Multiple Choice

Identify the letter of the choice that best completes the statement or answers the question.

1. Of the following statements, which response BEST describes factors that influence the development of personality?
   A. Events in early development form all of a person's personality.
   B. Psychological factors such as poverty or wealth do not contribute to an individual's personality.
   C. Genetic factors are the only true markers of personality.
   D. None of the above statements are correct.

2. In Maslow's Hierarchy of Needs, _____ needs are being met when we feel loved and appreciated.
   A. safety
   B. physical
   C. social
   D. self-actualization

3. When this level of Maslow's hierarchy is achieved, an individual has a sense of being in control.
   A. Physical
   B. Self-esteem
   C. Social
   D. Self-actualization

4. _____ is the process of interpreting information gathered from our surroundings.
   A. Expectations
   B. Perceptions
   C. Self-esteem
   D. Consensus

5. _____ is one of the primary levels of Maslow's hierarchy.
   A. Hunger
   B. Fatigue
   C. Past experiences
   D. Age

6. _____ are (is) a psychological influence on how we perform.
   A. Senses
   B. Number of experiences
   C. Expectations
   D. Health

7. Young adults are moving from the _____ concept concerning education, job, home, and family.
   A. us to them
   B. I to we
   C. you to them
   D. them to them

8. Fear is a(n) _____ reaction to _____ danger.
   A. abnormal, perceived
   B. normal, perceived
   C. abnormal, genuine
   D. normal, genuine

9. An emotional response that alerts the body to take appropriate action to protect itself from danger is _____.
   A. fight or flight
   B. fright or freeze
   C. flee or be
   D. none of the above

10. Of the following which is NOT a phobia category?
    A. Interference
    B. Simple
    C. Social
    D. Agoraphobia

11. _____ is the feeling of apprehension, uneasiness, or uncertainty about a situation.
    A. Fear
    B. Anxiety
    C. Phobia
    D. Stress

12. Symptoms of anxiety include all of the following EXCEPT _____.
    A. inability to sleep
    B. self-doubt
    C. difficulty breathing
    D. direct eye contact

13. During periods of _____, our natural body defense systems weaken, fatigue takes over, and we become more susceptible to disease.
    A. fear
    B. stress
    C. anxiety
    D. elation

14. Research has proved that many _____ disorders are caused by the effects of stress.
    A. psychosomatic
    B. physiological
    C. psychiatric
    D. terminal

15. Long-term stress can cause any or all of the following disorders EXCEPT _____.
    A. headache
    B. ulcers
    C. muscle tension
    D. hypertension

16. If a person cannot recognize a real problem or situation, or chooses not to face it head-on, a _____ may be used to cope with it.
    A. psychosomatic disorder
    B. defense mechanism
    C. phobia
    D. terminal illness

17. _____ is a defense mechanism that allows a patient to deal with the shock of death.
    A. Denial
    B. Anger
    C. Bargaining
    D. All of the above

18. _____ is the process of making deals with anyone in sight, including the physician, a higher power, and/or family members when dealing with grief.
    A. Denial
    B. Anger
    C. Bargaining
    D. All of the above

19. _____ is coming to terms with dying or the loss of a loved one
    A. Denial
    B. Acceptance
    C. Depression
    D. Anger

20. Putting yourself in another person's situation is called (a) _____.
    A. defense mechanism
    B. empathy
    C. sympathy
    D. socialism

21. _____ is considered daydreaming inappropriately.
    A. Displacement
    B. Projection
    C. Fantasy
    D. Compensation

22. Inventing excuses or reasons for one's behavior is called _____.
    A. compensation
    B. rationalization
    C. repression
    D. sublimation

23. A co-worker who feels shy may talk too much or too loudly in an attempt to not be seen as shy. This is called _____.
   A. rationalization
   B. aggression
   C. displacement
   D. overcompensation

24. Physically or emotionally pulling away from people and/or conflict is called _____.
   A. conversion reaction
   B. sublimation
   C. withdrawal
   D. repression

25. An example of a simple phobia might include _____.
   A. fear of being ridiculed
   B. fear of snakes
   C. fear of public speaking
   D. fear of crowds

Sentence Completion

Complete each sentence or statement.

1. _____ is a package of services and a team of people helping patients and their families during the last months of a terminal illness.

2. Studies have shown that if a family's psychological and _____ needs are met in addition to the treatment of the patient's disease, the dying process is less distressing for all concerned.

3. _____ is a change for many people because their children are independent, often leaving home, and a void is created.

4. We recall _____ when we perform similar tasks: "I've never been very good at it" versus "With some help, I am ready to tackle this."

5. Physical needs are met when the body is in _____.

Short Answers

1. List in order of importance for survival Maslow's Hierarchy of Needs.

    _____

    _____

    _____

    _____

2. Explain why it is important to YOU to have a good self-esteem.

    _____

    _____

    _____

    _____

3. Contrast the differences between fear, phobia, anxiety, and stress.

    _____

    _____

    _____

    _____

4. List and describe six defense mechanisms.

    _____

    _____

    _____

    _____

    _____

CRITICAL THINKING

Tanya was hired by Dr. Ortega, an oncologist, 2 months ago. Many of Dr. Ortega's patients are terminally ill, and four patients have passed away this week. Tanya is not sure that she can cope personally with so many terminally ill patients. Tanya's mother died of breast cancer last year, which was one of the reasons that Tanya originally wanted to work for an oncologist. After a particularly upsetting day, Dr. Ortega asked Tanya to meet with her in her office, after the last appointment of the day. Dr. Ortega asked Tanya how she is handling the loss of the patients. "It has been very difficult. I am not sure that I am working through it. We talked about death and dying in school, but other than my mother passing away from cancer last year, I have never been around anyone else who has died." Dr. Ortega and Tanya talked for quite awhile about ways for Tanya to work through the loss of her mother and come to terms with her overall feelings of death and then how she can best be supportive of the clinic's patients and families. Dr. Ortega gave Tanya a list of books on death and dying to read on her own and a homework assignment to write her own obituary if she were to die tomorrow and a second one if she were to die of old age at 93. Tanya thanked Dr. Ortega for being so understanding and promised to read the books, and even though she was extremely uncomfortable with writing her own obituary, she agreed to try.

A. Write your own obituary as if you were to die tomorrow.

B. Write your own obituary as if you were to die of old age at 93.

INTERNET RESEARCH

Keyword: Medical Phobias. Research three Web sites and list five medical phobias. Cite the source of your information.

WHAT WOULD YOU DO?

If you have accomplished the objectives in this chapter, you will be able to make better choices as a medical assistant. Take a look at this situation and decide what you would do.

Sara Ann is a 22-year-old single mother and a medical assistant. She has no assistance at home with child care or with any of the chores necessary to keep up a household. Sara Ann works as many hours as she can to support herself and her two children in the best way possible. On top of all of this, going to school has added major financial problems for Sara Ann.

On many days, Sara Ann is tired and frustrated, and wonders just how she will get through the day. Because of her lack of self-esteem and the lack of help, anxiety and stress are affecting the way Sara Ann deals with co-workers. Sara Ann's anxiety level often leads her to label patients. In addition, Sara Ann has difficulty adapting to any variation in the daily schedule.

Because Sara Ann feels close to some patients with whom she has spent time in the medical office, she often discusses her personal problems with these patients. Also, Sara Ann must handle some of her personal business (banking, errands) while at work because she does not leave work early enough to do these things when the businesses are open.

Sara Ann is experiencing a lot of stress, which is having an impact on her performance at work. If you were in Sara Ann's situation, what would you do to reduce stress?

1. How are Sara Ann's reactions to her work understandable under the circumstances? What reactions are related to the anxiety and loss of self-esteem?

_____

_____

_____

_____

_____

_____

2. How are Sara Ann's reactions typical for someone who is not coping with personal or professional worlds?

_____

_____

_____

_____

3. What are some of the reactions that you would expect from Sara Ann's fellow employees about her behavior?

_____

_____

_____

4. Where on Maslow's Hierarchy of Needs would you place Sara Ann? Why did you place her at that level?

_____

_____

_____

_____

5. Because Sara Ann has no one at home for emotional or financial support, how would you, as a patient, feel if she told you about her problems? Are her actions of involving patients ethical? Why?

_____

_____

_____

_____

APPLICATION OF SKILLS

1. Select one defense mechanism from Table 5-5 and create a situational example of how a patient may exhibit the behaviors associated with the mechanism regarding an illness (two-paragraph minimum, single spaced).

2. Conduct research on the Internet or local library for methods of stress reduction. Select one method that appeals to you. Over the next 2 days, practice the method of stress reduction you selected at least once. Describe the method and your experience. Was it beneficial? Would you use it again?

3. Based on Maslow's Hierarchy of Needs, describe how to best respond to the following situations addressing physical and emotional needs.

   A. Angry patient: self-esteem

   _____

   _____

   _____

   B. Newly diagnosed terminal illness: safety

   _____

   _____

   _____

   C. Positive pregnancy test: survival and self-actualization

   _____

   _____

   _____

CHAPTER QUIZ

Multiple Choice

Identify the letter of the choice that best completes the statement or answers the question.

1. Coming to terms with an issue (e.g., impending death or loss) is _____.
   A. depression
   B. anxiety
   C. acceptance
   D. compensation

2. The body's response to threat is called _____.
   A. fight or flight
   B. bargaining
   C. rationalization
   D. overcompensation

3. The part of the personality that includes values and standards designed to promote proper behavior is called (the) _____.
   A. id
   B. ego
   C. superego
   D. self-esteem

4. _____ is a defense mechanism in which there is an unconscious rejection of an unacceptable thought, desire, impulse, and placing blame on someone else.
   A. rationalization
   B. denial
   C. subconscious
   D. projection

5. The _____ is the part of the brain associated with basic unconscious biological drives.
   A. id
   B. ego
   C. superego
   D. self-esteem

6. _____ was an Austrian physician who was interested in the development of the mind in order to treat psychological problems.
   A. Maslow
   B. Jung
   C. Hippocrates
   D. Freud

7. _____ is a medical specialty that deals with the treatment and prevention of mental illness.
   A. Psychology
   B. Psychiatry
   C. Physiology
   D. Oncology

8. The first level of Maslow's hierarchy and the foundation of a person's motivational drive is _____.
   A. security needs
   B. social needs
   C. physical needs
   D. self-esteem

9. The need to be all that you can be is called _____.
   A. social
   B. self-esteem
   C. self-defeating
   D. self-actualization

10. Self-esteem can fluctuate throughout the day based on the challenges a person faces.
    A. True
    B. False

11. _____ is (are) the process of interpreting information gathered from our surroundings.
    A. Subconscious
    B. Perception
    C. Assumptions
    D. Past experiences

12. Physiological influences of what we sense and feel and how we perform include all of the following EXCEPT _____.
    A. fatigue
    B. age
    C. gender
    D. senses

13. _____ are irrational fears of objects, activities, or situations.
    A. Phobias
    B. Defense mechanisms
    C. Rationalizations
    D. Psychiatric responses

14. _____ is the fear of blood.
    A. Agoraphobia
    B. Hemophobia
    C. Claustrophobia
    D. Arachnophobia

15. _____ is the fear of water.
    A. Apiphobia
    B. Hydrophobia
    C. Agoraphobia
    D. Phagophobia

16. Glossophobia is the fear of speaking in public.
    A. True
    B. False

17. Physical symptoms of stress include all of the following EXCEPT _____.
    A. forgetfulness
    B. chronic upset stomach
    C. headaches
    D. chills or heavy sweating

18. Depression is a psychological symptom of stress.
    A. True
    B. False

19. Behaving aggressively toward someone who cannot fight back as a substitute for anger toward the source of frustration is called _____.
    A. compensation
    B. displacement
    C. fantasy
    D. projection

20. Exaggerated and inappropriate behavior of a person in one area to handle inadequacy in some other area is called _____.
    A. aggression
    B. intellectualization
    C. sublimation
    D. overcompensation

CHAPTER SIX

Understanding Patient Behavior

VOCABULARY REVIEW

Matching: Match each term with the correct definition.

A. adulthood

B. childhood

C. cultural diversity

D. infancy

E. mental growth

F. physical growth

G. psychosocial growth

H. development

_____ 1. Part of the human life span including birth through the first year

_____ 2. Individual's emotional and social development

_____ 3. Individual's cognitive development

_____ 4. Part of the human life span concerned with an individual during early, middle, and later years in life

_____ 5. Mix of ethnicity, race, and religion in a given population

_____ 6. Individual's growth and development in physical size and motor and sensory skills

_____ 7. Part of human life span dealing with toddlers, preschoolers, school-age children, and adolescents

_____ 8. Progressive increases in the function of the body throughout a lifetime

THEORY RECALL

True/False

Indicate whether the sentence or statement is true or false.

_____ 1. Growth and change occur only throughout a human's adolescent years.

_____ 2. Medical assistants have a responsibility to their profession and to their patients to accept and respect the cultural beliefs of others even if they differ from their own.

_____ 3. Fear of pain and death are two very strong emotions for most people.

_____ 4. When a patient is fearful, talkative, withdrawn, or angry, the medical assistant should get the physician immediately to take care of the problem.

_____ 5. As a patient ages, the gastrointestinal tract slows down, learning is possible but slower, and drugs are processed more slowly.

Multiple Choice

Identify the letter of the choice that best completes the statement or answers the question.

1. There is a potential for ineffective communication when all of the following occur EXCEPT when
   _____.
   A. English is a second language
   B. the patient is angry, frightened, or in pain
   C. there are cultural differences
   D. direct eye contact is made

2. Which one of the following is NOT a category of change during growth and development of the human life span?
   A. Physical
   B. Socioeconomic
   C. Mental
   D. Psychosocial

3. Cognitive development occurs during _____ growth.
   A. physical
   B. socioeconomic
   C. mental
   D. psychosocial

4. During infancy, a baby that coos when happy or smiles at age 6 weeks is demonstrating _____ growth.
   A. physical
   B. socioeconomic
   C. mental
   D. psychosocial

5. When caring for an infant (birth to 3 months), in the office or clinic, the medical assistant should
   _____.
   A. make eye contact when speaking to the infant
   B. focus on eating and sleeping habits
   C. encourage grasping toys and toys with sounds
   D. encourage playing with large blocks for stacking

6. A toddler (13 months to 3 years) typically grows slowly, gaining only _____ pounds and growing only
   3 inches.
   A. 1 to 2
   B. 3 to 4
   C. 5 to 10
   D. 10 to 15

7. An infant aged 8 to 12 months is capable of which of the following task(s)?
   A. Shaking head "no"
   B. Waving "bye-bye"
   C. Both A and B
   D. Neither A nor B

8. A 19- to 23-month-old is capable of which of the following task(s)?
   A. Kicking a ball
   B. Hopping
   C. Coloring within the lines
   D. None of the above

9. The medical assistant should engage a child aged 24 to 36 months by _____.
   A. encouraging cooing and happy sounds
   B. encouraging grasping toys and toys with sound
   C. encouraging play with large blocks for stacking
   D. none of the above

10. Wrinkles typically first appear on patients in the age range of _____ years.
    A. 19 to 45
    B. 45 to 59
    C. 70 to 79
    D. 80 and older

11. In some _____ cultures, direct eye contact is considered to be disrespectful.
    A. Asian
    B. Latin
    C. African American
    D. European

12. _____ can cause more misunderstandings than any other form of communication.
    A. Foods
    B. Clothing
    C. Gestures
    D. Physical space

13. A(n) _____ is a universal gesture accepted by every culture.
    A. wave
    B. OK sign
    C. cry
    D. smile

14. Which one of the following is NOT an area of cultural difference?
    A. Eye contact
    B. Emotions
    C. Nontraditional/traditional healthcare
    D. All of the above

15. _____ is NOT a common response patients have toward illness, injury, or pain?
    A. Joy
    B. Anger
    C. Talkativeness
    D. Withdrawing

16. When dealing with an angry patient, it would NOT be productive to _____.
    A. remain calm and professional
    B. mimic the patient's level of anger
    C. listen, because some patients just need to vent
    D. agree with the patient; after all, you may be wrong

17. In the United States, the color black is a sign of mourning; in certain Asian cultures, the color _____ indicates mourning.
    A. yellow
    B. blue
    C. white
    D. purple

18. Bone mass begins to decrease in which age group?
    A. 20 to 25 years
    B. 30 to 35 years
    C. 40 to 45 years
    D. 45 to 59 years

19. Muscle efficiency peaks in the late _____.
    A. teens
    B. 20s
    C. 30s
    D. 40s

20. Minor motor skills greatly improve in which age group?
    A. Birth to 8 months
    B. 8 to 12 months
    C. 13 to 18 months
    D. 19 to 23 months

Sentence Completion

Complete each sentence or statement.

1. As a toddler becomes a(n) _____, expectations about physical, mental, and psychosocial

   characteristics and abilities are raised.

2. A(n) _____ development in infancy is a reaction to sound, motion, and light.

3. Involve _____ when demonstrating procedures for home care and have them practice

   the procedures.

4. A child of _____ to _____ months old will smile at himself or herself in the

   mirror.

5. A child of _____ to _____ years old can learn to print his or her name.

Short Answers

1. List and describe the three areas of change during growth and development that occur in a lifetime.

   _____

   _____

   _____

   _____

2. Explain why the medical assistant must understand the various body system changes involved in the
   aging process.

   _____

   _____

   _____

   _____

3. List five things a medical assistant can do when a patient becomes angry.

_____

_____

_____

_____

_____

4. Explain the importance of being knowledgeable about the cultural background of a patient.

_____

_____

_____

_____

CRITICAL THINKING

Simon lives in a large city and works as a medical assistant for a free health clinic with 15 physicians, 6 physician assistants, and 3 nurse practitioners on staff. Simon loves the fast pace of the practice. He enjoys working with the patients and their families and knows in his heart at the end of the day that he has given back to the community in which he grew up. The patient population is very diverse. Patients are from numerous ethnicities, with different religious beliefs, medical traditions, educational backgrounds, and age groups. The patients are very poor, and many are homeless. The practice's philosophy states that any person in the need of medical attention who comes through the door will receive treatment to the best of the facility's abilities. Some of the patients are on state-assisted programs or Medicare; many more of them pay on a sliding fee scale or do not pay at all. Simon speaks fluent Spanish and has learned several medical phrases in five languages, like "Where does it hurt?" "How long have you felt this way?" "What have you taken to help?" and "Did it help?" He cannot always understand the answers, but by watching the patient's nonverbal communication, he is able to form a basic understanding of what is going on. Simon has been able to learn the basics of many of the different cultures of his patients, and the patients respect Simon for his dedication.

A. Learn two medical phrases in Spanish and two medical phrases in another language of your choice that is not your primary language. Write them down and be able to repeat them verbally in class.

B. How do you think Simon learned about his patients' cultures?

C. List five nonverbal communication techniques for understanding "I am in pain here."

INTERNET RESEARCH

Keyword: Growth and Development in Infancy. Research three Web sites and list one physical, one mental, and one psychosocial development that occurs during infancy that is not listed in your textbook. Cite the source of your information.

WHAT WOULD YOU DO?

If you have accomplished the objectives in this chapter, you will be able to make better choices as a medical assistant. Take a look at this situation and decide what you would do.

Juan, 40 years old, has moved to the United States. His family is still in Mexico, but he hopes to find a good job soon and pay for them to come to the United States. Because Juan does not speak English very well, he has had difficulty finding employment and a place to live. Lately, he has been staying at a shelter for homeless people. His educational background is limited, and his broken English makes communicating difficult. Few Hispanic people live in the area where he has settled. Juan has lost 10 pounds, his vision is declining, and he has noticed that he is not hearing as well as he used to. Because of his constant weight loss and the vision problems, he decided to visit the local medical office. He has heard the office provides services to those who cannot pay.

When Juan arrives at the office, his clothing is worn and torn. The new medical assistant tells Juan that he cannot be seen at the office unless he can pay for his visit before he is seen. She does not explain her statement, and because of his broken English, Juan does not ask further questions. He thinks that the physician will not see him and leaves the office very upset. He decides to start taking herbal medications and to try home remedies. He now believes that seeing a physician in America just is not worth the trouble and embarrassment. Several weeks later, Juan is hospitalized with dehydration, starvation, and severe reactions to the herbal drugs.

This situation did not have to result in Juan's being hospitalized. If you were the new medical assistant, what would you have done differently?

1. **What part does age play in the symptoms that Juan is experiencing? Could the symptoms be related to the illnesses as well? Explain.**

   _____

   _____

   _____

   _____

2. **What influence did differing cultural backgrounds have in this situation?**

   _____

   _____

   _____

   _____

3. **How would the situation have turned out if the new medical assistant had studied cultural differences? What activities would help the medical assistant in understanding diversity?**

_____

_____

_____

_____

4. **What factors led to Juan's withdrawal from medical care until he was hospitalized?**

_____

_____

_____

_____

5. **As the medical assistant, how would you approach Juan differently?**

_____

_____

_____

_____

APPLICATION OF SKILLS

1. Select one age group of growth and development. Interview two individuals (parents or guardians, depending on the age group selected) that fall within the age group you selected. Using the development charts in the textbook, ask or assess each individual (parent or guardian) if they have met or accomplished each guideline listed in all three categories: physical, mental, and psychosocial.

2. Research on the Internet or local library a culture other than your own. (You may ask an individual of that culture to provide you with information.) Write two or three sentences addressing the following areas. Cite your source(s) of information.

   A. History

   B. Food

   C. Music

   D. Medical traditions

   E. Clothing

   F. One holiday celebration unique to their culture

CHAPTER QUIZ

Multiple Choice

Identify the letter of the choice that best completes the statement or answers the question.

1. _____ is the part of the human life span concerned with an individual during early, middle, and later years in life.
   A. Physical growth
   B. Adulthood
   C. Infancy
   D. Mental growth

2. An individual's emotional and social development is called _____.
   A. cultural diversity
   B. physical growth
   C. psychosocial growth
   D. mental growth

3. _____ is the mix of ethnicity, race, and religion in a given population.
   A. Social standards
   B. Cultural diversity
   C. Socioeconomic status
   D. Self-esteem

4. _____ is NOT a common patient response to illness.
   A. Anger
   B. Talkative
   C. Withdrawn
   D. Calmness

5. Dexterity decreases in patients aged _____.
   A. 10 to 12 months
   B. 20 to 15 years
   C. 40 to 49 years
   D. 60 to 69 years

6. Toilet training should be completed by the age of _____ months.
   A. 6
   B. 12 to 18
   C. 20 to 24
   D. 24 to 36

7. An infant aged _____ months explores by banging, dropping, and throwing.
   A. 0 to 3
   B. 4 to 7
   C. 10 to 12
   D. 24 to 36

8. At what age should the medical assistant start to observe a child's behavior and interaction with peers?
   A. 13 to 18 months
   B. 19 to 23 months
   C. 24 to 36 months
   D. At no age is this appropriate

9. At what age should a child be able to drink from a cup?
   A. 10 to 12 months
   B. 13 to 18 months
   C. 19 to 23 months
   D. 24 to 36 months

10. During what age is a child most susceptible to unfavorable experiences that can lead to mistrust and hamper attempts to trying new things?
    A. 1 to 2 years
    B. 3 to 5 years
    C. 6 to 8 years
    D. 10 to 12 years

11. During the years of _____, peer pressure becomes a major issue in the child's life.
    A. childhood
    B. adolescence
    C. early adulthood
    D. geriatrics

12. Wrinkles typically first appear during the ages of _____ years.
    A. 20 to 29
    B. 30 to 39
    C. 45 to 59
    D. 64 to 69

13. The psychosocial occurrence of retirement typically occurs during what age group?
    A. 35 to 39 years
    B. 40 to 50 years
    C. 50 to 55 years
    D. 60 to 69 years

14. Does a feeling of self-worth have any impact on how a person approaches life span changes?
    A. Yes
    B. No

15. Religion, race, ethics, economics, and social upbringing have little, if any, impact on a patient's behavior.
    A. True
    B. False

16. In some cultures, it is believed that poor health is a punishment from a higher power.
    A. True
    B. False

17. Typically, financial and employment concerns do NOT contribute to the overall wellness of an individual.
    A. True
    B. False

18. A medical assistant must become very proficient in stereotyping their patients as quickly as possible to ensure they receive the best health care.
    A. True
    B. False

19. In the United States, the color _____ is a sign of mourning; whereas in certain cultures, the color white means mourning.
    A. black
    B. yellow
    C. white
    D. purple

20. Cognitive development occurs during _____ growth.
    A. physical
    B. socioeconomic
    C. mental
    D. psychosocial

CHAPTER **SEVEN**

Effective Communication

VOCABULARY REVIEW

Matching: Match each term with the correct definition.

A. active listening

B. adjective

C. adverb

D. conjunction

E. distracter

F. feedback

G. grammar

H. interjection

I. noun

J. preposition

K. pronoun

L. punctuation

M. sentence

N. subject

O. verb

_____ 1. Verbal or nonverbal indication that a message was received

_____ 2. Word used to describe a noun or pronoun

_____ 3. Word used to begin a prepositional phrase

_____ 4. Word used to express strong feelings or emotion

_____ 5. Word in a sentence that expresses action or a state of being

_____ 6. Occurs when a listener maintains eye contact and provides responses to the speaker

_____ 7. Word used to join words or groups of words

_____ 8. Marks within and between sentences that separate, emphasize, and clarify the different ideas within a sentence or group of sentences

_____ 9. Study of words and their relationship to other words in a sentence

_____ 10. Something that prevents the sender or receiver from giving full attention to the message

_____ 11. Word used to name things, including people, places, objects, and ideas

_____ 12. Word used to describe a verb, an adjective, or an another adverb

_____ 13. Word used to take the place of a noun

_____ 14. Group of words that express a complete thought

_____ 15. Part of a sentence that expresses action or a state of being

THEORY RECALL

True/False

Indicate whether the sentence or statement is true or false.

_____ 1. The goal of communication is to clearly exchange information between a sender and a receiver.

_____ 2. Public space is considered to be 2 to 4 feet apart.

_____ 3. Active listening involves hearing what the speaker is saying but not listening with enough effort to become personally, intensely involved in what is being said.

_____ 4. In order to express a complete thought, a sentence must contain at least one noun and one pronoun.

_____ 5. A fax machine converts written material or pictures into electronic impulses that are transmitted by telephone lines to other locations with similar equipment.

Multiple Choice

Identify the letter of the choice that best completes the statement or answers the question.

1. Nonverbal communication comprises approximately _____ percent of all communication.
   A. 10
   B. 40
   C. 75
   D. 90

2. Which one of the following is NOT an important part of delivering messages?
   A. Not using slang terms
   B. Rate of speech that is neither too fast nor too slow
   C. Voice inflection
   D. Ability to multitask while delivering the message

3. _____ is a communication distracter.
   A. Quiet environment
   B. Incorrect use of grammar
   C. Climate-controlled temperature
   D. Quiet music in the background

4. When communicating with a patient, it is best to ask _____ questions.
   A. open-ended
   B. closed-ended

5. Interpreting body language is an important part of _____ communication.
   A. verbal
   B. nonverbal

6. Two typical nonverbal signals that our eyes send are pupil size and _____.
   A. iris color
   B. direction of gaze
   C. posture
   D. both A and B

7. _____ is NOT a nonverbal response.
   A. Singing
   B. Smiling
   C. Physical appearance
   D. Both B and C

8. Numbers may be used as nouns or _____.
   A. verbs
   B. adjectives
   C. adverbs
   D. pronouns

9. _____ is an automated answering device.
   A. Voice mail system
   B. Facsimile
   C. E-mail
   D. None of the above

10. Which of the following is a disadvantage of voice mail?
    A. People can call all day or at any hour to leave a message.
    B. Length of message is reduced because communication is one-way.
    C. Some people want to speak to a person immediately.
    D. Messages can be retrieved from other locations.

11. Which of the following is NOT an item that can be included on a Web site?
    A. Practice philosophy
    B. Hours of operation
    C. Billing and insurance information
    D. All of the above could be included

12. Advantages of a Web site include all of the following EXCEPT that _____.
    A. it saves patients the time and effort of calling the office
    B. a Web site can be quickly updated
    C. it can provide answer to FAQs (frequently asked questions)
    D. patients may not have access to the Internet

13. Faxes (*are* or *are not*) considered forms of original and legal documents.
    A. are
    B. are not

14. A disadvantage of e-mail messages is that _____.
    A. e-mail is available 24 hours a day
    B. messages are sent and received rapidly
    C. messages once sent are often not retrievable
    D. verification can be made that a message was sent and received

15. A _____ sentence expresses only one thought.
    A. subject
    B. simple
    C. complex
    D. compound

16. Numbers that begin a sentence should be spelled out even if they are greater than _____.
    A. 3
    B. 5
    C. 7
    D. 9

17. Which one of the following is correctly spelled?
    A. abcess
    B. abscess
    C. absces
    D. abbscess

18. Which one of the following is correctly spelled?
    A. negligence
    B. nagligance
    C. negligance
    D. neglligence

19. Which one of the following is correctly spelled?
    A. theif
    B. percieve
    C. concieve
    D. believe

20. Always use a _____ when sending a fax.
    A. typewriter
    B. letter of introduction
    C. cover sheet
    D. reference page

Sentence Completion

Complete each sentence or statement.

1. Do not send _____ information via e-mail.

2. The acronym _____ outlines the six steps to becoming a better listener.

3. I (always/all ways) go to the park after school.

4. In (awhile/a while) we will go to the beach.

5. (Its/It's) not likely the order will arrive today.

Short Answers

1. State the goal of the communication process.

   _____

   _____

   _____

2. List and describe the three components of the communication process.

   _____

   _____

   _____

3. List the three components of effective listening.

   _____

   _____

   _____

4. Explain the importance of choosing the correct words.

   _____

   _____

   _____

CRITICAL THINKING

Cassandra brought her mother, Elizabeth Seneca, to her doctor's appointment this morning. Mrs. Seneca has been feeling poorly for the past 4 days. Cassandra does not know what exactly is wrong. Kym, the medical assistant, takes Cassandra and her mother into the exam room and notices bruises on Mrs. Seneca's arm. Mrs. Seneca glances quickly around the room and sits with a sigh in the chair. She straightens her skirt and brushes at an invisible speck repeatedly. Kym asks Mrs. Seneca how she is feeling today. Cassandra answers immediately, "She is not eating, she barely sleeps, and she won't even go outside for some fresh air." Mrs. Seneca twists an almost shredded tissue in her hands. Kym looks directly at Mrs. Seneca and asks again how she is feeling. Mrs. Seneca looks up briefly. Kym notices that her pupils are large and that her mouth is set in a firm, thin line. Mrs. Seneca mumbles a response almost under her breath. Kym moves closer to Mrs. Seneca to hear her better, and Mrs. Seneca moves back farther on her chair. Kym steps away. "Are you in pain?" Kym asks. There still is no response. Kym washes her hands and gathers the equipment together to take Mrs. Seneca's pulse, respiration, and blood pressure. When she reaches out to take Mrs. Seneca's arm to help her roll up her sleeve, Mrs. Seneca quickly looks at her daughter and then back at the floor and at the same time bats away Kym's hand.

A. In your opinion, what do you think is going on with Mrs. Seneca?

B. What verbal communication leads you to your opinion?

C. What nonverbal communication leads you to your opinion?

D. What should be Kym's next step? Why?

INTERNET RESEARCH

Keyword: Interpreting Body Language. Research three Web sites. Create a list of 10 body language indicators. Describe what they indicate and how you can use this knowledge as a medical assistant. Cite the source(s) of your information.

WHAT WOULD YOU DO?

If you have accomplished the objectives in this chapter, you will be able to make better choices as a medical assistant. Take a look at this situation and decide what you would do.

Panina is a former resident of the Middle East who moved to the United States with her husband, Abed, 6 months ago. Naturally, she brings with her the cultural and ethnic contexts of her homeland. Panina awakens one morning with a pain in her breast. She becomes concerned and calls a physician's office for an appointment. Because she has difficulty understanding the English language, she misunderstands the appointment time, and Panina and Abed arrive at the office an hour late. Abed demands to accompany his wife to the exam room. Therese, the medical assistant, tells Abed that they are late for the appointment and that he must stay in the waiting room while Panina is being examined. Panina, refusing eye contact with Therese, begins to cry. Abed becomes upset and tells Therese that the only way Panina will be examined is if he accompanies her to the room to explain to the male doctor what is wrong with her. Therese refuses, and Panina and Abed leave the office, threatening to tell all their friends how this office "just does not care about patients at all."

Effective communication helps eliminate misunderstandings. If you were the medical assistant in this situation, how could you have used your understanding of effective communication skills to help?

1. **What role did Panina and Abed's cultural and ethnic background play in the misunderstandings in the physician's office? What role did communication skills play in the misunderstandings?**

   _____

   _____

   _____

2. **What distracters may have caused the lack of communication between Panina and Therese?**

   _____

   _____

   _____

3. **What nonverbal communication between Panina and Therese could have been recognized and used to diffuse the negative situation that occurred in the physician's office?**

   _____

   _____

   _____

4. **Why is an understanding of ethnicity and cultural differences so important in the medical field?**

   _____

   _____

   _____

5. **What body parts are involved in the communication of body language?**

   _____

   _____

   _____

APPLICATION OF SKILLS

1. Underline the SUBJECT in each of the following sentences.
   A. We will open the office at 8:00 A.M.
   B. The physician is in a meeting at the hospital.
   C. Sharon stayed late to inventory the supplies.
   D. The committee will adjourn and reconvene tomorrow.

2. Underline the VERB in each of the following sentences.
   A. Sam ran quickly down the hall to grab the crash cart.
   B. Tomorrow, we will begin the new research project.
   C. Chelsea booked the reservations for the medical conference.
   D. Mrs. Jones seems to be unconscious.

3. Underline the PRONOUN(s) in each of the following sentences
   A. She looked nauseated.
   B. Please pass me the stapler.
   C. Will they be done in the exam room soon?
   D. I would like to go over the end-of-month reports this afternoon.

4. Underline the ADJECTIVE(s) in each of the following sentences.
   A. This new brand of antibacterial soap smells like fresh lemons.
   B. The physician ordered two new oak computer desks for his office and two black leather chairs.
   C. The medical assistant just hired has exceptional skills.
   D. The casting room was left in a huge mess.

5. Underline the ADVERB(s) in each of the following sentences.
   A. Mrs. Thompson carefully removed the bandages from Lincoln's infected toe.
   B. We nearly didn't make the 1:00 o'clock flight.
   C. Angela lazily thumbed through an old magazine in the waiting room.
   D. Next year we are certainly going to need a larger office.

6. Underline the PREPOSITION(s) in each of the following sentences.
   A. The new clinic is just around the corner.
   B. Henry will have to go over to the hospital before he can file the insurance forms.
   C. Mickey reached across the minor surgery tray and contaminated the sterile field.
   D. Tressa, please go behind the curtain and change into the patient gown I left for you.

7. Underline the CONJUNCTION(s) in each of the following sentences.
   A. I ordered three pairs of turquoise scrubs and two of the raspberry ones as well.
   B. He could change Mr. Crinshaw's medication, but he is concerned that it will not be as effective.
   C. Since Sara stopped eating fast food, she has lost 15 pounds, but she is still 50 pounds overweight.
   D. The biopsy was delayed because the patient was not fasting.

8. Underline the INTERJECTION(s) in each of the following sentences.
   A. Stop! That really hurts.
   B. Perfect! Just a few more stitches and we will be all done.
   C. Oh, we will need a second opinion before we operate.
   D. Wonderful, Diane, you did a great job today; thank you.

9. Using Table 7-4 as a guideline, punctuate the following sentences.
   A. Where are my new scrubs I wanted to wear them today and if I cant find them were going to be late
   B. Have you seen their lab equipment theyre going to be hiring next week I would really like to work there
   C. Dr Xaxon the world renowned physician performed the procedure impeccably
   D. Katherine has given up smoking about five times but she cannot seem to break the habit

CHAPTER QUIZ

Multiple Choice

Identify the letter of the choice that best completes the statement or answers the question.

1. _____ is NOT a component of the communication process.
   A. Organization
   B. Message
   C. Sender
   D. Receiver

2. Based on statistics, _____ percent of all communication is nonverbal.
   A. 10
   B. 25
   C. 75
   D. 90

3. The way a message is delivered is NOT as important as the message itself.
   A. True
   B. False

4. A _____ is anything that causes the sender or receiver of a message to not give full attention to the message.
   A. detractor
   B. distracter
   C. distortion
   D. deformation

5. Assessing _____ from the receiver allows you to determine if the message was understood the way it was intended.
   A. opinions
   B. responses
   C. feedback
   D. all of the above

6. _____ involves hearing what the speaker is saying, but not listening with enough effort to become personally involved in what is being said.
   A. Passive listening
   B. Active listening
   C. Aggressive listening
   D. Unconscious listening

7. Acceptable personal space is used for those times of closeness and is typically _____ feet apart.
   A. 12 to 25
   B. 10 to 15
   C. 1½ to 2½
   D. 1 to 1½

8. _____ help(s) separate, emphasize, and clarify the different ideas within sentences and between groups of sentences.
   A. Capitalization
   B. Punctuation marks
   C. Proofreading marks
   D. Adjectives

9. A word that shows action in a sentence is a(n) _____.
   A. subject
   B. noun
   C. adverb
   D. verb

10. A(n) _____ converts written material or pictures into electronic impulses that are transmitted by telephone lines and recorded magnetically and can be printed as a hard copy.
    A. voice mail
    B. e-mail
    C. facsimile
    D. telephone call

11. "The hemostats fell to the floor with a clang." Select the VERB.
    A. fell
    B. to the
    C. hemostats
    D. with

12. "The three medical assistants all went to lunch together yesterday." Select the SUBJECT.
    A. yesterday
    B. three
    C. medical assistants
    D. lunch

13. "Dr. Xaxon, the world-renowned physician, performed the procedure impeccably." Select the ADJECTIVE.
    A. Dr. Xaxon
    B. world-renowned physician
    C. performed
    D. procedure

14. "Good grief! What now?" Select the INTERJECTION.
    A. Good grief
    B. What
    C. now
    D. All of the above

15. "Quickly! We are very nearly there, Thom." Select the ADVERB.
    A. Quickly
    B. are
    C. very nearly
    D. Thom

16. Which one of the following sentences is punctuated correctly?
    A. In 3 weeks' time we'll have to begin school again.
    B. After surviving this ordeal the patient felt relieved.
    C. He replied "I have no idea what you mean."
    D. Its such a beautiful day that Ive decided to take the day off.

17. Which one of the following sentences is punctuated correctly?
    A. The problems involved in this operation are I think numerous.
    B. Yes Helen did mention that all three of you were coming to the medical conference.
    C. The patient used to live at 1721 Gretchen Avenue Kansas City MO but has since moved to 3rd Street West Holland Way Dubuque Iowa.
    D. Chris did not see how he could organize, write, and proofread the paper in only 2 hours.

18. Which one of the following sentences is punctuated incorrectly?
    A. Having cut the roses she decided to bring them to her friend in the hospital.
    B. Jillian, who had worked in the dress shop all summer, hoped to work there again during the Christmas holidays.
    C. "Oh no" Max exclaimed, "I think that Dr. Holmes wanted Mrs. Jenson's file immediately."
    D. I hope that someday, we can redecorate the reception area.

19. Which statement is correctly written?
    A. Wear are my new scrubs? I wanted to where them today, and if I can't find them wear going to be late.
    B. Were are my new scrubs? I wanted to wear them today, and if I can't find them where going to be late.
    C. Where are my new scrubs? I wanted to wear them today, and if I can't find them we're going to be late.
    D. Where are my new scrubs? I wanted to we're them today, and if I can't find them we're going to be late.

20. Which statement is correctly written?
    A. Have you seen their lab equipment? They're going to be hiring next week. I would really like to work there.
    B. Have you seen there lab equipment? Their going to be hiring next week. I would really like to work their.
    C. Have you seen they're lab equipment? Their going to be hiring next week. I would really like to work there.
    D. Have you seen their lab equipment? Their going to be hiring next week. I would really like to work they're.

CHAPTER **EIGHT**

Communicating With Patients

VOCABULARY REVIEW

Matching: Match each term with the correct definition.

A. litigation

B. holistic

C. maturation

D. rapport

_____ 1. A growth-and-development process involving a patient's physical, social, and emotional functioning

_____ 2. Lawsuit

_____ 3. Effective relationship that considers both the physical and emotional needs

_____ 4. Involving all health needs of the patient, including physical, emotional, social, economic, and spiritual needs

THEORY RECALL

True/False

Indicate whether the sentence or statement is true or false.

_____ 1. Communicating effectively with patients is a key factor in providing quality care.

_____ 2. Patient complaints should be handled directly by the physician.

_____ 3. Patients with disabilities expect sympathy and special considerations.

_____ 4. When communicating with children, use wording and methods that are appropriate to their age.

_____ 5. Use both verbal and nonverbal clues to assess a patient's ability to read and comprehend information.

Multiple Choice

Identify the letter of the choice that best completes the statement or answers the question.

1. _____ does NOT apply when expecting a patient to comply with treatment plans.
   A. Patient's physical state
   B. Patient's emotional state
   C. Patient's educational background
   D. None of the above, because all do apply

2. Which one of the following is NOT important in effective communication for patient teaching?
   A. Assessing patient's readiness to learn
   B. Including patient's family or support group in treatment plans
   C. Patient's dietary habits
   D. Providing time for questions

3. Developmentally delayed patients are those who are behind in _____.
   A. maturation
   B. intelligence
   C. education
   D. physical abilities

4. When communicating with children, do all of the following EXCEPT _____.
   A. use technical terms to explain all procedures
   B. use dolls and pictures to enhance communication
   C. allow children to handle "safe" medical equipment.
   D. encourage them to talk about themselves

5. The ability to process new information and to apply it appropriately in a given setting reflects a patient's _____ functioning.
   A. verbal
   B. nonverbal
   C. mental
   D. emotional

6. Which one of the following is NOT an effective means of communicating with a patient who is hearing impaired?
   A. Directly face the patient when speaking.
   B. Speak louder and more quickly.
   C. Use visual examples.
   D. Both A and B

7. All of the following are appropriate ways to communicate effectively with patients EXCEPT to _____.
   A. involve the patient's family in decision-making
   B. argue with the patient about his or her beliefs that conflict with their medical treatment
   C. provide honest feedback
   D. Both B and C

8. _____ healthcare deals with all of the health needs of the patient.
   A. Allopathic
   B. Holistic
   C. Generic
   D. Western

9. Three of the following statements pertain to considerations that should be made when accommodating patients with physical disabilities. Which one does NOT pertain?
   A. Restate directions and instructions frequently.
   B. Do not rush special needs patients.
   C. Special needs patients may require assistance in the bathroom.
   D. Be careful ushering a special needs patient through doorways.

10. Which one of the following does NOT apply when working with patients who are visually impaired?
    A. Use written material with large print.
    B. Face the patient directly when speaking.
    C. Give verbal clues when necessary.
    D. Alert patients before touching them.

Sentence Completion

Complete each sentence or statement.

1. The medical assistant must use the skills he or she has learned about human relations and behavior to develop a working _____ with patients.

2. Finding better ways to _____ with patients results in quality service and patient care.

3. A patient may _____ if he or she perceives the quality of the service to be unsatisfactory.

4. _____ occurs when the patient is unhappy with the performance of the support staff in a medical facility.

5. Use _____ language when responding to a complaint, and reassure the patient that the complaint will be investigated.

Short Answers

1. Explain the concept of holistic care.

   _____

   _____

2. Explain the importance of handling patient complaints effectively.

_____

_____

3. List seven ways to effectively communicate with a patient who has a hearing impairment.

_____

_____

_____

_____

4. List six considerations for communicating effectively with elderly patients.

_____

_____

_____

_____

_____

_____

APPLICATION OF SKILLS

1. Select a partner in class for this activity. Partner A should be blindfolded, while Partner B navigates Partner A through a half-hour of lunch time. Then they switch places for an additional half-hour. Pay particular attention to effectively communicating with the blindfolded partner. Write one paragraph journaling the experience from both perspectives, being the caregiver and then being the visually impaired.

2. Using cotton balls or earplugs, perform the above activity but this time as a hearing impaired person.

CRITICAL THINKING

Using the paragraphs written in the Application of Skills section, exchange papers with your partner.

A. How did your partner feel about you as the caregiver and your ability to effectively communicate?

_____

_____

_____

_____

B. What did you learn from performing this activity that will help you to become a better medical assistant?

_____

_____

_____

_____

C. Have you ever assisted a physically challenged individual in the past? If so, what have you learned from that experience? If not, look for an opportunity to do so within the next 2 days and then answer the above question.

_____

_____

_____

_____

_____

INTERNET RESEARCH

Keyword: Americans With Disabilities Act. Locate the answer to following question, "Who is a 'qualified individual with a disability'?" Cite the source(s) of your information.

WHAT WOULD YOU DO?

If you have accomplished the objectives in this chapter, you will be able to make better choices as a medical assistant. Take a look at this situation and decide what you would do.

Mr. Joplin is a spry 82-year-old and still lives in his own home. His wife died about a year ago, but Mr. Joplin has no severe medical problems and is able to care for himself. He does have visual problems caused by cataracts in his left eye, as well as joint stiffness related to his age. John, the medical assistant, approaches Mr. Joplin to escort him to the examining room. John shouts at Mr. Joplin as if he has a hearing difficulty, then walks away without assisting Mr. Joplin from the chair. When John reaches the door, he looks over his shoulder, rolls his eyes, and shouts, "Do you need some help?" Mr. Joplin looks away and refuses any assistance. Dr. Smith examines Mr. Joplin and asks John to explain the treatment so Mr. Joplin will comply. John hurriedly tells Mr. Joplin one time what is expected, then returns him to the waiting room. Several days later, Mr. Joplin calls the office to tell the receptionist to cancel his next appointment because he is going to find a new physician.

John's poor communication skills caused Dr. Smith to lose Mr. Joplin as a patient. If you were the medical assistant in this situation, what would you have done to communicate more effectively with Mr. Joplin?

1. **Did John need to speak in a loud voice to Mr. Joplin, or did he stereotype Mr. Joplin because of his age and visual impairments?**

_____

_____

_____

_____

2. **Did John show professionalism? List three ways that John could have improved his interaction with Mr. Joplin.**

_____

_____

_____

_____

3. **What body language did John display that exhibited negative thoughts about Mr. Joplin?**

_____

_____

_____

_____

4. **What role did Mr. Joplin's age play in this interaction?**

_____

_____

_____

_____

5. **What steps could John have taken to show that he really wanted Mr. Joplin to comply with the physician's treatment plan?**

_____

_____

_____

_____

6. **What role did the receptionist play in this scenario? What should she have done when Mr. Joplin canceled his appointment?**

_____

_____

_____

_____

CHAPTER QUIZ

Multiple Choice

Identify the letter of the choice that best completes the statement or answers the question.

1. The growth and development process involving patient's physical, social, and emotional functioning is called _____.
   A. holistic health care
   B. litigation
   C. Americans With Disabilities Act
   D. maturation

2. Communicating ineffectively with patients is a key factor in providing quality care.
   A. True
   B. False

3. All of a patient's needs influence his or her behavior and compliance with treatment.
   A. True
   B. False

4. Which one of the following is NOT a means of assessing a patient's understanding or a method to improve communication?
   A. Communicating in technical/medical terms
   B. Asking patients to write down questions
   C. Identifying any communication barriers
   D. Not being afraid to say, "I don't know"

5. Which one of the following is NOT a category of reasons for which patients complain?
   A. Administrative complaints
   B. Medical complaints
   C. Laboratory complaints
   D. All of the above are complaint categories

6. Take all complaints seriously, but write down only the facts that feel important to you.
   A. True
   B. False

7. Always inform the physician and/or office manager of any statements made by the patient that reflect a negative attitude.
   A. True
   B. False

8. A large number of _____ result from careless actions or comments made by physicians and office staff when patients complain.
   A. warnings
   B. threats
   C. lawsuits
   D. thank-you cards

9. All treatment plans must allow patients to maintain their _____ and help establish trust in the healthcare team.
   A. self-esteem
   B. modesty
   C. confidence
   D. All of the above

10. You must get rid of all positive beliefs so they do not affect your communication with or care for patients.
    A. True
    B. False

11. A medical assistant must answer only questions within their scope of training. With the physician's guidance, he or she may explain the reasons for the needed changes and the importance of compliance.
    A. True
    B. False

12. A medical assistant must never accept the patient's decisions regarding medical care if it is not in alignment with his or her personal beliefs.
    A. True
    B. False

13. When working with patients with special needs, it is extremely important to ask if they would like assistance before assuming they are incapable of performing a task.
    A. True
    B. False

14. In working with visually impaired patients, you must NEVER _____.
    A. provide verbal directions
    B. yell so they will hear you more clearly
    C. alert the patient before touching them
    D. all of the above

15. Patients with disabilities do NOT expect sympathy or special considerations.
    A. True
    B. False

16. A person is diagnosed as mentally challenged when he or she functions at a higher-than-normal intellectual level.
    A. True
    B. False

17. Developmentally delayed patients are those behind in maturation.
    A. True
    B. False

18. Very few communities actually have support groups or special day care centers equipped to handle mentally handicapped or developmentally delayed individuals.
    A. True
    B. False

19. A medical assistant is expected to be an active listener and to understand and anticipate the patient's needs.
    A. True
    B. False

20. An unhappy patient is more likely to sue.
    A. True
    B. False

CHAPTER NINE

Understanding Medical Terminology

✗ VOCABULARY REVIEW

Matching: Match each term with the correct definition.

A. combining form

B. combining vowel

C. consonant

D. diagnostic

E. diminutive

F. eponym

G. homonym

H. operative

I. plural

J. prefix

K. root word

L. suffix

M. symptomatic

N. synonym

O. vowel

__K__ 1. Core meaning of a word *main*

__F__ 2. Name of a specific person, place, or thing for which something is being named

__O__ 3. Speech sound used to pronounce words (a, e, i, o, u, and sometimes y)

__B__ 4. Vowel added to a root word before any prefixes or suffixes

__A__ 5. Root word with a vowel added to make pronunciation easier

__G__ 6. Word that has the same pronunciation but a different spelling and meaning than another word

__I__ 7. Noun that refers to two or more

__M__ 8. Having to do with the characteristics of a particular disease

__D__ 9. Having to do with recognizing or identifying diseases in the body

__N__ 10. Root word, prefix, or suffix that has the same or nearly the same meaning as a given word, prefix, or suffix

__H__ 11. Having to do with an action or operation

__C__ 12. Speech sound used to pronounce words that include all letters except a, e, i, o, u, and sometimes y

__J__ 13. Word part placed at the beginning of a root word to change its meaning

__L__ 14. Word part or series of word parts added to the end of a root word to change the meaning

__E__ 15. Small; a small version of something

THEORY RECALL

True/False

Indicate whether the sentence or statement is true or false.

___F___ 1. The vast majority of medical terms have German and French origins.

___T___ 2. We use medical terminology because we can use one word for something that might otherwise take many words to describe.

___T___ 3. All medical terms have at least one root word.

___T___ 4. All medical terms must contain at least one prefix.

___T___ 5. Phonetics help make the pronunciation of medical terms easier.

Multiple Choice

Identify the letter of the choice that best completes the statement or answers the question.

1. In general, when a medical term has a vowel followed by a ___C___ the vowel receives a short pronunciation and a *breve* is placed over the vowel.
   A. second vowel
   B. consonant
   C. "y"
   D. All of the above apply

2. Some consonants are referred to as having a _SOFT_ or _hard_ sound.
   A. short, long
   B. quick, sharp
   C. soft, hard
   D. None of the above

3. When forming a plural of most English words, add a(n) ___A___.
   A. s
   B. 's
   C. es
   D. 'es

4. For nouns ending in a "y" preceded by a consonant, change the "y" to a(n) ___C___ and add "es."
   A. a
   B. e
   C. i
   D. o

5. The synonym meaning "lung" is ___D___.
   A. plur/o -pleura
   B. pulmon/o -pneumo
   C. respirat/o -respirata
   D. lung/o -lunga

6. __D__ is an example of an eponym.
   A. Pinkeye
   B. Athlete's foot
   C. McBurney point
   D. All of the above

7. The suffix that means "the study of" is __D__.
   A. -ologist
   B. -oscopy
   C. -ic
   D. -ology

8. The term that means "the heart is located in the right hemothorax" is __B__.
   A. cardiomegaly
   B. dextrocardia
   C. cardiopathy
   D. cardiac

9. __A__ means "feverish" or "having a fever."
   A. Febrile
   B. Afebrile
   C. Disfebrile
   D. Anafebrile

10. "Death of cells or tissues through injury or disease" is called __C__.
    A. macrosis
    B. narcolepsy
    C. necrosis
    D. cryptorchidism

11. The term meaning "above the pubis" is __A__.
    A. suprapubic
    B. supranasal
    C. supracostal
    D. supraventricular

12. Bluish discoloration of the skin and mucous membranes from lack of oxygen is called __B__.
    A. erythroderma
    B. cyanosis
    C. chromatoderma
    D. leukoplakia

13. "Xanthroderma" means __C__.
    A. blue skin
    B. white skin
    C. yellow skin
    D. none of the above

14. "Ferrous" means __B__.
    A. nitrogenous waste in the blood
    B. relating to or containing iron
    C. excretion of excessive amounts of sodium in the urine
    D. colorless, odorless gas formed from carbon and oxygen

15. Muscular tissue of the heart is ___C___.
    A. adipose tissue
    B. epithelium
    C. myocardia
    D. epicardia

16. The prefix meaning "half, one side or partial" is ___D___.
    A. bi-
    B. milli-
    C. multi-
    D. hemi-

17. The prefix of the word "multicellular" is ___A___.
    A. multi-
    B. cell
    C. cellular
    d. -ar

18. A condition or disease affecting a large population is called a(n) ___B___.
    A. pandemic
    B. epidemic
    C. endemic
    D. peridemic

19. The process of removing the calcium from bones is called ___C___.
    A. deactivation
    B. catabolism
    C. decalcification
    D. endocalcification.

20. A person who specializes in the study of diseases is called a(n) ___B___.
    A. endocrinologist
    B. pathologist
    C. anesthesiologist
    D. cardiologist

Sentence Completion

Write the correct term in the blank for each prefix, suffix, or word root.

1. _Blood_ hemat/o

2. _Chemical_ chem/o

3. _gland_ aden/o

4. _hidden_ crypt/o

5. _Cancer_ carcin/o

6. _double_ dipl/o

7. _without_ exo-

8. _Water_ hydro-

9. _abnormally_ scler/o _hard_

10. _Pertaining_ noct/o _To The night_

11. _above_ super- ?

12. _heat_ therm/o _heat_

13. _grey_ glauc/o

14. _White_ leuk/o ?

15. _Stainble_ chromat/o _by dye_

16. _yellow_ xanth/o

17. _Chronic_ cirrh/o _inflammation of Liver RRcsu [Txellow skin & eyes_

18. _chloride_ chlori- ?

19. _oxygen_ ox-

20. _Fat_ adip/o

21. _muscle_ my/o

22. _connecTn_ sarc/o

23. _above_ epi- ?

24. _nervous_ nuer/o

25. _Twice_ bi-

26. _1/00_ centi- _on hundredth_

27. _1000_ kilo-

28. _1/000,000_ micro- _one millionth_

29. _1/000_ milli- _one Thousandth_

30. _many_ multi-

31. _none_ nulli-

32. _First_ primi-

33. _Three_ tri-

34. _one_ mono- ?

35. _Taking away_ ab-

36. _without_ ana-

37. _Inside_ endo-

38. _inBetween_ inter-

39. _around_ para-

40. _behind_ post-

41. _below_ sub-

42. _Lowblood pressure_ hypo-

43. _across_ trans-

44. _against_ anti-

45. _difficult_ dys-

46. _Fast_ tachy-

47. _decrease_ -ic

48. _state of being condition_ -ism

49. _one who specializes_ -logist

50. _constant standing_ -stasis

51. _pain_ -algia

52. _sarcoid_ -oid

53. _breaking down_ -lysis

54. _enlargment_ -megaly

55. _Breathing_ -pnea

56. _discharge_ -rrhea

57. _narrowing_ -stenosis

58. _Record_ -gram

59. _Process of_ -graphy

60. _inFlamation_ -itis

61. _presence of inflammation_ -iasis

62. _soft Thing_ -malacia

63. _Tumor_ -oma

64. _abnormal Condition_ -osis

65. _excess cells_ -plasia

66. _discharge_ -rrhagia

67. _Process oF examing with_ -scopy a scope _From Blood vessels_

68. _Rupture_ -rrhexis

69. _surgical Puncture_ -centesis

70. _excision_ -ectomy

71. _Fixing_ -pexy

72. _surgical Repair_ -plasty

73. _sucture_ -rrhaphy

74. _Creation of_ -stomy _a new opening_

75. _incision_ -tomy

76. _crushing of_ -tripsy

77. _One who is_ -ist _specialized in a treatment_

78. _begining_ -gen _origin_

79. _blood condition_ -emia

80. _Stone_ -lith

Short Answers

1. Explain the importance of using correct medical terminology.

The patient will get the right treatment, will lose trust in health care Team, Insurance will not pay, and lawsuits could result

2. List and define the four word parts used in medical terminology. Pg. 128

1-Root word: The main meaning of a word

2 Prefix: Root word placed at the begining of the word To change its meaning.s

3- suffix: word part or series of word parts added To the end of The Root word to change its meaning

4-Combining form: Root word with a Vowel added

3. Define and give an example of an antonym, a homonym, and a synonym.

an antonym: Root word, prefix, or suffix, that has the opposite meaning of another word. Pnea   dyspnea

homonym: have the same pronounciation but different spelling meaning. Right   dextro

Synonyms: have same meaning ex. pulmono/o   Pneumo

4. Explain why it is not important to memorize every medical term.

by dividing words into parts will be easier To Figure The meaning

CRITICAL THINKING

Underline the medical terms and medical abbreviations in the following paragraph. (Underline a word or an abbreviation only once, for a total of 28 terms.)

Susan Simmons, a 52-year-old woman, was transported by ambulance to the hospital in acute abdominal distress, severe pain in the RLQ, with guarding. Patient's BP 140/76 P 92 R 20 all WNL. An HCG, Hct, Hgb, and sed rate were ordered by the physician. The HCG test was negative, Hct and Hgb were WNL, and the sed rate was slightly elevated. The patient affirms nausea but denies vomiting. Upon further examination the physician noted rebound tenderness over the RLQ. An abdominal ultrasound was ordered to rule out appendicitis and a KUB was ordered to rule out renal calculi, or cystitis. The ultrasound revealed an enlarged appendix.

An ECG and IV were performed, and a bleeding time was performed by the phlebotomist. The anesthesiologist and surgeon met with the patient, and it was determined the patient would be scheduled for an appendectomy STAT. The surgery was successful and proceeded without incident. The patient tolerated the procedure well and was sent to recovery.

INTERNET RESEARCH

Keyword: Medical Terminology. Use an Internet search to define medical terms and/or abbreviations in the above scenario.

WHAT WOULD YOU DO?

If you have accomplished the objectives in this chapter, you will be able to make better choices as a medical assistant. Take a look at this situation and decide what you would do.

Dr. Smith has a medical assistant who does the medical transcription of her patient notes. The following is a note the medical assistant has transcribed on Susie Ramos:

"Seen in the office today for arteriaslcerosis and hipertension. Mrs. Ramos complained of feeling dizzy with some fertigo for three days. On questioning, Mrs. Ramos did state that she was febrille two days ago with some gastroentestinal symptomes such as darhea and nausea. She also complained of aralgia and laryngetes. On examination the toncils are red and swollen. Her blood pressure is controlled by medication. There are no complaints of chest pain or anjina, nor does she have dispnea, although she does have some orthapnea. She does have some syanosis of the hands and feet, but does not complain of pain in these areas. Her sinuses are painful. Her current diagnosisses are sinisitus, athuroscleroisis, possible streptocokki infection, gastrointeritis, and faringitis."

1. **There are 20 mistakes in the use of medical terminology in this dictation. Find the mistakes and then define each of the medical terms found in the paragraph.**

   _____

   _____

   _____

   _____

2. **Explain why using and spelling the correct medical term is important in the medical record.**

   _you could harm the patient_____

   _____

   _____

   _____

3. Why does the medical assistant need to study medical terminology? How does a solid understanding of medical terminology benefit the care that patients receive?

as a medical assistant you will hear & see a lot of the words, so this will give the patient a professional care

APPLICATION OF SKILLS

1. Create 15 medical terms using the following word parts.
   -ology
   onc/o
   -itis
   my/o
   cardi/o
   melan/o
   -oma
   neur/o
   epi-
   -etctomy
   peri-
   -al
   dys-
   -algia
   path/o
   -graphy

2. Write the definitions for the following medical terms.
   A. cardiopathy   _____
   B. echocardiogram   _____
   C. endoscope   _____
   D. intrabronchial   _____
   E. osteomalacia   _____
   F. homeostasis   _____
   G. adipose   _____
   H. neuropathology   _____
   I. tracheostenosis   _____
   J. adenopathy   _____
   K. diplococcus   _____

CHAPTER QUIZ

Multiple Choice

Identify the letter of the choice that best completes the statement or answers the question.

1. A word root, prefix, or suffix that has the opposite meaning of another word is a(n) _____.
    A. eponym
    B. antonym
    C. diminutive
    D. synonym

2. A word that has the same pronunciation but a different spelling and meaning than another word is a(n) _____.
    A. homonym
    B. eponym
    C. diminutive
    D. synonym

3. What is the medical term for inflammation of a joint?
    A. Arthralgia
    B. Arthrodynia
    C. Arthritis
    D. Arthroscopy

4. A(n) _____ is added to the root word before any prefix or suffix to make pronunciation easier.
    A. consonant
    B. "e"
    C. "i"
    D. combining vowel

5. A _____ is a word part that is sometimes placed at the beginning of a root work to change its meaning.
    A. combining vowel
    B. prefix
    C. suffix
    D. none of the above

6. When analyzing medical words, begin with the suffix, then proceed to the root and prefix.
    A. True
    B. False

7. Which one of the following is the correct pleural for the word "lumen"?
    A. luminol
    B. lumina
    C. lumines
    D. luminia

8. Which one of the following is the correct pleural for the word "sarcoma"?
    A. carinoma
    B. sarcomita
    C. sarcomitis
    D. sarcomata

9. Part of the small intestine is the _____.
   A. ileum
   B. ilium
   C. ilaum
   D. iloum

10. _____ is an eponym.
    A. Fahrenheit
    B. Babinski reflex
    C. Rake retractor
    D. Forceps

11. The correct medical term for the study of blood is _____.
    A. hemopoiesis
    B. circulatology
    C. cardiology
    D. hematology

12. A pair of cocci bacteria are called _____.
    A. monococci
    B. diplococci
    C. streptococci
    D. staphylococci

13. The outermost layer of a developing embryo is called an _____.
    A. exoderm
    B. ectoderm
    C. endoderm
    D. ergoderm

14. Disorder with sudden attacks of deep sleep is _____.
    A. nyctophobia
    B. noctophobia
    C. narcolepsy
    D. all of the above

15. An accumulation of fluid in a body cavity is called hydrocele.
    A. True
    B. False

16. The medical term for "blood poisoning" is _____.
    A. uremia
    B. choloremia
    C. streptemia
    D. septicemia

17. The medical term for "an abnormal redness of the skin" is _____.
    A. erythroderma
    B. leukoderma
    C. xanthoderma
    D. cyanosis

18. The medical term for "low potassium in the blood" is _____.
    A. hypercalcium
    B. hyperkalemia
    C. hypocalcium
    D. hypokalemia

19. The medical term for "fat tissues" is _____.
    A. lipase
    B. adipose
    C. adipose
    D. lipose

20. Therapy based on the theory "like cures like" is called _____.
    A. isotonic
    B. homeostasis
    C. homeopathy
    D. isostasis

CHAPTER TEN

Basic Anatomy and Physiology

VOCABULARY REVIEW

Matching: Match each term with the correct definition.

A. anatomy

B. physiology

C. anterior

D. inferior

E. posterior

F. supine position

G. midsagittal plane

H. membrane

I. viscera

J. abdominopelvic cavity

K. pelvic

L. quadrants

M. mediastinum

N. thoracic cavity

O. cranial cavity

P. cervical

Q. meninges

R. spinal cord

S. vertebra

RR   1. Recessive gene disorder of the exocrine glands causing the excretion of thick mucus into the lungs

H   2. Specialized tissue that covers an organ surface or lines a body cavity or is located between a space

_____ 3. Condition or anomaly that a baby is born with; is not necessarily inherited from the parents

E   4. Back, behind

_____ 5. Muscle of the heart

B   6. Study of the function of an organism

_____ 7. Having the same amount of solutes as another

I   8. Organs of any cavity

S   9. Bony structure of the spinal column

_____ 10. Quality of a membrane that allows some materials to pass through and not others

_____ 11. Threadlike strand inside the nucleus that contains genetic information

D   12. That which is below

M   13. Area located behind the sternum and in front of the lungs; houses trachea, esophagus, and large blood vessels

T. axial

U. appendicular

V. molecule

W. cell

X. organelle

Y. anabolism

Z. chromosomes

AA. genes

BB. mitochondria

CC. nucleus

DD. semipermeable

EE. diffusion

FF. hemolyze

GG. isotonic

HH. phagocytosis

II. mitosis

JJ. malignant

KK. gametes

LL. congenital

MM. familial

NN. hereditary

OO. sign

PP. symptom

QQ. Down syndrome

RR. cystic fibrosis

SS. dyspnea

TT. muscular dystrophy

_CC_ 14. Tissue that carries electrical impulses to body structures

_G_ 15. Vertical cut through the body that divides the body into equal anterior and posterior sections

_J_ 16. Cavity between the diaphragm and the pelvic floor

_T_ 17. Having to do with the area of the body that includes the head, neck, and torso

_____ 18. To burst open due to taking on too much water

_____ 19. Organelle that functions as the control center of a cell and contains the chromosomes

_A_ 20. Study of the structure of an organism

_L_ 21. Clinical division of the abdominal area into four parts

_____ 22. Cellular activity of combining simple substances to form more complex substances

_____ 23. Cell division of body cells

_____ 24. Chromosomal disease that occurs because of a duplication of number 21 chromosome

_Q_ 25. Tissues that provide a protective covering for the brain and the spinal cord

_____ 26. Tissue that covers the body and internal cavities

_K_ 27. Having to do with the area of the pelvis

_F_ 28. Describes the body when lying on the back with the face up

_____ 29. Sex cells

_____ 30. X-linked recessive muscular wasting disease

_N_ 31. Chest area

UU. sickle cell anemia

VV. epithelial tissue

WW. nervous tissue

XX. endocrine gland

YY. myocardium

ZZ. matrix

_____ 32. Substance within a cell that provides strength

_C_ 33. In or referring to the front

_O_ 34. Cavity that holds the brain and is formed by the skull

_____ 35. Organelles that produce the energy within the cell called ATP

_R_ 36. Nerve tissue surrounded by the spinal column

_____ 37. Movement of a substance from an area of higher concentration to one of lower concentration

_____ 38. Two or more atoms

_P_ 39. Having to do with the spinal area in the neck

_____ 40. Gland that secretes its substance through a duct

_____ 41. Condition passed to a baby by its parents

_____ 42. Fundamental unit of living tissue; made up of atoms and molecules

_____ 43. Something that the patient can tell you about but that cannot be measured or seen

_____ 44. Cancerous

_____ 45. Structure contained within the cytoplasm of a cell; each one has a specific function

_____ 46. Cellular process of taking in or digesting waste material

_____ 47. Hereditary unit containing inherited material and carried within chromosomes

_____ 48. Something that can be seen or measured

_____ 49. Difficulty in breathing; shortness of breath

_U_ 50. Having to do with the area of the body that includes the upper and lower extremities

_____ 51. Occurring within a family

_____ 52. Inherited disease that causes the red blood cells to be crescent shaped

THEORY RECALL

True/False

Indicate whether the sentence or statement is true or false.

___T___ 1. The body is assumed to be in a correct or true anatomical position when the individual is standing erect and facing forward.

___T___ 2. The anterior and lateral cavities are the two main spaces that contain the internal organs of the human body.

___F___ 3. The diaphragm is the structure dividing the abdominal and pelvic cavities.

_____ 4. Bone tissue has fibers and a hard mineral substance that provides for protection and support of the body.

_____ 5. The final organizational level in the human body consists of the body systems.

Multiple Choice

Identify the letter of the choice that best completes the statement or answers the question.

1. A vertical cut through the body that divides the body into anterior and posterior sections is called the _____.
   A. frontal plane
   B. midsagittal plane
   C. transverse plane
   D. coronal plane

2. The _____ position describes the body lying on the belly with the face down.
   A. supine
   B. prone
   C. transverse
   D. recumbent

3. The _____ cavity contains organs that maintain homeostasis when the body is exposed to internal and external stimuli.
   A. thoracic
   B. pleural
   C. ventral
   D. pericardial

4. The abdominal cavity is lined with a double-folded membrane called the _____.
   A. parietal peritoneum
   B. visceral peritoneum
   C. mesentery
   D. pericardium

5. The center square of the abdominal region is _____.
   A. hypochondriac
   B. iliac
   C. epigastric
   D. umbilical

6. Which quadrant contains part of the small and large intestines, left ureter, and the left ovary and left fallopian tube in the female?
   A. RUQ
   B. LUQ
   C. RLQ
   D. LLQ

7. Which one of the following is NOT a division of the spinal column?
   A. Cranial
   B. Cervical
   C. Lumbar
   D. Coccygeal

8. The _____ skeleton consists of the upper and lower extremities.
   A. afferent
   B. axial
   C. appendicular
   D. appendable

9. The smallest part of the body is a(n) _____.
   A. molecule
   B. compound
   C. chemical
   D. atom

10. The fundamental unit of all living things is (the) _____.
    A. cell
    B. molecules
    C. chemicals
    D. atom

11. Red blood cells live for approximately _____.
    A. 12 hours
    B. 120 days
    C. 12 months
    D. 120 minutes

12. Which one of the following is NOT one of the three main parts of a cell?
    A. cytoplasm
    B. organelles
    C. nucleus
    D. cell membrane

13. Organelles carry out several life functions that include all of the following EXCEPT _____.
    A. immune response and hormone replacement
    B. growth and reproduction
    C. nourishment and waste removal
    D. reacting and adapting to change

14. The cell membrane is composed of _____.
    A. acids and bases
    B. salts and sugars
    C. proteins and lipids
    D. none of the above

15. Each chromosome contains thousands of _____.
    A. nucleoli
    B. mitochondria
    C. ribosomes
    D. genes

16. Which one of the following is an example of passive transport?
    A. Diffusion
    B. Osmosis
    C. Filtration
    D. All of the above

17. _____ is the random movement of dissolved particles that move from an area of higher concentration to an area of lower concentration.
    A. Diffusion
    B. Osmosis
    C. Filtration
    D. None of the above

18. _____ occurs when particles are pushed through a membrane by a mechanical pressure.
    A. Diffusion
    B. Osmosis
    C. Filtration
    D. None of the above

19. _____ is when a stationary cell engulfs and digests droplets of a fluid ("cell drinking").
    A. Phagocytosis
    B. Pinocytosis
    C. Mitosis
    D. Meiosis

20. A person has a total of _____ chromosomes.
    A. 23
    B. 46
    C. 92
    D. an unlimited amount

Sentence Completion

Write the correct term in the blank for each prefix, suffix, or word root.

1. The brain and spinal cord are one continuous structure that is covered by _____.

2. _____ occurs when cancer cells break away from the tumor and travel to other parts of the body.

3. _____ are sex cells.

4. _____ is an example of a chromosomal disease that occurs in males when an extra X chromosome is present at birth.

5. _____ is an X-linked recessive bleeding disorder caused by a missing coagulation factor.

6. Cells of _____ tissue fit tightly together and have only small amounts of intercellular substance holding them.

7. _____ are ductless and discharge their hormones into the tissue fluid to be absorbed by the capillaries in the body.

8. _____ tissue contracts, or shortens, allowing movement.

9. _____ is a benign tumor of the epithelium.

10. Smooth or _____ muscles form the walls of hollow organs.

11. A _____ is a tumor usually found in involuntary muscles.

12. _____ tissue helps anchor muscle to bone, or connects bone to bone.

13. _____ supports the rings of the bronchi, which aid in keeping open the airway.

14. _____ is the most highly organized tissue in the body.

15. An _____ is composed of two or more types of tissues that allow it to perform a specific function or functions.

Short Answers

1. Describe the progression from an atom to a system.

   _____

   _____

   _____

2. List five things that can cause genes to mutate.

   _____

   _____

   _____

3. List the 10 body systems and describe the functions of each.

   _____

   _____

   _____

   _____

   _____

   _____

   _____

   _____

   _____

   _____

4. List the four main types of body tissues and describe the functions of each.

   _____

   _____

   _____

   _____

   _____

CRITICAL THINKING

Create an analogy that explains the active and passive transport processes. Explain these concepts to a family member or friend. Write the analogy and one paragraph explaining if the friend or family member understood the concept using your analogy.

INTERNET RESEARCH

Keyword: Cellular Division. Locate an Internet site that explains the process of cellular division. Identify the five phases with a brief explanation of what occurs in each phase.

_____

_____

_____

_____

_____

_____

_____

_____

_____

_____

WHAT WOULD YOU DO?

If you have accomplished the objectives in this chapter, you will be able to make better choices as a medical assistant. Take a look at this situation and decide what you would do.

John Choi is a medical assistant in a primary care facility. Barb Quinn arrives and complains of pain that she thinks is in her stomach. She states that she has had vomiting with blood and diarrhea. She also complains of difficulty in eating, stating that she just does not want anything to eat, "I have to force myself to eat." After the examination, Dr. Elory tells Ms. Quinn that based on her symptoms, he is suspicious of a cancer in her abdomen. Dr. Elory orders several diagnostic tests that will be completed the next day. Dr. Elory tells Ms. Quinn that he will call as soon as he has her test results.

John needs to chart the pain using the correct cavity for the stomach, the region of the abdominopelvic area, and the correct quadrant of the abdominal area. In what body system would John know the stomach is found?

1. How might John explain to Ms. Quinn what her symptoms mean in relation to anatomy and physiology?

_____

_____

_____

2. What is cancer?

_____

_____

3. What does cell division have to do with cancer?

_____

_____

_____

4. If Ms. Quinn had complained of pain in the left upper quadrant, what organs might have been involved?

_____

_____

5. If the pain was in the umbilical region, what could this mean?

_____

_____

6. What does pain in the right lower quadrant indicate as a possible organ involvement?

_____

_____

7. If Ms. Quinn had complained of shortness of breath, in what cavity would you expect the discomfort to be? What organ systems would be found in this cavity? What separates this cavity from the abdominopelvic cavity?

_____

_____

_____

_____

_____

8. What is the difference between a sign and a symptom when discussing illness? What are the symptoms in the above scenario? What is a subjective finding and what is an objective finding in the patient's medical history?

_____

_____

_____

_____

_____

_____

_____

9. What symptoms indicate a disturbance of the homeostasis of Ms. Quinn's body?

_____

_____

_____

APPLICATION OF SKILLS

Label the diagrams.

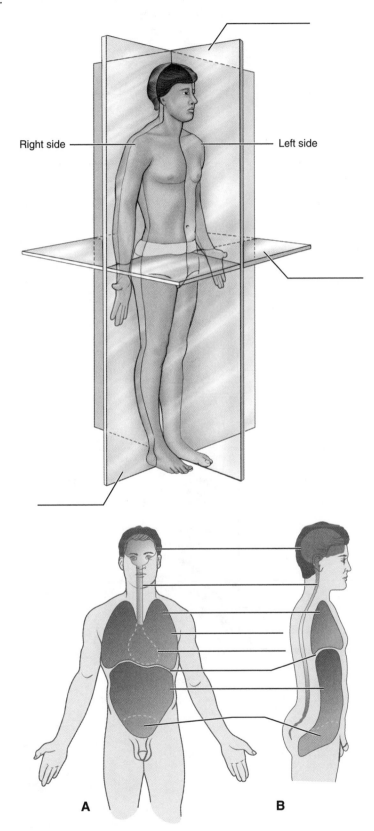

Right side

Left side

A

B

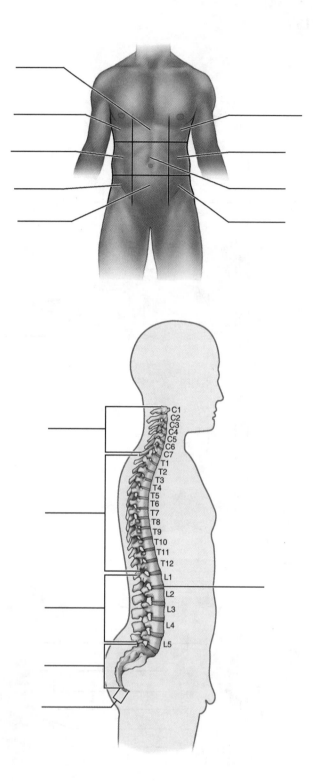

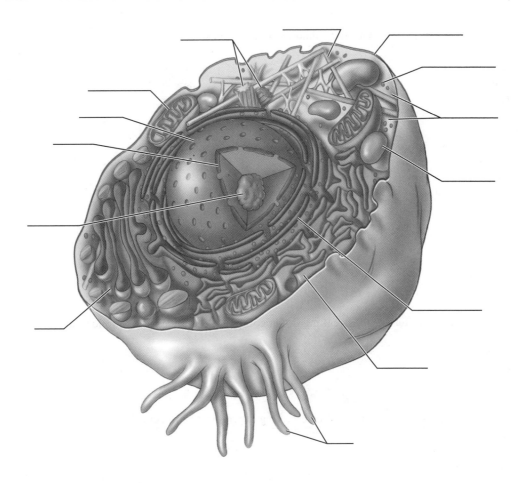

CHAPTER QUIZ

Multiple Choice

Identify the letter of the choice that best completes the statement or answers the question.

1. _____ is a vertical cut that divides the body into right and left portions.
   A. frontal
   B. midsagittal
   C. lateral
   D. transverse

2. The main muscle of breathing that lies between the thoracic and abdominal cavities is called the _____.
   A. pleura
   B. sternocleidomastoid
   C. diaphragm
   D. costal muscle

3. The _____ cavity contains the teeth and tongue.
   A. buccal
   B. orbital
   C. lacrimal
   D. periodontal

4. _____ means having to do with the spinal area in the neck.
   A. Coccygeal
   B. Cervical
   C. Thoracic
   D. Lumbar

5. The _____ is the outer layer of the heart sac.
   A. pericardial membrane
   B. epicardial membrane
   C. parietal thoracic membrane
   D. none of the above

6. _____ means having to do with the spinal area between the ribs and the ilium.
   A. Lumbar
   B. Thoracic
   C. Cervical
   D. None of the above

7. _____ is the cellular activity of breaking down complex substances into simple matter.
   A. Anabolism
   B. Catabolism
   C. Cannibalism
   D. Phagocytosis

8. A _____ is an organelle responsible for breaking down larger molecules.
   A. lysosome
   B. ribosome
   C. Golgi apparatus
   D. Mitochondrion

9. A substance that carries genetic information and is considered to the "blueprint" of the cell is called _____.
   A. RNA
   B. DNA
   C. ATP
   D. PKU

10. _____ are organelles involved in cellular division.
    A. Mitochondria
    B. Ribosomes
    C. Centrioles
    D. Nucleoli

11. _____ means "not cancerous."
    A. Benign
    B. Malignant
    C. Metastatic
    D. None of the above

12. A(n) _____ solution has more than solutes than any other.
    A. isotonic
    B. hypotonic
    C. hypertonic
    D. none of the above

13. A _____ is a condition or an anomaly that a baby is born with; it is not necessarily inherited.
    A. congenital
    B. hereditary
    C. genetic
    D. all of the above

14. A(n) X-linked disorder that causes malformation of the skull is _____.
    A. hydrocephalus
    B. cleft palate
    C. Turner syndrome
    D. Klinefelter syndrome

15. _____ is an X-linked recessive muscular wasting disease.
    A. Tay-Sachs disease
    B. PKU
    C. Turner syndrome
    D. Muscular dystrophy

16. The _____ is the main muscle of the heart.
    A. pericardium
    B. epicardium
    C. endocardium
    D. myocardium

17. Muscle fibers that are divided by bands of stripes called _____.
    A. nonstriated muscle
    B. striated muscle
    C. smooth muscle
    D. cardiac muscle

18. Tissue occurring outside the cell is called _____.
    A. dense tissue
    B. fibrous tissue
    C. extracellular tissue
    D. intracellular tissue

19. _____ nerves carry impulses from the senses to the brain.
    A. Afferent
    B. Efferent

20. Cells that provide support for nervous tissue are called _____ cells.
    A. glitter
    B. glial
    C. astro
    D. familial

CHAPTER **ELEVEN**

Circulatory System

VOCABULARY REVIEW

Matching: Match each term with the correct definition.

A. cardiovascular system

B. myocardium

C. atrium

D. ventricle

E. aorta

F. cardiac cycle

G. electrocardiogram

H. infarction

I. ischemia

J. cardiologist

K. vasoconstrict

L. aneurysm

M. embolus

N. hematopoiesis

O. erythropoiesis

P. macrophage

Q. hemolysis

R. type and cross-match

S. ecchymosis

_____ 1. When the blood vessel is made more narrow

_____ 2. Lower chambers of the heart

_____ 3. Systole and diastole that produce the heartbeat

_____ 4. Altered, weakened

_____ 5. Production of blood cells

_____ 6. Main muscle layer of the heart wall

_____ 7. Recording of the cardiac cycle

_____ 8. Disease-producing bacteria

_____ 9. Bruised or bluish area of skin caused by trauma to a blood vessel

_____ 10. Largest artery in the body

_____ 11. Breakup of red blood cells

_____ 12. Small, oval-shaped bodies of lymphoid tissue

_____ 13. Body system that consists of the heart and blood vessels

_____ 14. Death of tissue because of lack of blood to area

_____ 15. Proteins produced by T-cells and cells infected with viruses that block the ability of a virus to reproduce

T. interstitial fluid

U. lymph nodes

V. thymus gland

W. attenuated

X. interferons

Y. pathogens

Z. vaccination

_____ 16. Process of determining a person's blood type

_____ 17. Process of red blood cell formation

_____ 18. Upper chamber of the heart

_____ 19. Physician who specializes in the structure, function, and diseases of the heart

_____ 20. Cells responsible for destroying worn out red blood cells

_____ 21. Fluid between the cells of the tissue

_____ 22. Process of giving a small sample of the disease into the body

_____ 23. Lymphatic organ located in the mediastinum and a primary site for T-cell formation

_____ 24. Clot that moves through the bloodstream

_____ 25. Deficiency of a blood supply because of an obstruction

_____ 26. Weakness in the wall of an artery

THEORY RECALL

True/False

Indicate whether the sentence or statement is true or false.

_____ 1. The heart is a solid, muscular pump that averages 72 beats per minute.

_____ 2. The outer covering of the heart is a sac called the pericardium.

_____ 3. When the blood leaves the left atrium, it passes through the pulmonary semilunar valve.

_____ 4. The atrioventricular node is known as the body's natural pacemaker.

_____ 5. Capillaries are the smallest blood vessels of the human body.

Multiple Choice

Identify the letter of the choice that best completes the statement or answers the question.

1. The inner muscle layer of the heart is called the _____.
   A. myocardium
   B. endocardium
   C. pericaridum
   D. epicardium

2. The _____ is the partition between the two sides of the heart.
   A. chamber
   B. atria
   C. ventricle
   D. septum

3. The vein that brings blood low in oxygen from the head and upper limbs is called the _____.
   A. inferior vena cava
   B. aorta
   C. superior vena cava
   D. pulmonary artery

4. Movement of blood from the heart to the lungs and back is known as _____.
   A. fetal circulation
   B. coronary circulation
   C. systemic circulation
   D. pulmonary circulation

5. Death of tissue because of lack of blood to an area is called _____.
   A. ecchymosis
   B. ischemia
   C. infarction
   D. diaphoresis

6. _____ are white blood cells that react to the release of histamine in the body.
   A. Eosinophils
   B. Lymphocytes
   C. Basophils
   D. Neutrophils

7. _____ is a blood test that determines the percentage of each type of white blood cell present in a blood sample.
   A. Gram stain
   B. Differential count
   C. Platelet count
   D. Erythrocyte sedimentation rate

8. _____ is a hormone that is secreted by the thymus that helps to develop the T-cells.
   A. Trinomial 3
   B. Terexel
   C. Testosterone
   D. Thymosin

9. A _____ is a person with neither A nor B antigens in his or her blood.
   A. universal donor
   B. universal recipient

10. A _____ is a cell fragment responsible for clotting.
    A. protozoan
    B. petechiae
    C. platelet
    D. fibrin

11. Inborn immunity or natural immunity is called _____.
    A. acquired immunity
    B. active immunity
    C. genetic immunity
    D. nonspecific immunity

12. The blood carries _____ to target organs and removes excess fluids from body tissues.
    A. interferons
    B. hormones
    C. prothrombin
    D. stem cells

13. In the average adult male, the heart weighs _____ grams.
    A. 200
    B. 300
    C. 400
    D. 500

14. The purpose of the cardiac valves is to prevent _____ of blood into the atria.
    A. regurgitation
    B. deoxygenation
    C. hypertrophy
    D. none of the above

15. An abnormal heart sound is called a(n) _____.
    A. arrhythmia
    B. regurgitation
    C. diastole
    D. murmur

16. The _____ extend(s) along the outer walls of the ventricles. When the impulse passes through, the ventricles contract.
    A. bundle of His
    B. atrioventricular nodes
    C. ventricular septum
    D. Purkinje fibers

17. The _____ is an opening located in the septum between the atria of the fetal heart, allowing blood to be pumped to fetal tissue.
    A. cardiac fontanel
    B. semipulmonary artery
    C. foramen ovale
    D. none of the above

18. An average adult has _____ liters of blood.
    A. 2 to 4
    B. 4 to 6
    C. 5 to 7
    D. 6 to 8

19. _____, a pale yellow fluid, is approximately 90% water.
    A. Plasma
    B. Antibodies
    C. Antigens
    D. Whole blood

20. The human body has more _____ than _____.
    A. red blood cells, white blood cells
    B. white blood cells, red blood cells

21. Which of the following statements is correct?
    A. Granulocytes = neutrophils, lymphocytes, basophils
    B. Granulocytes = neutrophils, basophils, eosinophils
    C. Granulocytes = lymphocytes, monocytes, neutrocytes
    D. Granulocytes = lymphocyte, eosinophils, monocytes

22. Platelet factors combine with _____ and calcium to form thrombin, which cause(s) platelets to become sticky and form a plug.
    A. fibrinogen
    B. fibrin
    C. prothrombin
    D. coagulants

23. Which one of the following situations could cause hemolytic disease of the newborn?
    A. Rh-positive mother + Rh-positive father
    B. Rh-negative mother + Rh-negative father
    C. Rh-positive mother + Rh-negative father
    D. Rh-negative mother + Rh-positive father

24. Which one of the following is NOT a component of the lymphatic system?
    A. Lymphatic fluid
    B. Lymph node
    C. Gallbladder
    D. Tonsils

25. What heart condition causes fever, malaise, chest pain that increases with inspiration or heartbeat, dyspnea, and tachycardia?
    A. Myocardial infarction
    B. Pericarditis
    C. Atrial stenosis
    D. Patent ductus arteriosus

Sentence Completion

Complete each sentence or statement.

1. _____ occurs when the heart muscle is unable to pump blood efficiently, causing the heart to enlarge and the lungs to fill with blood.

2. A(n) _____ is a blood clot that travels, frequently lodging in a blood vessel.

3. Urea, uric acid, and amino acids are examples of _____ substances carried in the blood.

4. _____ are a type of blood cell that is the first responder to an infection or damaged site. It is phagocytic in nature.

5. _____ are the smallest type of white blood cell.

6. _____ is a megaloblastic anemia resulting in a decrease of hydrochloric acid.

7. _____ is caused by the protozoan *Plasmodium*.

8. _____ is the medical term for "hemolytic disease of the newborn."

9. _____ is a syndrome that is caused by a virus that attacks an individual's entire immune system.

10. The drug classification for captopril is _____.

Short Answers

1. What are the two main types of immunity?

   _____

   _____

2. List three diseases of the immune system, and describe the etiology, signs and symptoms, diagnosis, therapy, and interventions for each.

_____

_____

_____

_____

_____

_____

_____

3. Describe the considerations associated with the testing of AIDS patients.

_____

_____

_____

_____

4. List the three types of blood cells, and describe the functions of each.

_____

_____

_____

_____

_____

_____

_____

_____

_____

CRITICAL THINKING

One of your patients has recently received a diagnosis of HIV. Create a dialogue between you, as the medical assistant, and the patient regarding his recent diagnosis. If you are unfamiliar with this diagnosis, research it. If you were the patient, what questions would you ask? What would you want to know?

_____

_____

_____

_____

_____

_____

_____

_____

_____

_____

_____

_____

INTERNET RESEARCH

Keyword: (Use the name of the condition or disease you select to write about).

Select one condition or disease from one of the following tables: Table 11-2, 11-4, 11-8, 11-9, or 11-10. Write a two-paragraph report regarding the condition or disease you selected, listing the etiology, signs and symptoms, diagnosis, therapy, or interventions. Cite your source. (You may not use the information on the tables exclusively for your report.) Be prepared to give a 2-minute oral presentation should your instructor assign you to do so.

WHAT WOULD YOU DO?

If you have accomplished the objectives in this chapter, you will be able to make better choices as a medical assistant. Take a look at this situation and decide what you would do.

Dr. Kim Kea is going to examine Mr. Stan Baleaut today for a routine follow-up examination for high blood pressure and possible coronary artery disease. Mr. Baleaut tells Erin, the medical assistant, that he has some abdominal pain in his right lower quadrant that he wants Dr. Kea to check out. As Erin takes Mr. Baleaut's blood pressure, she obtains a reading of 142/88 and a pulse rate of 92. Dr. Kea examines Mr. Baleaut and orders a stat CBC with a differential count as a way of ruling out a diagnosis of appendicitis. As Erin is completing the blood draw, Mr. Baleaut has several questions. He wants to know the following:

1. What causes systolic blood pressure, and what is happening when this is measured? Diastolic pressure?

   _____

   _____

   _____

   _____

2. What is the pulse rate measuring?

   _____

   _____

3. What is the route of the conduction system through the heart?

   _____

   _____

   _____

4. In the past, Mr. Baleaut has worn a Holter monitor and now wants to know why this was necessary when he had an ECG.

   _____

   _____

   _____

   _____

5. What is a myocardial infarction, and what are the symptoms that Mr. Baleaut needs to know?

   _____

   _____

   _____

   _____

6. What is congestive heart failure, and what are the symptoms that Mr. Baleaut needs to know?

   _____

   _____

   _____

   _____

The blood tests return with the following lab results:

Hgb 14.6   Hct 46.1   WBC 15,200   RBC 5.3   Segs 75

Bands 1%   Eos 0%   Basos 0%   Mono 2%   Lymphs 22%   Platelets 350,000

7. Which of these results are abnormal, and which indicate a possible acute infection?

_____

_____

_____

_____

Finally, Dr. Kea has asked Mr. Baleaut about his immunizations and when he last had a tetanus shot.

8. Why is it important for Mr. Baleaut to continue to have tetanus immunizations? Do tetanus immunizations provide natural or artificial acquired immunity?

_____

_____

_____

_____

_____

APPLICATION OF SKILLS

1. Label the diagrams.

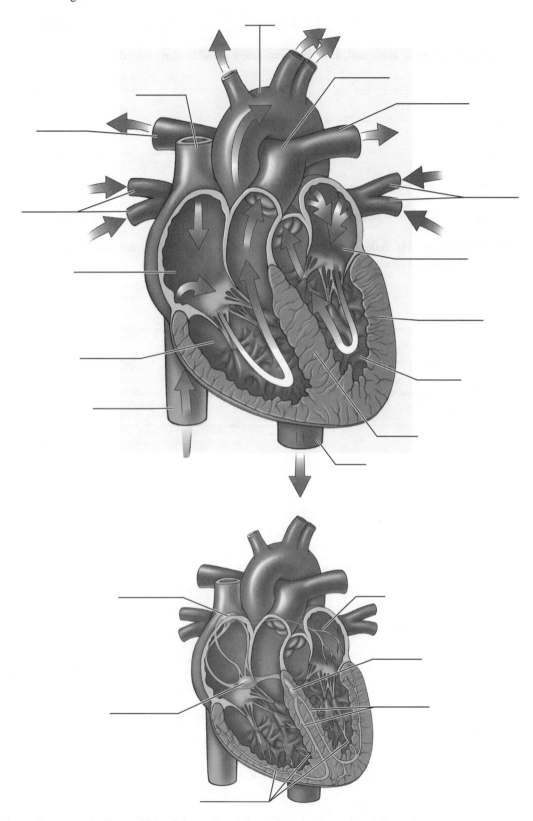

2. Trace the systemic flow of blood from the right atrium back to the right atrium.

CHAPTER QUIZ

Multiple Choice

Identify the letter of the choice that best completes the statement or answers the question.

1. The outermost layer of the heart wall is called the _____.
   A. myocardium
   B. epicardium
   C. pericardium
   D. endocardium

2. The combining form for "blood vessel" is _____.
   A. cardi/o
   B. atri/o
   C. angi/o
   D. varic/o

3. The upper chambers of the heart are called _____.
   A. arterioles
   B. ventricles
   C. venules
   D. atria

4. The space between the lungs where the heart, esophagus, and trachea lie is called the _____.
   A. mediastinum
   B. diaphragm
   C. apex
   D. septum

5. The _____ are the tricuspid and bicuspid valves, which prevent the blood in the ventricles from backing up into the atria when the ventricles contract.
   A. chorea tendineae
   B. cardiac valves
   C. pulmonary valves
   D. none of the above

6. A specialized group of cardiac cells that function as the heart's natural pacemaker are called the _____.
   A. SA node
   B. AV node
   C. bundle of His
   D. Purkinje fibers

7. _____ is the movement of blood through the heart.
   A. Systemic circulation
   B. Pulmonary circulation
   C. Coronary circulation
   D. Fetal circulation

8. The _____ is the heart valve that prevents backflow of blood into the right ventricle.
   A. mitral valve
   B. pulmonary semilunar valve
   C. tricuspid valve
   D. aortic semilunar valve

9. _____ is enlargement of the heart.
   A. Cardiomegaly
   B. Hypertrophy
   C. Sequel
   D. Hypoxia

10. A(n) _____ is a weakness in the wall of an artery.
    A. thrombus
    B. ischemia
    C. infraction
    D. aneurysm

11. _____ are the largest white blood cells and are phagocytic.
    A. Neutrophils
    B. Lymphocytes
    C. Basophils
    D. None of the above

12. _____ are the main cells from which all cells develop.
    A. Leukocytes
    B. Erythrocytes
    C. Stem cells
    D. Basal cells

13. The _____ is an organ that stores and destroys RBCs and produces agranulocytes.
    A. pancreas
    B. thymus
    C. liver
    D. spleen

14. _____ is immunity provided by antibodies being passed through the placenta or mother's milk.
    A. Genetic immunity
    B. Passive immunity
    C. Active immunity
    D. Acquired immunity

15. _____ is death of the tissue of the heart muscle caused by lack of oxygen to the tissues.
    A. Myocardial infarction
    B. Angina pectoris
    C. Congestive heart failure
    D. Pericarditis

16. _____ is progressive thickening of the inner walls of a vessel leading to an occlusion.
    A. Congestive heart failure
    B. Atherosclerosis
    C. Arteriosclerosis
    D. Pericarditis

17. _____ is(are) an abnormal occurrence of swollen and twisted veins to the legs and anus.
    A. Embolus
    B. Occlusion
    C. Varicosities
    D. Phlebitis

18. _____ protect the body by reacting to the release of histamine during an allergic reaction.
    A. Lymphocytes
    B. Eosinophils
    C. Monocytes
    D. Neutrophils

19. _____ is decreased clotting capability of the blood.
    A. Thrombocytopenia
    B. Leukemia
    C. Vitamin K deficiency
    D. Erthyroblastosis fetalis

20. _____ is an overproduction of RBCs by the bone marrow.
    A. Thrombocytopenia
    B. Vitamin K deficiency
    C. Polycythemia
    D. Leukemia

CHAPTER TWELVE

Respiratory System

VOCABULARY REVIEW

Matching: Match each term with the correct definition.

A. respiration

B. expiration

C. inspiration

D. cilia

E. sinuses

F. adenoids

G. nasopharynx

H. pharynx

I. epiglottis

J. trachea

K. bronchi

L. alveoli

M. pleura

N. phrenic nerve

O. pons

P. cardiopulmonary resuscitation

Q. spirometer

R. asphyxia

S. pulmonary edema

_____ 1. Nosebleed

_____ 2. Occurs when there is an increase in CO_2 in tissues, thus oxygen deficiency

_____ 3. Tiny air sacs at the end of the bronchioles through which gases are exchanged

_____ 4. Process of taking air into the lungs

_____ 5. Lymph tissues located in the nasopharynx

_____ 6. Cavities in the skull connected with the nasal cavities

_____ 7. Passageway that conducts air to and from the lungs

_____ 8. Instrument used to measure breathing volumes

_____ 9. Process of inhaling oxygen to the lungs and exhaling carbon dioxide

_____ 10. Passageway of oxygen to the bronchioles

_____ 11. Passageway that transports air into the lungs and food and liquids into the esophagus

_____ 12. Incomplete lung expansion; lung collapse

_____ 13. Results in abnormal distention and destruction of the alveoli

T. pulmonary function tests

U. epistaxis

V. atelectasis

W. bronchodilators

X. emphysema

Y. pulmonary embolism

Z. tuberculosis

_____ 14. Top of the pharynx; extends from the posterior nares to the soft palate

_____ 15. Part of the brain stem responsible for automatic control of respiration

_____ 16. Process of air leaving the lungs

_____ 17. Serous membrane that provides moisture to prevent friction during movement

_____ 18. Collection of fluid in the lungs

_____ 19. Respiratory drugs that relax the bronchi

_____ 20. Hairlike projections derived from epithelial cells

_____ 21. Bacterial infection of the lungs, although this bacteria can affect other areas of the body

_____ 22. Emergency measure used when a person stops breathing and heart rate ceases

_____ 23. Flap that prevents food from entering the larynx and trachea

_____ 24. Nerve responsible for stimulating the diaphragm in breathing

_____ 25. Tests that measure how well the lungs intake and exhale air and how efficiently they transfer oxygen into the blood

_____ 26. Occurs when a clot dislodges and obstructs the pulmonary artery branch either partially or completely

THEORY RECALL

True/False

Indicate whether the sentence or statement is true or false.

_____ 1. The lower respiratory tract warms, moisturizes, and cleans the air that is taken in during expiration.

_____ 2. Ventilation is the cyclic process of moving air into and out of the lungs.

_____ 3. Bronchoscopy is an endoscopic procedure used to visually examine the bronchial tubes.

_____ 4. COPD is an acronym for coronary obstruction pulse deficient.

_____ 5. The heart is responsible for the process of respiration.

Multiple Choice

Identify the letter of the choice that best completes the statement or answers the question.

1. The upper respiratory tract includes all of the following EXCEPT _____.
   A. sinuses
   B. lungs
   C. pharynx
   D. larynx

2. _____ is a substance that decreases surface tension within the alveoli.
   A. Phlegm
   B. Pleura fluid
   C. Surfactant
   D. Interstitial fluid

3. The _____ is a muscular tube that is a passageway for food between the pharynx and the stomach.
   A. esophagus
   B. trachea
   C. bronchioles
   D. larynx

4. The medical term for the voice box is _____.
   A. nasopharynx
   B. pharynx
   C. larynx
   D. laryngopharynx

5. The area of the brain that controls conscious respiration is the _____.
   A. cerebellum
   B. cerebral cortex
   C. medulla oblongata
   D. pons

6. The medical term for "difficulty speaking" is _____.
   A. aphonia
   B. dysphonia
   C. dyspnea
   D. apnea

7. Radiographic method used to visualize the lungs is called a(n) _____.
   A. x-ray
   B. CT scan
   C. MRI
   D. PFT

8. A(n) _____ is a test that measures how well the lungs intake and exhale air.
   A. x-ray
   B. CT scan
   C. MRI
   D. PFT

9. _____ is an acute respiratory disorder in children.
   A. Croup
   B. Epistaxis
   C. Laryngitis
   D. Sinusitis

10. The medical term for the common cold is _____.
    A. croup
    B. laryngitis
    C. pertussis
    D. rhinitis

11. Which one of the following is not a sinus of the respiratory system?
    A. Frontal
    B. Ethmoidal
    C. Temporal
    D. Sphenoidal

12. _____ are lymphatic tissues that filter out bacteria and viruses, preventing their entry into the respiratory tract.
    A. Lymph nodes
    B. Tonsils
    C. Lymphatic vessels
    D. Cilia

13. The epiglottis is attached to the base of the _____.
    A. palatine tonsils
    B. nasal septum
    C. tongue
    D. oropharynx

14. The right lung has _____ lobes.
    A. 2
    B. 3
    C. 4
    D. none of the above

15. When atmospheric pressure is _____ than the pressure within the lungs, inspiration occurs.
    A. greater
    B. less

16. Air is inspired when the diaphragm is stimulated by _____.
    A. hormones
    B. carbon dioxide
    C. glucose
    D. phrenic nerve

17. Oxygen + glucose → carbon dioxide + water + energy, where ATP is energy + heat for biological systems is the formula for _____.
    A. exchange of gases during cell respiration
    B. hypoxia
    C. hyperventilation
    D. none of the above

18. The combining form for "lung" is _____.
    A. bronch/o
    B. lung/o
    C. rhin/o
    D. pneum/o

19. The suffix for "breathing" is _____.
    A. -phonia
    B. -pnea
    C. -oxia
    D. none of the above

20. An antitussive _____.
    A. promotes expulsion of mucus from the respiratory tract
    B. blocks histamine production
    C. suppresses the cough reflex
    D. reduces congestion

21. Robitussin is an example of a(n) _____.
    A. antihistamine
    B. antitussive
    C. decongestant
    D. expectorant

22. SARS first appeared in Asia in February _____.
    A. 1998
    B. 2001
    C. 2003
    D. none of the above

23. The pulmonary function test that measures the amount of air taken into and out of the lungs during respiration is called _____.
    A. TV
    B. ERV
    C. TLC
    D. IRV

24. A high-pitched breathing associated with obstructed airway heard during inspiration is called _____.
    A. rales
    B. wheezes
    C. stridor
    D. rhonchi

25. _____ is a viral infection of the upper respiratory tract.
    A. Pharyngitis
    B. Rhinitis
    C. Influenza
    D. Pneumonia

Sentence Completion

Complete each sentence or statement.

1. _____ is caused by a virus and usually follows an upper respiratory infection.

2. The intervention for _____ is to receive an immunization at 2, 4, and 6 months of age.

3. _____ results in abnormal distention and destruction of the alveoli.

4. _____ starts out as an URI but progresses with chills, dyspnea, and purulent sputum.

5. _____ measures the amount of air that remains in the lungs after a maximal expiration.

6. _____ is a bacterial infection of the lungs, requiring mandatory reporting to the county public health office.

7. _____ is the abbreviation for adult respiratory distress syndrome.

8. According to WHO 8,098 people became ill with SARS: _____ of these people died.

9. The average vital capacity in a healthy adult is _____ mL.

10. _____ occurs when air enters the spaces between the pleural spaces.

Short Answers

1. List the four main structures in the lower respiratory tract and describe the function of each.

   _____

   _____

   _____

   _____

2. Explain the purpose (the function) of the respiratory system.

_____

_____

_____

3. Explain the importance of pulmonary function tests such as spirometry in the diagnosis of respiratory problems.

_____

_____

_____

_____

4. List 10 common signs and symptoms of respiratory diseases and disorders.

_____

_____

_____

APPLICATION OF SKILLS

Label the diagrams.

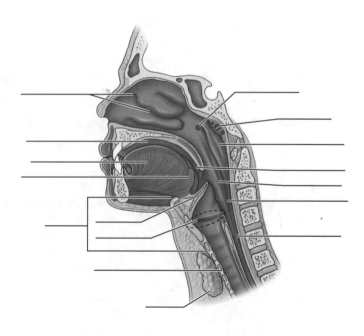

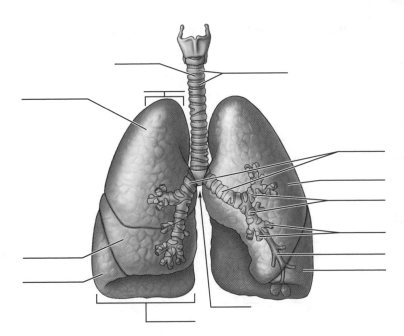

CRITICAL THINKING

1. Bill Johnson is a 52-year-old male patient who smokes two packs of cigarettes a day. Mr. Johnson has been diagnosed with emphysema, and the physician has asked you, the medical assistant, to discuss the alternatives with him to quit smoking. Describe at least three alternatives, listing their advantages and disadvantages.

2. Write one sentence appropriately using each respiratory abbreviation listed in the textbook.

INTERNET RESEARCH

Keyword: (Use the name of the condition or disease you select to write about).

Select one condition or disease from Table 12-3. Write a two-paragraph report regarding the condition or disease you selected, listing the etiology, signs and symptoms, diagnosis, therapy, and interventions. Cite your source. (You may not use the information on the table exclusively for your report.) Be prepared to give a 2-minute oral presentation should your instructor assign you to do so.

WHAT WOULD YOU DO?

If you have accomplished the objectives in this chapter, you will be able to make better choices as a medical assistant. Take a look at this situation and decide what you would do.

Mr. Chazara, with a long history of smoking both cigarettes and cigars, has been diagnosed with chronic obstructive pulmonary disease (COPD) with constriction of the bronchi. He is dyspneic with stridor and wheezing. When he is seen by the physician, an order is written for spirometry testing. The testing is positive for a mild loss of vital capacity and for moderately decreased forced expiratory volume. Because of the decreases in lung capacity, an order is also written for arterial blood gas measurements (ABGs). In addition, Mr. Chazara has sinus congestion and a productive cough, but has no fever; he needs medications for the congestion and the loss of lung function.

1. What is the cause and effect of long-term cigarette and cigar smoking on the lungs?

   _____

   _____

   _____

2. What does the diagnosis of chronic obstructive pulmonary disease mean?

   _____

   _____

3. What effect does the upper respiratory infection of sinus congestion and the productive cough have on COPD?

   _____

   _____

4. Why would you expect Mr. Chazara to be dyspneic with stridor and wheezing? Explain what each of these medical terms mean.

   _____

   _____

   _____

   _____

5. What is spirometry testing?

   _____

   _____

6. What do increased residual volume and decreased vital capacity indicate?

   _____

   _____

   _____

   _____

7. **Why would a bronchodilator be prescribed?**

_____

_____

_____

8. **Why would an expectorant rather than an antitussive be prescribed?**

_____

_____

_____

9. **Why would an arterial blood gas measurement be ordered?**

_____

_____

_____

CHAPTER QUIZ

Multiple Choice

Identify the letter of the choice that best completes the statement or answers the question.

1. The external openings of the nose are called _____.
    A. nostrils
    B. sinuses
    C. septum
    D. cilia

2. The passageway that conducts air to and from the lungs is called the _____.
    A. esophagus
    B. trachea
    C. bronchioles
    D. laryngopharynx

3. The combining form for "diaphragm" is _____.
    A. spir/o
    B. phren/o
    C. adenoid/o
    D. diaphragm/o

4. The pressure of outside air is called _____.
    A. external respiration
    B. internal respiration
    C. osmotic pressure
    D. atmospheric pressure

5. The flap that prevents food from entering the larynx and trachea is called the _____.
   A. alveoli
   B. surfactant
   C. epiglottis
   D. epistaxis

6. The area of the brain responsible for automatic control of respiration is the _____.
   A. medulla
   B. pons
   C. cerebral cortex
   D. cerebellum

7. _____ is a series of x-ray pictures taken at different angles creating cross-sectional pictures of the organ.
   A. Chest x-ray
   B. Computerized tomography
   C. Magnetic resonance imaging
   D. Pulmonary function tests

8. _____ is an abnormal enlargement of the ends of the fingers due to low oxygen levels in the blood.
   A. hemoptysis
   B. dysphonia
   C. asphyxia
   D. clubbing

9. The medical term for "difficulty breathing" is _____.
   A. dysphonia
   B. apnea
   C. dyspnea
   D. aphonia

10. The medical term for "inadequate oxygen in tissues" is _____.
    A. asphyxia
    B. hypoxia
    C. hemoptysis
    D. pneumothorax

11. _____ are the crackling sounds heard during inspiration using auscultation.
    A. Rales
    B. Rhonchi
    C. Wheezes
    D. Stridor

12. The medical term for "inflammation of the throat" is _____.
    A. croupitis
    B. laryngitis
    C. pharyngitis
    D. rhinitis

13. A combination of respiratory diseases including chronic bronchitis, asthma, and emphysema is called _____.
    A. CPR
    B. PET
    C. CBAE
    D. COPD

14. A bacterial infection of the lungs that can also affect other areas of the body is _____.
    A. pleurisy
    B. pulmonary embolism
    C. SIDS
    D. tuberculosis

15. _____ measures the amount of air that can be exhaled after maximum inhalation.
    A. Tidal volume
    B. Residual volume
    C. Vital capacity
    D. Total lung capacity

16. _____ measures the amount of air that remains in the lungs after a maximal expiration.
    A. Tidal volume
    B. Residual volume
    C. Vital capacity
    D. Total lung capacity

17. _____ is the term for incomplete lung expansion; lung collapse.
    A. Asphyxia
    B. Atelectasis
    C. Hemoptysis
    D. Hypoxia

18. The medical term for "blood in the pleural cavity" is _____.
    A. hemothorax
    B. pneumothorax
    C. hemoptysis
    D. hemostasis

19. The medical term for "whooping cough" is _____.
    A. croup
    B. bronchitis
    C. pertussis
    D. influenza

20. A(n) _____ is the medication given to patients with asthma.
    A. antibiotic
    B. antitussive
    C. immunization
    D. bronchodilator

CHAPTER THIRTEEN

Digestive System

VOCABULARY REVIEW:

Matching: Match each term with the correct definition.

A. digestion

B. alimentary canal

C. bolus

D. uvula

E. mastication

F. enzyme

G. peristalsis

H. chyme

I. gastroenteritis

J. mesentery

K. peritoneum

L. stomach

M. vagus nerve

N. villi

O. vermiform appendix

P. defecation

Q. liver

R. hepatic duct

_____ 1. Duct from the liver to the gallbladder

_____ 2. Serous membrane that lines the walls of the abdominal cavity and folds over and protects the intestines

_____ 3. Reflux into the esophagus of stomach acids and food

_____ 4. Digestive tract; extends from the mouth to the anus

_____ 5. Wavelike motions that propel food through the digestive tract

_____ 6. Enlarged, saclike portion of the alimentary canal; one of the main organs of digestion

_____ 7. Small mass of tissue hanging from the soft palate at the back of the mouth

_____ 8. Organ that secretes bile; active in the formation of certain blood proteins and the metabolism of carbohydrates, fats, and proteins

_____ 9. Inflammation of the liver caused by a viral infection

_____ 10. Food broken down by chewing and mixed with saliva

_____ 11. Protein produced by living organisms that causes biochemical changes

S. insulin

T. metabolism

U. constipation

V. flatulence

W. jaundice

X. regurgitation

Y. hepatitis

Z. volvulus

_____ 12. Vascular projections of the small intestine for absorption of nutrients

_____ 13. Membrane that attaches itself to the small and large intestines and holds them in place

_____ 14. Difficulty in defecation caused by hard, compacted stool; lack of water absorption in the large intestine

_____ 15. Colon twisting on itself

_____ 16. Chewing

_____ 17. Physical and chemical breakdown of food

_____ 18. Attached to the cecum

_____ 19. Digestive gas

_____ 20. Inflammation of the stomach and intestines

_____ 21. Energy production after the absorption of nutrients

_____ 22. Elimination of feces

_____ 23. Hormone functions to regulate the metabolism of carbohydrates and fats, especially the conversion of glucose to glycogen, which lowers the blood glucose level

_____ 24. Semiliquid contents of the stomach after it has been mixed with stomach acid

_____ 25. Controls secretions of hydrochloric acid, as well as many other responsibilities

_____ 26. Yellowish discoloration of the skin due to a breakdown of bilirubin

THEORY RECALL

True/False

Indicate whether the sentence or statement is true or false.

_____ 1. The alimentary canal is a muscular tube that extends from the mouth to the anus and is approximately 30 feet long.

_____ 2. The liver is the largest organ in the body.

_____ 3. The trachea carries the bolus to the stomach via the process of peristalsis.

_____ 4. The duodenum is where the final breakdown of nutrients takes place.

_____ 5. The LES allows chyme to exit into the small intestine.

Multiple Choice

Identify the letter of the choice that best completes the statement or answers the question.

1. _____ is the process of taking nutrition into the body.
   A. Absorption
   B. Elimination
   C. Ingestion
   D. None of the above

2. Which one of the following is not one of the four areas of the taste buds of the tongue?
   A. Sweet
   B. Metallic
   C. Salty
   D. Sour

3. The top portion of the stomach is called the _____.
   A. fundus
   B. rugae
   C. body
   D. frenulum

4. The combining form for "mouth" is _____.
   A. cheil/o
   B. enter/o
   C. pylor/o
   D. stomat/o

5. A large pouch forming the first part of the large intestine is called the _____.
   A. cecum
   B. appendix
   C. colon
   D. jejunum

6. The suffix for "digestions" is _____.
   A. -emesis
   B. -pepsia
   C. -stalsis
   D. -phage

7. _____ is fluid that is secreted by the liver, stored in the gallbladder, and discharged into the duodenum.
   A. Chyme
   B. Bolus
   C. Feces
   D. Bile

8. The suffix for "hernia" is _____.
   A. -cele
   B. -clysis
   C. -pexy
   D. -ose

9. The medical abbreviation that means "before meals" is _____.
   A. BE
   B. BM
   C. AC
   D. NPO

10. The second part of the small intestine, responsible for absorption, is the _____.
    A. duodenum
    B. jejunum
    C. vermiform appendix
    D. cecum

11. An organ that has both endocrine and exocrine functions is the _____.
    A. liver
    B. spleen
    C. pancreas
    D. appendix

12. The medical term for "forceful expulsion of the stomach contents" is _____.
    A. emesis
    B. dyspepsia
    C. flatulence
    D. ascites

13. The process of converting smaller molecules into larger molecules is called _____.
    A. cannibalism
    B. metabolism
    C. catabolism
    D. anabolism

14. Frequent bowel movements of loose, watery stools is _____.
    A. flatulence
    B. ascites
    C. emesis
    D. none of the above

15. Dilated veins in the rectum and anus are called _____.
    A. caries
    B. hemorrhoids
    C. varicose veins
    D. glossitis

16. The medical term for gallstones is _____.
    A. cholelithiasis
    B. choledocolithotomy
    C. cholecystitis
    D. diverticulitis

17. _____ are usually benign growths that can be attached to the mucosal lining of the colon.
    A. Hemorrhoids
    B. Polyps
    C. Caries
    D. None of the above

18. Telescoping of one part of the intestine into another is called _____.
    A. diverticulitis
    B. gastroenteritis
    C. intussusception
    D. celiac sprue

19. A(n) _____ is a lesion of the mucosal lining of the stomach or intestine.
    A. pyloric stenosis
    B. volvulus
    C. ulcer
    D. celiac sprue

20. The medical term for "vomiting blood" is _____.
    A. gastritis
    B. intussusception
    C. ascites
    D. hematemesis

21. _____ is a viral infection of the parotid glands.
    A. Melena
    B. Mumps
    C. Measles
    D. Ulcers

22. Which one of the following is NOT a stage of digestion?
    A. Ingestion
    B. Respiration
    C. Absorption
    D. Elimination

23. When food is chewed and mixed with saliva, it becomes known as _____.
    A. bolus
    B. chyme
    C. feces
    D. phlegm

24. The oral ingestion of a suspension for imaging of the esophagus is what type of diagnostic test?
    A. Cholecystography
    B. Barium enema
    C. Barium swallow
    D. Endoscopy

25. When permanent teeth replace baby teeth, there are four _____.
    A. canines
    B. molars
    C. bicuspids
    D. none of the above

Sentence Completion

Complete each sentence or statement.

1. The _____ leads from the gallbladder into the common bile duct.

2. The first set of teeth is called _____.

3. Gastric juices contain the enzyme _____.

4. _____ is the inability for the body to process dairy products.

5. The _____ is the part of the intestinal tract that moves up the right side of the body toward the lower part of the liver.

6. The _____ is continuous with the sigmoid colon and measures about 5 inches in length.

7. The liver, _____, and pancreas all empty their secretions into the duodenum.

8. _____ cause the evacuation of the bowel by increasing bulk of the feces, softening the stool, or lubricating the intestinal wall.

9. Bile leaves the gallbladder through the _____.

10. _____ is the abbreviation for "nothing by mouth."

Short Answers

1. Explain the purpose of the digestive system.

   _____

   _____

   _____

2. List the four stages of the digestive process.

   _____

   _____

   _____

3. Explain the role of the mouth in digestion.

   _____

   _____

   _____

4. Explain the role of the stomach in digestion.

   _____

   _____

   _____

CRITICAL THINKING

1. Using Box 13-2 in the textbook, create a patient history using a minimum of 10 of the terms on the list.

2. Clarence Johansen is 67 years old and has been encouraged by his wife to have a colon check-up. The physician ordered a standard cleansing diet and is going to perform a sigmoidoscopy this afternoon. Explain to Mr. Johansen what is a sigmoidoscopy. Explain why and how the procedure is performed.

INTERNET RESEARCH

Keyword: (Use the name of the condition or disease you select to write about).

Select one condition or disease from Table 13-2. Write a two-paragraph report regarding the condition or disease you selected, listing the etiology, signs and symptoms, diagnosis, therapy, and interventions. Cite your source. (You may not use the information on the tables exclusively for your report.) Be prepared to give a 2-minute oral presentation should your instructor assign you to do so.

WHAT WOULD YOU DO?

If you have accomplished the objectives in this chapter, you will be able to make better choices as a medical assistant. Take a look at this situation and decide what you would do.

Saril Paratel, age 69, was brought to the physician's office with fever and pain in the right lower quadrant of her abdomen. The pain has lasted for 3 days and has become progressively worse over the past 36 hours. The pain originally started in the umbilical area, but over time moved to McBurney's point. Last night she had nausea and vomiting. She has not had a bowel movement for 4 days. Saril had dyspepsia for several days prior to this episode of pain. She has also noticed that fatty foods tend to cause flatulence with some pain in her right upper quadrant, radiating into her back at the right shoulder. No history of hematemesis is given, but malaise has been present for several weeks. When asked about diarrhea, Saril answers that her stools 5 days ago were soft, formed, and frequent, so yes, she had diarrhea. The white blood cell count ordered by the physician is reported as WBC 15,600 with a differential of 67% neutrophils, 6% bands, 25% lymphs, 0% basos, 1% monos, and 1% eos. The physician refers Saril to a surgeon because he wants her to be evaluated for possible appendicitis and to rule out the cause of the right upper quadrant pain.

1. **What gastrointestinal organs are found in the right lower quadrant?**

   _____

   _____

2. **Where is McBurney's point?**

   _____

3. **What is appendicitis?**

   _____

   _____

   _____

4. **What is hematemesis, and why would this be important in this case study?**

   _____

   _____

   _____

5. **What is the difference between emesis and regurgitation?**

   _____

   _____

   _____

6. **Did Saril really have diarrhea? Explain your answer.**

_____

_____

_____

_____

7. **What did the white blood cell count indicate?**

_____

_____

8. **How did the white cell differential confirm that Saril might have appendicitis?**

_____

_____

_____

9. **What organs of digestion are found in the right upper quadrant?**

_____

_____

_____

10. **What disease processes might be seen with right upper quadrant pain that radiates into the right back at the shoulder with associated flatulence?**

_____

_____

_____

_____

APPLICATION OF SKILLS

1. Label the diagrams.

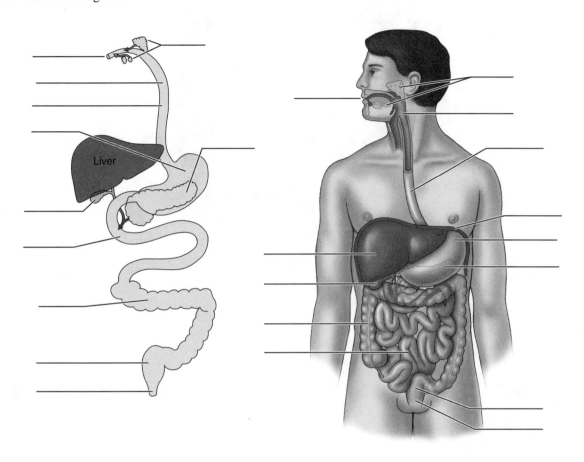

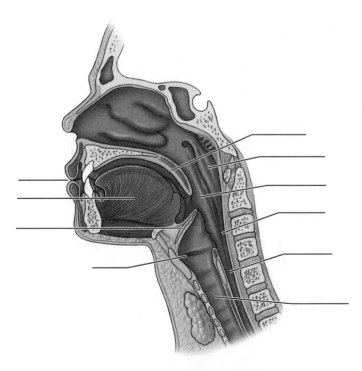

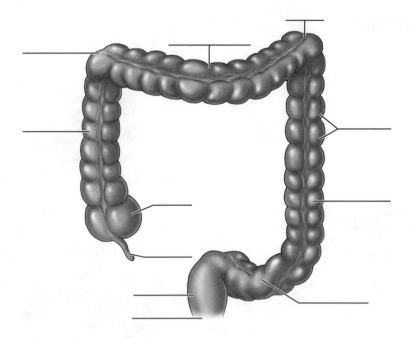

2. Trace a hamburger through the alimentary canal.

CHAPTER QUIZ

Multiple Choice

Identify the letter of the choice that best completes the statement or answers the question.

1. A toothache is a symptom of _____.
   A. glossitis
   B. caries
   C. gingivitis
   D. thrush

2. The therapy for GERD is _____.
   A. to elevate the head of the bed 4 to 6 inches
   B. the removal of plaque and antibiotic therapy
   C. a bland diet to reduce acid
   D. a gluten-free diet

3. _____ is the narrowing of the pyloric sphincter.
   A. Intussusception
   B. Pyloric stenosis
   C. Endoscopy
   D. Pyloricectomy

4. _____ is an inflammation of small outpouches in the colon.
   A. Gastritis
   B. Colitis
   C. Diverticulitis
   D. Hepatitis

5. _____ is an inflammation of the liver caused by a viral infection and contracted by coming in contact with an infected person's blood or body fluids.
   A. HIV
   B. Hepatitis C
   C. Crohn disease
   D. Hepatitis B

6. _____ is a loss of appetite.
   A. Anorexia
   B. Dyspepsia
   C. Colic
   D. Ascites

7. _____ is a yellowish discoloration of skin due to the lack of breakdown of bilirubin in the blood.
   A. Hematemesis
   B. Melena
   C. Jaundice
   D. Cirrhosis

8. _____ cause evacuation of the bowel by stimulating nerves in the intestines, resulting in increased peristalsis.
   A. Antacids
   B. Antiemetics
   C. Cathartics
   D. Laxatives

9. _____ is the physical and chemical change nutrients undergo after absorption.
   A. Metabolism
   B. Anabolism
   C. Catabolism
   D. Hemabolism

10. The _____ is(are) the largest organ of the body.
    A. heart
    B. liver
    C. lungs
    D. stomach

11. Which one of the following vitamins is NOT stored in the liver?
    A. A
    B. B_{12}
    C. C
    D. E

12. Which one of the following is NOT an accessory organ of the digestive system?
    A. Appendix
    B. Pancreas
    C. Gallbladder
    D. Liver

13. _____ occurs when the stomach protrudes through the diaphragm into the chest cavity.
    A. An ulcer
    B. Spastic colon
    C. Appendicitis
    D. A hiatal hernia

14. Which one of the following is the correct spelling for the medical term meaning "inflammation of the gallbladder"?
    A. Koleecystitis
    B. Cholesisitis
    C. Cholecystitis
    D. Coaleesystitis

15. _____ are usually benign growths that can be attached to the mucosal lining of the colon.
    A. Hemorrhoids
    B. Polyps
    C. Varices
    D. Ulcers

16. The _____ is the portion of the digestive tract that extends from the sigmoid colon to the anal canal
    A. descending colon
    B. duodenum
    C. ascending colon
    D. rectum

17. The medical term for "difficulty swallowing" is _____.
    A. dysphonia
    B. dysphagia
    C. dyspepsia
    D. dysuria

18. The second part of the small intestine responsible for absorption is the _____.
    A. jejunum
    B. rectum
    C. duodenum
    D. ileum

19. The _____ are the teeth located in the front of the mouth.
    A. molars
    B. canines
    C. incisors
    D. bicuspids

20. Absorption of nutrients takes place in the _____.
    A. stomach
    B. pancreas
    C. small intestine
    D. large intestine

CHAPTER **FOURTEEN**

Nervous System

VOCABULARY REVIEW

Matching: Match each term with the correct definition.

A. nerve

B. neurons

C. dendrites

D. myelin sheath

E. dermatome

F. synapse

G. brain

H. equilibrium

I. hypothalamus

J. meninges

K. oxytocin

L. thalamus

M. spinal column

N. reflex

O. gait

P. vertigo

Q. psychiatry

_____ 1. Manner of walking

_____ 2. Functional unit of a nerve that transmits impulses; located within the CNS

_____ 3. Bone structure that surrounds and protects the spinal cord

_____ 4. Medical science that deals with the origin, diagnosis, prevention, and treatment of developmental and emotional components of physical disorders

_____ 5. Pertains to the sense of touch

_____ 6. Loud/soft measurement of sound

_____ 7. Protective covering of the brain and spinal cord

_____ 8. Instrument used to view the retina

_____ 9. Surface area of the body where the afferent fibers travel from a spinal root

_____ 10. Covering of an axon

_____ 11. Small bones of the middle ear

_____ 12. Involuntary reaction that occurs because of a stimulus

_____ 13. Located in the skull; main functioning unit of the CNS that contains many neurons

_____ 14. Controls equilibrium

R. tactile

S. accommodation

T. ophthalmoscope

U. cerumen

V. eustachian tube

W. ossicles

X. decibels

Y. otolaryngologist

Z. semicircular canals

_____ 15. Adjustment that allows for vision at various distances

_____ 16. Bundle of fibers containing neurons and blood vessels

_____ 17. Yellow-brown substance produced by the sweat glands in the external ear

_____ 18. Dizziness

_____ 19. Specialist in the treatment of ear, nose, and throat diseases

_____ 20. Space from the end of one neuron to the beginning of the next neuron

_____ 21. Hormone that is stored in the posterior pituitary gland and needed for uterine contractions

_____ 22. Tube that connects the middle ear with the nasopharynx and acts to equalize pressure between the outer and middle ear

_____ 23. Responsible for relaying messages from parts of the body; monitors sensory stimuli

_____ 24. Receive nerve impulses

_____ 25. Balance

_____ 26. Controls activities of the pituitary gland; secretes oxytocin and ADH; regulates the autonomic nervous system

THEORY RECALL

True/False

Indicate whether the sentence or statement is true or false.

_____ 1. The endocrine system is the main communication and control system of the body.

_____ 2. There are 16 pairs of cranial nerves.

_____ 3. A general increase in nerve conduction occurs with age.

_____ 4. An ophthalmologist treats disorders of the eye.

_____ 5. Antiseptics are used to reduce growth of bacteria in the eye.

Multiple Choice

Identify the letter of the choice that best completes the statement or answers the question.

1. Phagocytic cells that do not transmit impulses and are located within the CNS are called _____.
   A. glial cells
   B. astrocytes
   C. ganglia
   D. None of the above

2. _____ are nerve cells that engulf cellular waste and destroy microorganisms in nerve tissue.
   A. Astrocytes
   B. Ependymal cells
   C. Microglial cells
   D. Oligodendroglial cells

3. The _____ is known as the little brain.
   A. brain stem
   B. cerebellum
   C. diencephalon
   D. cerebrum

4. The middle layer of the meninges is called the _____.
   A. dura mater
   B. pia mater
   C. arachnoid
   D. none of the above

5. _____ are(is) (a) chemical substance(s) that cause(s) a nerve impulse.
   A. Neurotransmitters
   B. Aqueous humor
   C. Oxytocin
   D. Cerebrospinal fluid

6. The combining form for "brain" is _____.
   A. neur/o
   B. dur/o
   C. rhiz/o
   D. encephal/o

7. The suffix for "hearing" is _____.
   A. -acusis
   B. -geusia
   C. -kinesia
   D. -otia

8. _____ are used to produce sleep.
   A. Analgesics
   B. Hypnotics
   C. Sedatives
   D. Anesthetics

9. _____ soften and break down ear wax.
   A. Antiinfectives
   B. Vasodilators
   C. Ceruminolytics
   D. Anxiolytics

10. Paxil is an example of an _____.
   A. antimanic
   B. antipsychotic
   C. anxiolytic
   D. antidepressant

11. What roman numeral is the trigeminal nerve?
   A. III
   B. IV
   C. V
   D. X

12. The _____ nerve controls salivation, swallowing, and taste.
   A. olfactory
   B. trochlear
   C. glossopharyngeal
   D. hypoglossal

13. A _____ headache occurs unilaterally and involves an eye, temple, cheek, and forehead. These headaches start during sleep and can last for several weeks.
   A. tension
   B. cluster
   C. migraine
   D. none of the above

14. A(n) _____ is the surgical puncture performed to remove CSF for examination.
   A. spinal tap
   B. angiography
   C. myelography
   D. electoneuromyography

15. A test that measures muscle activity and aids in diagnosing neuromuscular problems is called a(n) _____.
   A. electroencephalogram
   B. angiogram
   C. electromyogram
   D. nerve conduction study

16. A(n) _____ seizure begins with an outcry and movements that are first tonic and then clonic.
   A. petit mal
   B. myoclonic
   C. partial
   D. grand mal

17. _____ occurs when a blood vessel ruptures or a blood clot occludes a blood vessel, which decreases blood flow to the brain.
   A. ALS
   B. CVA
   C. MS
   D. TIA

18. _____ is inflammation of the brain and spinal cord coverings.
    A. Meningitis
    B. Parkinson's disease
    C. Multiple sclerosis
    D. Alzheimer's disease

19. Neuralgia of the fifth cranial nerve is called _____.
    A. Alzheimer's disease
    B. Tic doulourex
    C. transient ischemic attack
    D. shingles

20. Which one of the following is NOT an extrinsic eye muscle?
    A. Superior rectus
    B. Lateral rectus
    C. Superior oblique
    D. Ciliary

21. Which eye muscle elevates or rolls the eyeball upward?
    A. Superior rectus
    B. Medial rectus
    C. Superior oblique
    D. Inferior oblique

22. _____ is used to measure intraocular pressure.
    A. Amsler grid
    B. Gonioscopy
    C. Tonometry
    D. All of the above

23. _____ occurs when the aqueous humor does not drain properly and the intraocular pressure increases and compresses the choroid layer, diminishing blood supply to the retina.
    A. Cataract
    B. Glaucoma
    C. Strabismus
    D. Myopia

24. _____ is a refraction error caused by the abnormal curvature of the cornea and lens.
    A. Astigmatism
    B. Ptosis
    C. Strabismus
    D. Hyperopia

25. _____ is a buildup of excess fluid in the semicircular canals, which places excess pressure on the canals, vestibule, and cochlea.
    A. Otosclerosis
    B. Mastoiditis
    C. Meniere disease
    D. None of the above

Sentence Completion

Complete each sentence or statement.

1. The functional unit of the nervous system is the _____.

2. _____ is the progressive hearing loss occurring in old age.

3. _____ is an impaired perception of reality.

4. A(n) _____ test measures patient's ability to integrate intellectual and emotional fears.

5. _____ is an irreversible impairment of intellectual activities.

6. _____ is a disorder marked by severe mood swings from hyperactivity to sadness.

7. _____ behavior demonstrates a lack of empathy and sensitivity to the needs of others.

8. _____ is a severe anxiety following trauma. Impairment affects daily living.

9. A(n) _____ test compares bone conduction and air conduction of sound using a tuning fork.

10. _____ is a continuous sheath around the myelin.

Short Answers

1. Describe the organization of the nervous system and identify its two main divisions.

_____

_____

_____

_____

2. List the main divisions of the central nervous system.

_____

_____

_____

3. Describe the functions of the sympathetic and parasympathetic nervous system.

_____

_____

_____

_____

_____

4. Explain the purpose of the sensory system.

_____

_____

_____

_____

_____

APPLICATION OF SKILLS

1. Label the diagrams.

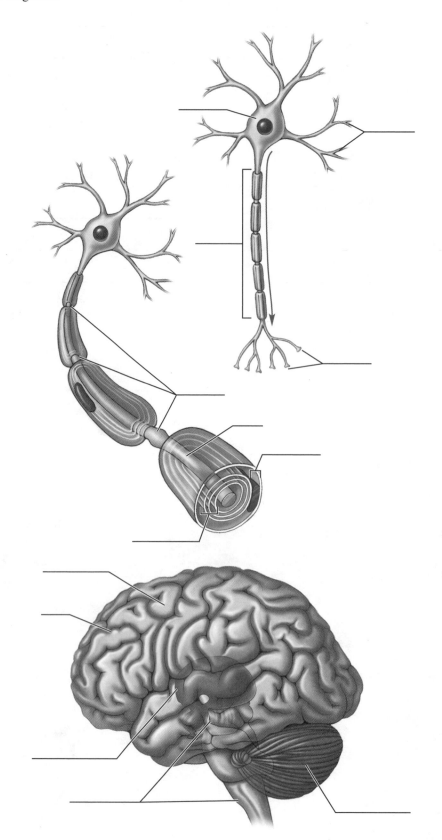

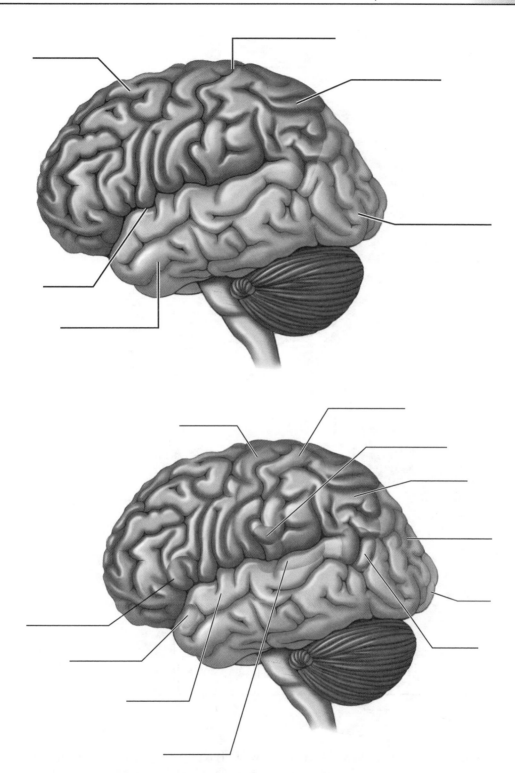

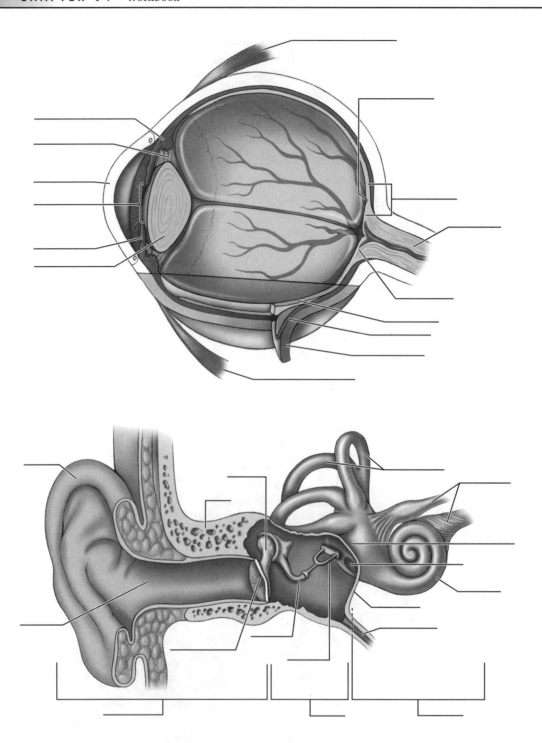

2. Wear a blindfold for 2 hours to completely block your vision. Participate in all of your regular activities—get dressed, brush your teeth, do household chores, etc. Write one paragraph describing your experience. Identify the points that you can now share with a recently blind patient or a patient who is losing his or her eyesight.

CRITICAL THINKING

1. Describe a past event that caused your sympathetic and parasympathetic nervous system to respond.

2. Clara Evanston is an 83-year-old patient who has been gradually exhibiting signs of Alzheimer's disease. Her husband is her primary caregiver and is finding it increasingly difficult to manage her care. On Clara's recent office visit, Mr. Evanston asked you to explain the progression of Clara's symptoms and what suggestions you have for her care. Explain to Mr. Evanston the progression of symptoms and what suggestions you would give him. Research Alzheimer's disease as needed.

INTERNET RESEARCH

Keyword: (Use the name of the condition or disease you select to write about).

Select one condition or disease from Tables 14-4, 14-8, and 14-10. Write a two-paragraph report regarding the condition or disease you selected, listing the etiology, signs and symptoms, diagnosis, therapy, and interventions. Cite your source. (You may not use the information on the tables exclusively for your report.) Be prepared to give a 2-minute oral presentation should your instructor assign you to do so.

WHAT WOULD YOU DO?

If you have accomplished the objectives in this chapter, you will be able to make better choices as a medical assistant. Take a look at this situation and decide what you would do.

Sally Jones, age 72, complained of dizziness with a loss of sensation on the left side that lasted only for a few minutes over the past few weeks. She also had a headache that lasted only during the paresthesia. She has a long history of moderately controlled hypertension for which she has taken antihypertensives, "When I thought about them." Dr. Smith was concerned that she might be having TIAs. He prescribed a vasodilator and a mild analgesic for the headache when he saw her last week. Today she was brought to the emergency room with sudden left-side hemiplegia and a headache, but no aphasia. Except for the hypertension, Ms. Jones has been in relatively good health for her age. On admission, her blood pressure was 210/120 and she was semialert. Dr. Smith ordered a CT scan, and it showed an infarct to the right frontotemporal lobes. Ms. Jones was admitted to the hospital for observation and possible treatment.

1. **What is a TIA? Why was that a precursor to the condition for which Ms. Jones was admitted to the hospital?**

   _____

   _____

   _____

2. **Why were the dizziness, loss of sensation, and the headache over the past few weeks important in making a diagnosis of TIA?**

   _____

   _____

   _____

3. Why did Dr. Smith give Ms. Jones vasodilators?

_____

_____

_____

4. What is paresthesia? What is aphasia? What is hemiplegia?

_____

_____

_____

_____

_____

5. Why was the control of blood pressure important in the prevention of illness?

_____

_____

6. Why is the paralysis on the left side of the body when the right side of the brain is involved? Why does Ms. Jones not have aphasia?

_____

_____

_____

_____

7. Why did Dr. Smith order a CT scan rather than an MRI?

_____

_____

_____

8. What is a common name for the disease process for which Dr. Smith is treating Ms. Jones?

_____

_____

9. **What type of problems would you expect Mrs. Jones to have since the infarct is in the frontal and temporal lobes?**

_____

_____

_____

_____

CHAPTER QUIZ

Multiple Choice

Identify the letter of the choice that best completes the statement or answers the question.

1. The _____ of a nerve cell carries impulses to other neurons and body tissue.
   A. nodes of Ranvier
   B. dendrites
   C. synapse
   D. axon

2. _____ neurons transmit nerve impulses from the CNS to muscles and glands.
   A. Efferent
   B. Integrative
   C. Afferent
   D. None of the above

3. Star-shaped nerve cells that hold blood vessels, closer to nerve cells, and transport water and slats between nerve cells are called _____.
   A. microglial cells
   B. oligodendroglial cells
   C. astrocytes
   D. ependymal cells

4. A sterile watery fluid formed within the ventricles of the brain is _____.
   A. CNS
   B. CSF
   C. PNS
   D. PSF

5. A(n) _____ reflex extends the foot when the tendon at the heel is tapped.
   A. abdominal
   B. Achilles
   C. Babinski
   D. plantar

6. _____ is the inability to focus one's attention for short periods or for engaging in quiet activities, or both.
   A. ADHD
   B. COPD
   C. Colic
   D. Kernig sign

7. _____ occurs when a blood vessel ruptures or a blood clot occludes a blood vessel that decreases blood flow to the brain.
   A. TIA
   B. ALS
   C. CVA
   D. OCD

8. _____ is an acute inflammation of the dorsal root ganglia of a dermatome.
   A. Meningitis
   B. Shingles
   C. Tic douloureux
   D. Encephalitis

9. _____ is a feeling of persistent sadness.
   A. Depression
   B. Anxiety
   C. Narcissism
   D. Paranoia

10. A(n) _____ is a test that records neuromuscular activity by electrical stimulation.
    A. CT scan
    B. MRI
    C. EEG
    D. EMG

11. _____ is a disorder characterized by a preoccupation with inner thoughts and marked unresponsiveness to social contact.
    A. Delusional disorder
    B. Autism
    C. Obsessive-compulsive disorder
    D. Munchausen's syndrome

12. _____ is the anterior portion of the sclera; also means "transparent—allows light through."
    A. Iris
    B. Chorioid
    C. Lens
    D. Cornea

13. Which one of the following is NOT a muscle of the eye?
    A. Oblique
    B. Canthus
    C. Rectus
    D. All of the above are muscles of the eye

14. _____ occurs when the lens loses its ability to change shape during accommodation for close objects.
    A. Presbycusis
    B. Strabismus
    C. Presbyopia
    D. Hyperopia

15. The _____ is the external flap of the ear.
    A. pinna
    B. auricle
    C. both A and B
    D. none of the above

16. The medical term for pinkeye is _____.
    A. chalazoin
    B. conjunctivitis
    C. strabismus
    D. hordeolum

17. _____ is a buildup of excess fluid in the semicircular canals, which places excess pressure on the canals, vestibule, and cochlea.
    A. Meniere disease
    B. Vertigo
    C. Otosclerosis
    D. Presbycusis

18. Which one of the following is NOT an ossicle?
    A. Malleus
    B. Incus
    C. Stapes
    D. All of the above are ossicles

19. The _____ of the ear lies below the vestibule and is shaped like a snail shell.
    A. labyrinth
    B. eustachian tube
    C. organ of Corti
    D. cochlea

20. There are _____ pairs of spinal nerves.
    A. 12
    B. 31
    C. 36
    D. 42

CHAPTER **FIFTEEN**

Skeletal System

VOCABULARY REVIEW

Matching: Match each term with the correct definition.

A. cartilage

B. epiphyseal plate

C. ossification

D. foramen

E. periosteum

F. cranium

G. fontanels

H. paranasal sinuses

I. sella turcica

J. sutures

K. nasal conchae

L. vomer

M. spinous process

N. vertebra

O. sternum

P. process

Q. amphiarthroses

R. orthopedic

S. bone scan

_____ 1. Joint with slight movement

_____ 2. Pertaining to treatment of the bones and joints

_____ 3. Outer covering of the bone that provides nourishment to the bone

_____ 4. Immovable joints

_____ 5. Area of each end of a long bone responsible for bone growth

_____ 6. Air-filled spaces within the skull

_____ 7. Caused when more bone cells are destroyed than are made; a decrease in bone density

_____ 8. Extend out from vertebral bone to serve as attachments for the ribs

_____ 9. Repair of a fracture when the skin has been surgically opened

_____ 10. Elastic substance attached to the end of some bones

_____ 11. Use of nuclear medicine to detect pathologies of bone

_____ 12. Pertaining to the study and analysis of human work devices that affect the anatomy

_____ 13. Breastbone

T. open reduction

U. subluxation

V. osteomyelitis

W. osteoporosis

X. metastasized

Y. crepitation

Z. ergonomic

_____ 14. Skull; fusion of 8 cranial bones with 14 facial bones that protect the brain

_____ 15. Cancer that has spread from its original site to a new site

_____ 16. Calcification of bone

_____ 17. Hole or opening for passage of nerves, blood vessels, and ligaments

_____ 18. Partial dislocation of a joint

_____ 19. Joints rubbing against each other

_____ 20. Forms the lower wall between the nostrils; nasal septum

_____ 21. Soft spots; located between the cranial bones

_____ 22. Projection on a bone

_____ 23. Facial bones above the roof of the mouth and the walls of the nasal cavities

_____ 24. Infection of the bone marrow and bone

_____ 25. Bony projection in the sphenoid bone that holds the pituitary gland

_____ 26. Protects the spinal cord

THEORY RECALL

True/False

Indicate whether the sentence or statement is true or false.

_____ 1. The skeletal system is the bony framework of the body and is made up of 206 bones.

_____ 2. Proper levels of calcium in the bloodstream are maintained in the blood by the pituitary hormone.

_____ 3. Long bones are located only in the upper and lower extremities.

_____ 4. The largest bone in the face is the maxilla.

_____ 5. Articulations are joints where two or more bones come together.

Multiple Choice

Identify the letter of the choice that best completes the statement or answers the question.

1. The combining form for "bone" is _____.
   A. chondr/o
   B. bon/o
   C. oste/o
   D. none of the above

2. Naproxen is an _____ prescribed to relieve and control inflammation.
   A. antiinflammatory
   B. antibiotic
   C. antiarthritic
   D. analgesic

3. _____ is the visual examination of a joint with the use of a scope.
   A. Arthrography
   B. Myeloscopy
   C. Bone scan
   D. Arthroscopy

4. _____ is a disease of adults in which deficiency of calcium and vitamin D occurs.
   A. Rickets
   B. Osteomyelitis
   C. Osteomalacia
   D. Scurvy

5. _____ is a lateral curvature of the spine.
   A. Scoliosis
   B. Lordosis
   C. Kyphosis
   D. None of the above

6. The suffix meaning "to break" is _____.
   A. -cyto
   B. -clast
   C. -blast
   D. -malacia

7. Which one of the following is not a type of joint?
   A. Amphiarthroses
   B. Diarthroses
   C. Synarthroses
   D. Articulothroses

8. _____ are the long bones of the foot.
   A. Metatarsals
   B. Tarsals
   C. Metacarpals
   D. Carpals

9. The _____ is the longest and strongest bone in the body.
   A. ulnar
   B. tibia
   C. femur
   D. humerus

10. The _____ and the _____ are located behind the nose and eye sockets.
    A. xiphoid, manubrium bones
    B. incus, stapes bones
    C. sphenoid, ethmoid bones
    D. mandible, maxilla bones

11. Which of the following is NOT a distinct region of a long bone?
    A. Metaphysis
    B. Paraphysis
    C. Diaphysis
    D. Epiphysis

12. An example of _____ cartilage can be found in the outer ear.
    A. fibrous
    B. hyaline
    C. elastic
    D. retractable

13. A(n) _____ is a bone-reabsorbing cell.
    A. osteoblast
    B. osteoclast
    C. osteocyte
    D. none of the above

14. _____ is made of connective tissue and blood vessels.
    A. Bone marrow
    B. Periosteum
    C. Lamellae
    D. Compact bone

15. The bone that extends from the top of the eye orbits to the top of the head forming the forehead is called the _____.
    A. temporal bone
    B. parietal
    C. occipital
    D. frontal

16. The main shaft of a bone is called the _____.
    A. diaphysis
    B. epiphysis
    C. metaphysis
    D. paraphysis

17. The _____ bones are located within the eye orbits and along the side of the nose.
    A. palatine
    B. zygomatic
    C. lacrimal
    D. vomer

18. The first vertebra is called the _____ and supports the head.
    A. axis
    B. atlas
    C. sphenoid
    D. coccyx

19. Adults have _____ vertebrae.
    A. 12
    B. 26
    C. 33
    D. 42

20. The part of the sternum that is used as a landmark for CPR is the _____.
    A. manubrium
    B. body
    C. xiphoid process
    D. none of the above

21. The medical term for shoulder blades is _____.
    A. scapulae
    B. clavicles
    C. humerus
    D. ulna

22. The wrist has eight small bones called _____.
    A. metatarsals
    B. tarsals
    C. metacarpals
    D. carpals

23. Which one of the following is NOT a pelvic bone?
    A. Acetabulum
    B. Ilium
    C. Ischium
    D. Pubis

24. Which one of the following is the "heel" bone?
    A. Talus
    B. Calcaneus
    C. Navicular
    D. Cuboid

25. _____ is/are a capsule made up of tough, fibrous connective tissue and filled with synovial fluid.
    A. Vertebrae
    B. Meniscus
    C. Bursae
    D. Tendons

Sentence Completion

Complete each sentence or statement.

1. The _____ is a structural unit of the bone that receives nutrition and removes wastes.

2. The _____ contains the bones of the central section of the skeleton, which includes the bones of the head and trunk.

3. The bones of the spinal column, sphenoid, and ethmoid bones of the skull, sacrum, coccyx, and mandible are _____ [type] bones.

4. _____ is connective tissue attached to bone and does not contain mineral salts.

5. _____ bone marrow is responsible for the manufacture of red and white blood cells.

6. The _____ is the covering on the outer surface of a bone.

7. The _____ bone forms the back part of the cranial floor and is the covering for the back portion of the brain.

8. The medical term for cheek bones is _____.

9. The medical term for the fingers and toes is _____.

10. _____ joints allow for rotation.

Short Answers

1. List the four types of bone shapes and give an example of each.

_____

_____

_____

_____

2. List the five major functions of the skeletal system.

_____

_____

_____

_____

_____

3. List three types of joints.

_____

_____

_____

4. Describe the four main types of movement.

_____

_____

_____

_____

CRITICAL THINKING

1. Describe a past event that caused your sympathetic and parasympathetic nervous system to respond.

   Your favorite patient, Felicia Robinson, has been diagnosed with osteoporosis. She is 78 years old. Provide Felicia with information regarding this condition.

INTERNET RESEARCH

Keyword: (Use the name of the condition or disease you select to write about).

Select one condition or disease from Table 15-5. Write a two-paragraph report regarding the condition or disease you selected, listing the etiology, signs and symptoms, diagnosis, therapy, and interventions. Cite your source. (You may not use the information on the tables exclusively for your report.) Be prepared to give a 2-minute oral presentation should your instructor assign you to do so.

WHAT WOULD YOU DO?

If you have accomplished the objectives in this chapter, you will be able to make better choices as a medical assistant. Take a look at this situation and decide what you would do.

At the age of 14, Celia was injured in a skiing accident. She had a simple fracture of the end of the tibia and into the tarsals in her left leg. The fracture was located at the epiphyseal line. She also subluxated her knee in the same accident. The fracture was repaired with a closed reduction. After she wore a long leg cast for 8 weeks, an arthroscopy was performed on the knee to be sure the tendons and ligaments had not been torn or stretched because weight-bearing was difficult. Prior to the arthroscopy, an arthrogram was performed on the knee; this was negative. The arthroscopy was also negative. Over time, Celia seemed to recover from the fracture and had no problems until lately.

   Celia is now 52 and has pain in the ankle attributed to arthritis. She has also been diagnosed with early osteoporosis as a result of a bone density scan. The physician ordered analgesics for arthralgia and vitamin D and calcium supplements for osteoporosis. Celia expresses concern while talking with Steve, the medical assistant, that the osteoporosis and arthritis will only progress as she ages. She also has questions about some of the terms the physician used in talking with her.

1. **What is a simple fracture?**

   _____

   _____

   _____

   _____

2. **What is a closed reduction?**

   _____

   _____

   _____

   _____

3. **What is subluxation of a joint?**

   _____

   _____

   _____

   _____

4. **Where is the tibia? Where are the tarsals?**

_____

_____

_____

_____

5. **What type of bone is the tibia? What type of bones are the tarsals?**

_____

_____

_____

_____

6. **Why would a fracture at the epiphysis be important in a child or young adult?**

_____

_____

_____

_____

7. **What is an arthrogram? Arthroscopy?**

_____

_____

_____

_____

8. **Why would a bone scan be used in diagnosing osteoporosis?**

_____

_____

_____

_____

9. **Why would analgesics be ordered for arthritis?**

_____

_____

_____

_____

10. **What is arthralgia?**

_____

_____

_____

_____

11. **Why would vitamin D and calcium supplements be ordered for osteoporosis?**

_____

_____

_____

_____

12. **What are the dangers for Celia if the osteoporosis progresses?**

_____

_____

_____

_____

_____

APPLICATION OF SKILLS

1. Label the diagrams.

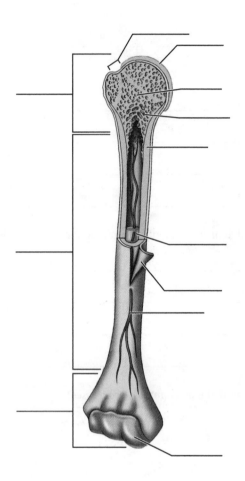

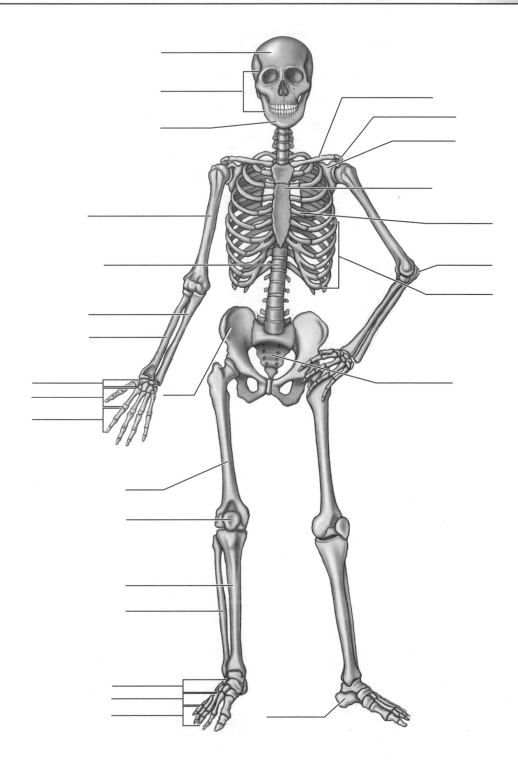

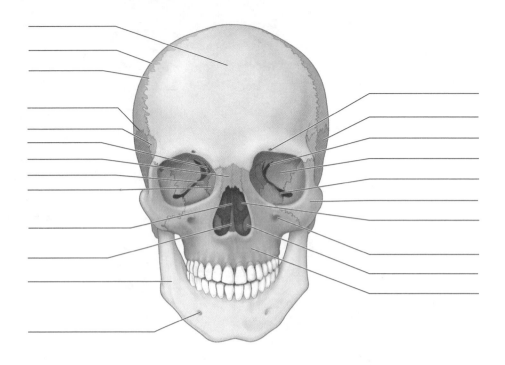

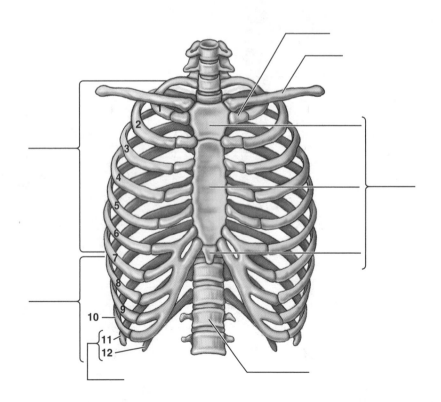

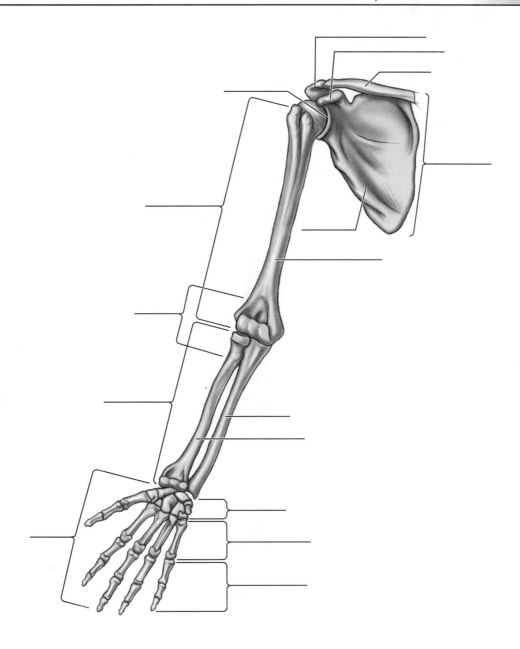

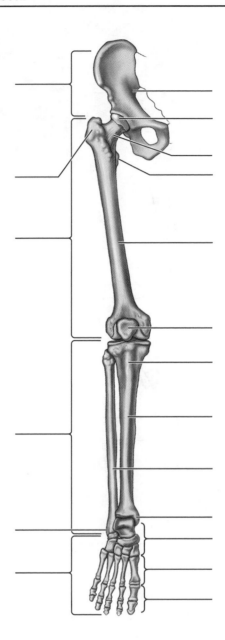

2. Using the classroom model of a human skeleton, identify each bone by sight.

CHAPTER QUIZ

Multiple Choice

Identify the letter of the choice that best completes the statement or answers the question.

1. _____ are bone-building cells.
   A. Osteoblasts
   B. Osteoclasts
   C. Osteocytes
   D. None of the above

2. The hormone that helps to maintain a proper level of calcium in the blood is _____.
   A. ADH
   B. LDH
   C. PTH
   D. none of the above

3. The _____ is the growth line for long bones in children.
   A. diaphysis
   B. epiphysis
   C. metaphysis
   D. paraphysis

4. The _____ vertebrae are the lower five verterbrae
   A. cervical
   B. thoracic
   C. lumbar
   D. sacral

5. The bone of the upper arm is called the _____.
   A. humerus
   B. radius
   C. femur
   D. ulna

6. The eight small bones of the wrist are called _____.
   A. tarsals
   B. metatarsals
   C. carpals
   D. metacarpals

7. A joint that allows flat surfaces to move across each other is a _____.
   A. hinge joint
   B. ball and socket
   C. condyloid joint
   D. gliding joint

8. _____ is motion that occurs when the extremity is moved away from the body.
   A. Abduction
   B. Adduction
   C. Flexion
   D. Circumduction

9. A fracture in which the bone protrudes through the skin is a(n) _____.
   A. open fracture
   B. closed fracture
   C. compound fracture
   D. greenstick fracture

10. When a bone breaks due to a twisting motion, it is called a _____.
    A. greenstick fracture
    B. spiral fracture
    C. compound fracture
    D. simple fracture

11. _____ is caused when more bone cells are destroyed than are made.
   A. Paget's disease
   B. Sarcoma
   C. Osteoarthritis
   D. Osteoporosis

12. _____ is the result of uric acid not being metabolized.
   A. Carpal tunnel syndrome
   B. Gouty arthritis
   C. Rheumatoid arthritis
   D. Ankylosis

13. A _____ is a depression or hollow space in a bone for attachments.
   A. foramen
   B. condyle
   C. fontanel
   D. fossa

14. A _____ is a narrow opening between parts of a bone that allows blood vessels or nerves to pass.
   A. fissure
   B. tuberosity
   C. foramen
   D. fossa

15. The medical term for "death of bone tissue" is _____.
   A. ostealgia
   B. osteonecrosis
   C. both A and B
   D. none of the above

16. The medical term for "swayback" is _____.
   A. lordosis
   B. kyphosis
   C. scoliosis
   D. necrophysis

17. _____ occurs when the spinal column in the lumbar and sacral area does not close properly.
   A. Paget's disease
   B. Gouty arthritis
   C. Rheumatoid arthritis
   D. Spina bifida

18. The combining form for "vertebrae" is _____.
   A. clavicul/o
   B. spin/o
   C. spondyl/o
   D. rachi/o

19. Antiarthritics relieve symptoms of _____.
    A. pain
    B. arthritis
    C. gout
    D. inflammation

20. A large, rounded knucklelike prominence that joins with another bone is called a _____.
    A. foramen
    B. fissure
    C. tuberosity
    D. condyle

CHAPTER SIXTEEN

Muscular System

VOCABULARY REVIEW:

Matching: Match each term with the correct definition.

A. adenosine triphosphate (ATP)

B. antagonistic

C. lactic acid

D. synergistic

E. tonus

F. fascia

G. Achilles tendon

H. aponeurosis

I. tendon

J. isometric

K. tetany

L. contractility

M. elasticity

N. insertion

O. origin

P. prime mover

Q. atrophy

R. cramps

S. electromyography

_____ 1. Enzyme in skeletal muscle that produces energy

_____ 2. Muscle anchored to a moving bone

_____ 3. Muscle tension increases, but the muscle does not shorten

_____ 4. Progressive weakness and atrophy of muscles

_____ 5. Fibrous sheath that covers, supports, and separates muscles

_____ 6. Twitching and cramping of a muscle due to low blood calcium

_____ 7. Painful muscle spasms

_____ 8. Strongest tendon in the body; attaches the calf muscle to the heel

_____ 9. Muscle that is responsible for movement when a group of muscles is contracting at the same time

_____ 10. Syndrome that causes chronic pain in the muscles and soft tissue surrounding the joints

_____ 11. Exerting an opposite action to that of another

_____ 12. Ability to shorten and thicken when stimulated.

_____ 13. Acting or working together

T. fibromyalgia

U. hernia

V. myalgia

W. myasthenia gravis

X. spasms

Y. sprain

Z. torticollis

_____ 14. White, cordlike structure that serves to connect muscle to bone

_____ 15. Ability of a muscle to return to its original length after stretching

_____ 16. Involuntary muscle twitches

_____ 17. When the intestines bulge through a weakness in a muscle wall

_____ 18. Slight tension in the muscle, which is always present, even at rest

_____ 19. Result of a shortened sternocleidomastoid muscle, causing the head and neck to tilt to one side

_____ 20. Wide, flat tendon that connects muscle to bone

_____ 21. Muscles anchored to nonmoving bones

_____ 22. Overstretching or tearing a ligament or joint

_____ 23. Waste product of muscle metabolism

_____ 24. Procedure that records the electrical activity of muscles

_____ 25. Wasting away of muscle tissues caused by nonuse over long periods of time

_____ 26. Muscle pain

THEORY RECALL

True/False

Indicate whether the sentence or statement is true or false.

_____ 1. The three main functions of muscles are to cause movement, provide support, and produce heat and energy.

_____ 2. Muscles arranged in synergistic pairs means that one muscle moves in one direction, and the antagonist causes movement in the opposite direction.

_____ 3. Chemical energy is used to make muscles contract.

_____ 4. Muscles are red because they contain myoglobin, and they have a rich blood supply.

_____ 5. The fixator is the muscle that is responsible for movement when a group of muscles are contracting at the same time.

Multiple Choice

Identify the letter of the choice that best completes the statement or answers the question.

1. The gluteus maximus is named for _____.
   A. origin/insertion
   B. size
   C. shape
   D. fiber direction

2. _____ move a bone away from the midline.
   A. Abductors
   B. Adductors
   C. Levators
   D. Flexors

3. _____ are ringlike muscles that close an opening.
   A. Abductors
   B. Flexors
   C. Sphincters
   D. Rotators

4. The muscles of mastication control the _____.
   A. eyelids
   B. mandible
   C. atlas
   D. vertebrae

5. Which one of the following is NOT an abdominal muscle?
   A. Lateral oblique
   B. External oblique
   C. Internal oblique
   D. Rectus abdominis

6. Stress-induced muscle tension can result in _____ and stiffness in the neck.
   A. sprain
   B. torticollis
   C. hernia
   D. myalgia

7. _____ is caused by a bacterium that enters the body through a deep open wound.
   A. Trichinosis
   B. Tetanus
   C. Torticollis
   D. Myalgia

8. The suffix that is means "weakness" is _____.
   A. -trophy
   B. -stenosis
   C. -asthenia
   D. -osis

9. The combining form for "muscle" is _____.
   A. fasci/o
   B. kines
   C. kinesi/o
   D. my/o

10. The abbreviation for nonsteroidal antiinflammatory drugs is _____.
    A. NSAIDs
    B. NADSs
    C. NSAIFs
    D. none of the above

11. The _____ is the smallest and deepest muscle of the buttocks.
    A. pectoralis minimus
    B. gluteus minimus
    C. adductor muscle
    D. internal oblique

12. The _____ is a fan-shaped muscle over the temporal bone.
    A. orbicularis oris
    B. zygomaticus
    C. masseter
    D. temporalis

13. The large muscle of the posterior neck and shoulder is called the _____.
    A. sternocleidomastoid
    B. frontalis
    C. trapezius
    D. external intercostals

14. The point of origin to insertion for the buccinator muscle is _____.
    A. temporal bone to mandible
    B. mandible and maxilla to skin around mouth
    C. cranial aponeurosis to eyebrows
    D. none of the above

15. The muscle that flexes the neck and rotates the head is called the _____.
    A. trapezius
    B. zygomaticus
    C. sternocleidomastoid
    D. internal intercostals

16. The point of origin to insertions for the biceps brachii is _____.
    A. clavicle and scapula to humerus
    B. ilium and lower vertebrae to femur
    C. vertebrae to humerus
    D. scapula to radius

17. The _____ forms muscle mass at the medial side of each thigh.
    A. rotator cuff
    B. gluteus maximus
    C. adductor muscles
    D. latissimus dorsi

18. The _____ dorsiflexes the foot.
    A. sartorius
    B. soleus
    C. iliopsoas
    D. tibialis anterior

19. A group of four muscles that form the fleshy mass of the anterior thigh is called _____.
    A. quadriceps femoris
    B. triceps brachii
    C. biceps femoris
    D. quadriceps femoris

20. The muscle that originates in the ischial tuberosity and inserts at the proximal tibia is called _____.
    A. sartorius
    B. hamstrings
    C. trapezius
    D. none of the above

21. _____ is a skeletal muscle relaxant.
    A. Mytelase
    B. Vicodin
    C. Flexeril
    D. Lodine

22. The medical term for "muscle pain" is _____.
    A. contusion
    B. myalgia
    C. myosis
    D. none of the above

23. _____ is a progressive weakening and atrophy of muscles.
    A. Myasthenia gravis
    B. Fibromyalgia
    C. Muscular dystrophy
    D. Tetany

24. Muscle _____ is an injury that involves overstretching or tearing of muscle fibers.
    A. strain
    B. sprain
    C. fracture
    D. all of the above

25. Which muscle is known as swimmer's muscle?
    A. Achilles tendon
    B. Sartorius
    C. Gastrocnemius
    D. Latissimus dorsi

Sentence Completion

Complete each sentence or statement.

1. _____ connect muscles to bone.

2. _____ is the skeletal muscle loss experienced by the aging population.

3. The _____ is known as the "praying muscle."

4. The medical term for the "kissing muscle" is _____.

5. _____ move a joint on its axis. The serratus anterior is an example.

6. The subclavius is an example of a(n) _____ muscle.

7. The _____ is the muscle of respiration.

8. The _____ are examples of muscle with three attachments.

9. _____ are muscles that help prime movers by stabilizing the movement.

10. _____ muscle is striated and involuntary.

Short Answers

1. State the three functions of muscles and explain the importance of each.

   _____

   _____

   _____

   _____

   _____

   _____

2. Explain the basic structure of muscle.

_____

_____

_____

_____

_____

3. Explain how a muscle contracts.

_____

_____

_____

4. List seven ways muscles can be named.

_____

_____

_____

_____

_____

_____

CRITICAL THINKING

1. Mrs. Greenbaum was given a prescription for an antiinflammatory for muscle pain in her back 6 months ago. However, she cannot remember the name of the medication, and her back is inflamed again and she would like the prescription refilled. What are five antiinflammatory medications that could have been Mrs. Greenbaum's prescription? (Reference the *Physicians' Desk Reference* as needed.)

2. Timothy injured his ankle playing hockey. The physician ordered a radiograph and determined the ankle was sprained. He applied a figure eight bandage and provided Timothy with a pair of crutches, instructing him to remain non–weight-bearing for 7 days. What other instructions would be given to a patient with a sprained ankle?

INTERNET RESEARCH

Keyword: (Use the name of the condition or disease you select to write about).

Select one condition or disease from Table 16-3 or another muscle-related condition or disease. Write a two-paragraph report regarding the condition or disease you selected, listing the etiology, signs and symptoms, diagnosis, therapy, and interventions. Cite your source. (You may not use the information on the tables exclusively for your report.) Be prepared to give a 2-minute oral presentation should your instructor assign you to do so.

WHAT WOULD YOU DO?

If you have accomplished the objectives in this chapter, you will be able to make better choices as a medical assistant. Take a look at this situation and decide what you would do.

Tommy has been playing sports for many years, since his childhood. He has used weights to increase and strengthen the muscles of his body. Tommy has often wondered just how the muscles of his body work to make him move and what happens when one muscle contracts. He knows that some muscles are involuntary and some are voluntary.

  This morning, Tommy was skiing and fell and twisted his ankle. The emergency physician told him that he had strained and sprained his ankle. In explanation, the physician also said that the extensors in the ankle had the greatest injury and the contusion was going to become worse if Tommy did not keep ice on the ankle overnight. Because of the severity of the injury, Tommy is to see an orthopedist in the morning. The orthopedist ordered antiinflammatory drugs and muscle relaxants.

  Tommy has some questions for the medical assistant about muscles, about what the antiinflammatory drugs will do, and about what this might have done to his muscles had he been older.

1. **How do muscles work to make the body move?**

   _____

   _____

   _____

2. **How do you define "synergistic muscles"?**

   _____

   _____

   _____

3. **How do you define "antagonistic muscles"?**

   _____

   _____

   _____

4. **What do voluntary muscles do in the body?**

_____

_____

_____

5. **Define "involuntary muscles."**

_____

_____

_____

6. **What is the difference between a sprain and a strain?**

_____

_____

_____

7. **What are the signs of a sprain?**

_____

_____

_____

8. **Why would antiinflammatory drugs and muscle relaxants be ordered?**

_____

_____

_____

9. **If Tommy were older, what would the physician expect the aging process to have done to his skeletal muscles?**

_____

_____

_____

10. **What are isotonic and isometric movements?**

_____

_____

_____

_____

_____

APPLICATION OF SKILLS

Label the diagrams.

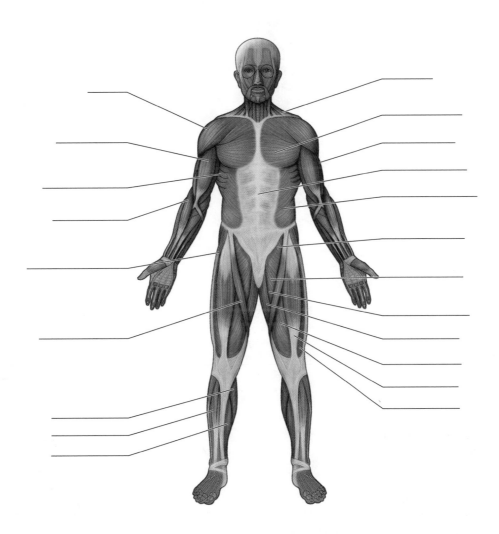

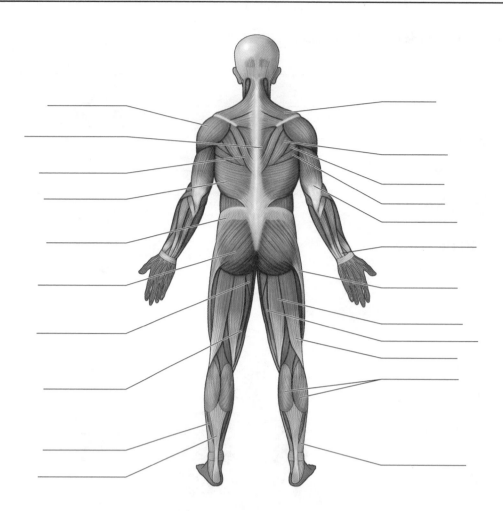

CHAPTER QUIZ

Multiple Choice

Identify the letter of the choice that best completes the statement or answers the question.

1. The enzyme in skeletal muscles that produce energy is _____.
   A. GH
   B. ATP
   C. ADH
   D. PTH

2. The strongest tendon in the body is the _____.
   A. Achilles tendon
   B. aponeurosis
   C. hamstrings
   D. none of the above

3. The medical term for "lacking muscle tone" is _____.
   A. atonic
   B. rigidity
   C. dystonic
   D. flaccid

4. Muscles that lower a bone are called _____.
   A. flexors
   B. depressors
   C. extensors
   D. fixators

5. Muscles that move a joint on its axis are called _____.
   A. extensors
   B. adductors
   C. rotators
   D. sphincters

6. The muscle of the shoulder shaped like an upside-down Greek letter D is _____.
   A. biceps
   B. iliopsoas
   C. deltoid
   D. pectoralis major

7. The wasting away of muscles caused by nonuse over long periods of time is called _____.
   A. atrophy
   B. dystrophy
   C. dystonic
   D. atonus

8. The medical term for "muscle and tendon inflammation" is _____.
   A. myalgia
   B. myosis
   C. atropy
   D. fibromyositis

9. Overstretching or tearing a ligament or joint is called _____.
   A. strain
   B. sprain
   C. myalgia
   D. dystrophy

10. The medical term for "wryneck" is _____.
    A. spasms
    B. cramps
    C. torticollis
    D. hernia

11. The _____ is a muscle located in the groin.
    A. latissimus dorsi
    B. quadriceps femoris
    C. semitendinosus
    D. iliopsoas

12. The _____ forms the curved calf of the leg.
    A. trapezius
    B. soleus
    C. buccinator
    D. masseter

13. The muscle that originates in the zygomatic arch and inserts to the mandible is the _____.
    A. frontalis
    B. sternocleidomastoid
    C. masseter
    D. orbicularis oculi

14. The muscle that closes the jaw is the _____.
    A. external intercostals
    B. temporalis
    C. zygomaticus
    D. frontalis

15. Muscle _____ cause involuntary muscle twitches.
    A. spasms
    B. cramps
    C. isotonic contractions
    D. none of the above

16. _____ is the procedure that records the electrical activity of muscles.
    A. EEG
    B. ECG
    C. EMG
    D. MRI

17. Skeletal muscles are described best by which one of the following?
    A. Striated and involuntary
    B. Smooth and involuntary
    C. Striated and voluntary
    D. Smooth and voluntary

18. _____ is the ability of a muscle to shorten and thicken when given proper stimulation.
    A. Irritability
    B. Contractility
    C. Elasticity
    D. Extensibility

19. _____ are specialized synergists that stabilize the origin of a prime mover.
    A. Rotators
    B. Extensors
    C. Levators
    D. Fixators

20. Triceps brachii are an example of _____ muscles.
    A. abductor
    B. levator
    C. extensor
    D. depressor

CHAPTER **SEVENTEEN**

Urinary System

VOCABULARY REVIEW

Matching: Match each term with the correct definition.

A. erythropoietin

B. uremia

C. antidiuretic hormone

D. filtration

E. kidney

F. nephron

G. retroperitoneal

H. urine

I. ureters

J. micturition

K. urinary bladder

L. urethral meatus

M. urethra

N. albuminuria

O. bacteriuria

P. incontinence

Q. blood urea nitrogen (BUN)

R. cystoscopy

S. intravenous pyelography

_____ 1. Inability to retain urine or feces

_____ 2. Hollow muscular sac that holds urine before it is excreted from the body

_____ 3. Process where substances are filtered out

_____ 4. Occurs when toxins accumulate in the blood

_____ 5. Progressive loss of nephrons, resulting in loss of renal function

_____ 6. Urethral opening to the outside of the body

_____ 7. Main functioning unit of the kidney

_____ 8. Measures the amount of nitrogenous waste in the circulatory system

_____ 9. Artificial kidney machine filters the patient's blood and returns the filtered blood back to the patient

_____ 10. Hormone responsible for reducing urine production

_____ 11. Bacteria in urine

_____ 12. Main organ of the urinary system

_____ 13. Medication that causes increased urine excretion

_____ 14. Hormone responsible for red blood cell production

T. KUB (kidney, ureters, and bladder)

U. urinalysis

V. acute renal failure (ARF)

W. dialysis

X. diuretics

Y. hemodialysis

Z. renal failure

_____ 15. Transports urine from the bladder to the outside of the body

_____ 16. Visual examination of the urinary bladder using a cystoscope

_____ 17. Located behind

_____ 18. Pair of muscular tubes that carry urine from the kidneys to the bladders

_____ 19. Renal failure occurring suddenly due to trauma

_____ 20. Presence of large amounts of protein in urine; usually sign of renal disease or heart failure

_____ 21. Process used to clean the blood of toxins

_____ 22. Imaging of the kidneys, ureters, and bladder without a contrast medium

_____ 23. Liquid and dissolved substances excreted by the kidneys

_____ 24. Physical, chemical, and/or microscopic examination of the urine

_____ 25. Urination

_____ 26. Imaging of the kidneys, ureters, and bladder with a contrast medium

THEORY RECALL

True/False

Indicate whether the sentence or statement is true or false.

_____ 1. Reabsorption retains essential elements the body needs to maintain pH and homeostasis.

_____ 2. The ureters extend from the bladder to the outside of the body.

_____ 3. The adrenal glands release the hormone aldosterone.

_____ 4. The cortex is the inner layer of the kidney.

_____ 5. The glomerulus is a group of capillaries responsible for filtering the blood.

Multiple Choice

Identify the letter of the choice that best completes the statement or answers the question.

1. The hormone responsible for blood pressure control is called _____.
   A. azotemia
   B. erythropoietin
   C. renin
   D. ADH

2. Cuplike edges of the renal pelvis that collect urine are called _____.
   A. Bowman's capsule
   B. calyces
   C. nephrons
   D. rugae

3. _____ is the backflow of urine from the bladder up into the ureters.
   A. Urinary reflux
   B. Micturition reflex
   C. Urination
   D. Filtration

4. _____ is a condition of having no urine production or output.
   A. Micturition
   B. Enuresis
   C. Anuresis
   D. Dysuria

5. _____ is the medical term for "excessive urination at night."
   A. Oliguria
   B. Polydipsia
   C. Ketonuria
   D. Nocturia

6. _____ occurs when a donor kidney is surgically placed in patients to function as their own.
   A. Incontinence
   B. Kidney transplant
   C. Peritoneal dialysis
   D. Hemodialysis

7. The combining form for "bladder" is _____.
   A. ureter/o
   B. vesic/o
   C. glomerul/o
   D. cyst/o

8. _____ are used as a genitourinary muscle relaxant.
   A. Diuretics
   B. Antispasmodics
   C. Analgesics
   D. Antihypertensives

9. _____ is a diuretic that increases urination.
   A. Lasix
   B. Macrobid
   C. Gantrisin
   D. Pyridium

10. In the process of urine formation, _____ is the step where wastes are eliminated into the collection duct in the form of urine.
    A. filtration
    B. reabsorption
    C. secretion of toxins
    D. excretion

11. _____ is increased urine production.
    A. Enuresis
    B. Dysuria
    C. Diuresis
    D. Oliguria

12. _____ is the medical term for "pus in the urine."
    A. Dysuria
    B. Pyuria
    C. Enuresis
    D. Polyuria

13. _____ is an abnormal presence of glucose in the urine.
    A. Albuminuria
    B. Oliguria
    C. Anuresis
    D. Glycosuria

14. Which of the following laboratory tests measures the amount of nitrogenous waste in the circulatory system?
    A. BUN
    B. KUB
    C. UA
    D. IVP

15. A(n) _____ is an imaging of the kidneys, ureters, and bladder with contrast media.
    A. KUB
    B. IVP
    C. BUN
    D. UA

16. The normal value for specific gravity of urine is which one of the following?
    A. 0.10 to 0.12
    B. 0.00 to 0.10
    C. 1.10 to 1.25
    D. 0.05 to 1.10

17. The medical term for "kidney stones" is _____.
    A. Cholelithiasis
    B. Cystolithiasis
    C. Pelvic calculi
    D. Renal calculi

18. Inflammation of the renal pelvis to include the connective tissue of the kidneys is called _____.
    A. glomerulonephritis
    B. pyelonephritis
    C. renalonephritis
    D. cystonephritis

19. _____ is an analgesic that produces an anesthetic effect on the lining of the urinary tract.
    A. Pyridium
    B. Lasix
    C. Macrobid
    D. Gantrisin

20. The combining form for "urea"; nitrogen is _____.
    A. vesic/o
    B. ure/o
    C. azot/o
    D. none of the above

21. Which one of the following is NOT a function of the kidneys?
    A. Filtration
    B. Reabsorption
    C. Excretion
    D. To produce leukocytes and secrete nitrites

22. Your blood passes through your kidneys approximately _____ times a day.
    A. 100
    B. 200
    C. 300
    D. 400

23. Because of the _____ in urine, some people tend to form kidney stones.
    A. solutes
    B. crystals
    C. leukocytes
    D. water

24. The part of the collection system where sodium is mainly reabsorbed is the _____.
    A. Bowman's capsule
    B. loop of Henle
    C. calyces
    D. distal convoluted tubule

25. Each kidney consists of approximately _____ nephrons.
    A. 1 million
    B. 100,000
    C. 3 million
    D. 300,000

Sentence Completion

Complete each sentence or statement.

1. The C-shaped structure that surrounds the glomerulus is the called the _____.

2. _____ can be performed with minimal equipment and in the patient's home. The procedure takes approximately 30 minutes and is done four times a day, 7 days a week.

3. _____ is an inflammation of the glomeruli.

4. _____ can be performed to remove calculi.

5. Blood enters the kidney through the _____.

6. _____ force urine into the bladder with the movements of their muscular walls.

7. The two kidneys are located _____ in the lumbar area of the spine.

8. The _____ is the urethral opening to the outside of the body.

9. The depression on the medial side of each kidney where the blood vessels, ureters, and nerves enter and exit the kidney is called the _____.

10. The main functioning units of the kidney are the _____.

Short Answers

1. State the five major functions of the urinary system.

_____

_____

_____

_____

_____

2. Explain the purpose of urine and describe urine formation.

_____

_____

_____

3. List 13 common signs and symptoms of urinary system disorders.

_____

_____

_____

_____

_____

_____

_____

4. Explain the purpose of dialysis and list two types.

_____

_____

_____

_____

CRITICAL THINKING

1. Samuel, a 27-year-old male patient, is complaining that it is painful to urinate, that he has to "go" all the time, and he cannot seem to control it; even during the night, he wakes up to go to the bathroom three or four times a night. He also has pain directly above the pubic bone. The physician orders a complete UA and a culture and sensitivity. You have the patient collect a urine sample and take it to the laboratory to perform the UA. Samuel's urine is cloudy, and on dipstick examination, you find the leukocytes and nitrites are increased. The microscopic examination confirmed the increase.

   What do you think the physician's diagnosis will be? What is the medical term for "having to go all the time, painful urination, and excessive urination at night"? What will be the most likely course of therapy? What should you, as the medical assistant, encourage the patient to do?

2. Obtain brochures from the kidney center or dialysis center in your area. (You may research on the Internet or the school's resource library if a center is not available in your area.) If a center is not available in your area, locate the closest facilities. Determine the services provided by the center, hours of operation, and location. This information will be beneficial when required to provide patients with the same or similar information.

INTERNET RESEARCH

Keyword: (Use the name of the condition or disease you select to write about).

Select one condition or disease from Table 17-3 or other urinary system–related condition or disease. Write a two-paragraph report regarding the condition or disease you selected, listing the etiology, signs and symptoms, diagnosis, therapy, and interventions. Cite your source. (You may not use the information on the tables exclusively for your report.) Be prepared to give a 2-minute oral presentation should your instructor assign you to do so.

WHAT WOULD YOU DO?

If you have accomplished the objectives in this chapter, you will be able to make better choices as a medical assistant. Take a look at this situation and decide what you would do.

Juanita is a regular patient in the medical office and has been in good health most of her life. At her office visit, she is complaining of pain in the flanks, in her thighs, in her lower abdomen, and in her back under her ribs. She also says that she has had burning and frequency of urination that has become progressively worse for about 2 weeks. Furthermore, she says when she has to go to the bathroom, she has to hurry or she will not make it. The burning is not on the perineum but occurs as she starts the flow of urine. These symptoms have only made her incontinence worse, and she now has nocturia. When asked if she can pinpoint anything new in her routine hygiene, she states that she has recently been using a perfumed soap on a regular basis to take her bath. On obtaining a urinalysis, hematuria is present. In addition, white blood cells are found on microscopic examination. The physician has prescribed medications for treating what he has diagnosed as urinary cystitis. Juanita would like to talk to the medical assistant to ask some questions

1. **Why do women have inflammation of the urinary tract more often than males?**

    _____

    _____

    _____

2. **What is hematuria? What is pyuria?**

    _____

    _____

    _____

3. **Would you expect Juanita to have pyuria because she has hematuria?**

    _____

    _____

    _____

4. **What is incontinence?**

_____

_____

_____

5. **What is the difference between incontinence and enuresis?**

_____

_____

_____

_____

6. **What is the name of the symptom that is used to describe feeling the need to urinate immediately?**

_____

7. **Why are urinary antiseptics used in treating urinary cystitis after antiinfective drugs have been prescribed?**

_____

_____

8. **What is urinary frequency?**

_____

_____

9. **What is nocturia?**

_____

_____

APPLICATION OF SKILLS

Label the diagrams.

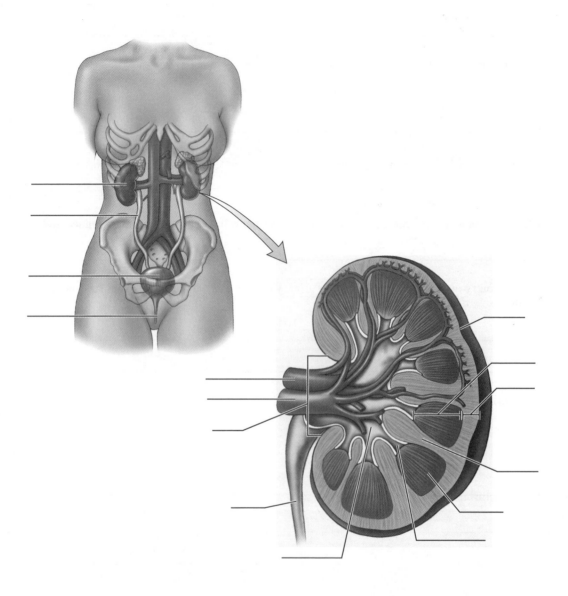

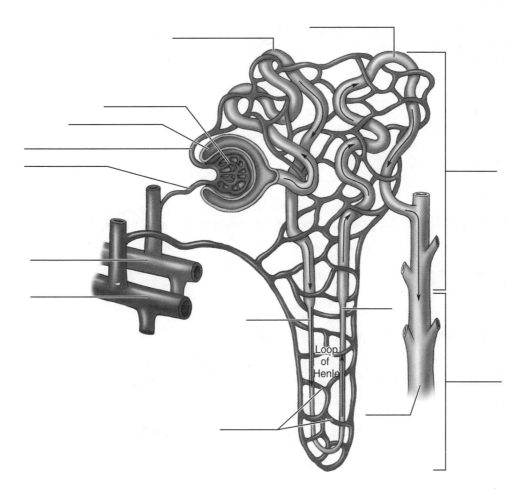

Loop
of
Henle

CHAPTER QUIZ

Multiple Choice

Identify the letter of the choice that best completes the statement or answers the question.

1. The medical term for "kidney stones" is _____.
   A. peritoneal calcui
   B. cystolithiasis
   C. renal calculi
   D. renolithiasis

2. The main functioning units of the kidneys are _____.
   A. ureters
   B. Bowman's capsules
   C. pyramids
   D. none of the above

3. The outer layer of the kidneys is called the _____.
   A. pyramid
   B. cortex
   C. medulla
   D. calyces

4. _____ is the hormone responsible for increased sodium reabsorption.
   A. Erythropoietin
   B. Aldosterone
   C. Antidiuretic hormone
   D. Renin

5. _____ occurs when toxins accumulate in the blood.
   A. Erythropoietin
   B. Bacteriuria
   C. Uremia
   D. Anuresis

6. The depression where blood vessels, nerves, and the ureters enter and exit the kidney is called the
   _____.
   A. hilum
   B. loop of Henle
   C. Bowman's capsule
   D. medulla

7. _____ are muscular folds that allow the bladder to expand.
   A. Calyces
   B. Rugae
   C. Pyramids
   D. Trigone

8. The _____ transports urine from the bladder to the outside of the body.
   A. ureters
   B. nephrons
   C. urethra
   D. glomeruli

9. _____ is painful or difficult urination.
   A. Anuresis
   B. Oliguria
   C. Enuresis
   D. Dysuria

10. An increase in the number of times urination occurs over a short period of time is called _____.
    A. urgency
    B. frequency
    C. immediacy
    D. none of the above

11. _____ are medications that increase urine excretion.
    A. Antispasmodics
    B. Analgesics
    C. Diuretics
    D. Pyuretics

12. _____ is the progressive loss of nephrons, resulting in loss of renal function.
    A. Renal failure
    B. Glomerulonephritis
    C. Cystitis
    D. Hematuria

13. The normal pH of urine is _____.
    A. 4.5
    B. 5.0
    C. 6.5
    D. 7.0

14. The main function of the kidneys is to filter _____ and other waste products from the blood.
    A. sodium
    B. urea
    C. glucose
    D. nutrients

15. The average daily production of urine is _____.
    A. 1 to 1.5 liters
    B. 1.5 to 2.5 liters
    C. 2 to 3 liters
    D. none of the above

16. _____ is an enzyme that reacts with a blood protein to form a substance that stimulates the adrenal gland to secrete aldosterone.
    A. Lipase
    B. Glucose
    C. Vitamin C
    D. Renin

17. The _____ narrow(s) to form the ureters, which empties into the bladder.
    A. renal pelvis
    B. hilum
    C. medulla
    D. pyramids

18. When urine flows from the bladder back into the ureters, this is known as urinary _____.
    A. regurgitation
    B. incontinence
    C. micturation
    D. reflux

19. A(n) _____ treats diseases and disorders of the urinary system.
    A. gynecologist
    B. endocrinologist
    C. urologist
    D. bacteriologist

20. Inflammation of the renal pelvis to include the connective tissue of the kidneys is called _____.
    A. pyelonephritis
    B. cystonephritis
    C. glomerulonephritis
    D. renalonephritis

CHAPTER EIGHTEEN

Reproductive System

VOCABULARY REVIEW

Matching: Match each term with the correct definition.

A. gametes

B. gonads

C. circumcision

D. insemination

E. prostate gland

F. spermatozoa

G. testosterone

H. areola

I. endometrium

J. estrogen

K. infertility

L. lactiferous ducts

M. mammary glands

N. perimetrium

O. follicle-stimulating hormone

P. human chorionic gonadotropin

Q. mammogram

R. menses

S. Papanicolaou (Pap) smear

_____ 1. Stage from the second week to the eighth week of gestation

_____ 2. Sperm cells

_____ 3. Radiographs of the breast

_____ 4. Reproductive cells; eggs and sperm

_____ 5. Process of expulsion of the fetus; child-birth

_____ 6. Gland that produces an alkaline fluid that neutralizes the acidity of the urethra and of the vaginal secretions

_____ 7. Joining of the egg and the sperm

_____ 8. Surgical removal of the prepuce

_____ 9. Hormone responsible for male sex characteristics

_____ 10. Surrounds the nipple; dark-colored skin

_____ 11. Cells scraped off the cervix are examined under a microscope for malignancy

_____ 12. Before birth

_____ 13. Inability to become pregnant

_____ 14. Monthly bloody discharge from the lining of the uterus

_____ 15. Sex glands; ovaries and testes

T. embryo

U. fertilization

V. parturition

W. prenatal

X. zygote

Y. gestational diabetes

Z. toxemia

_____ 16. Toxic condition in pregnancy that produces high blood pressure and decreased kidney function

_____ 17. Introduction of semen into the female

_____ 18. Hormone produced during pregnancy; responsible for the release of progesterone and estrogen to maintain the endometrium

_____ 19. Serous layer of the uterus

_____ 20. Fertilized egg; contains all the genetic material

_____ 21. Hormone that causes the egg to ripen in the Graafian follicle

_____ 22. Ducts that transport milk to each nipple

_____ 23. Inner lining of the uterus; holds the fertilized egg; vascular layer

_____ 24. Glands located within the breasts that are responsible for producing milk

_____ 25. Occurs when a pregnant woman is unable to metabolize carbohydrates; develops during the latter part of pregnancy and usually terminates with delivery

_____ 26. Hormone that prepares the uterus for the implantation of the fertilized egg and promotes female sex characteristics

THEORY RECALL

True/False

Indicate whether the sentence or statement is true or false.

_____ 1. The two main functions of the reproductive system are to produce offspring and to produce hormones.

_____ 2. Sperm mature and are stored in the epididymis.

_____ 3. Infertility is the inability to have or sustain an erection during sexual intercourse.

_____ 4. Progesterone is responsible for the development of both primary and secondary sex characteristics in females.

_____ 5. A typical menstrual cycle lasts 28 days.

Multiple Choice

Identify the letter of the choice that best completes the statement or answers the question.

1. A gland that produces a fluid that acts as a lubricant is called _____.
   A. Cowper's gland
   B. epididymis
   C. glans penis
   D. Graafian follicle

2. The _____ is a thick muscular layer of the uterus.
   A. endometrium
   B. myometrium
   C. perimetrium
   D. none of the above

3. The _____ is(are) where sperm are formed within the testes.
   A. prostate gland
   B. vas deferens
   C. epididymis
   D. seminiferous tubules

4. The male gonads is(are) called (the) _____.
   A. penis
   B. scrotum
   C. spermatozoa
   D. testes

5. The female gonads is(are) called _____ .
   A. uterus
   B. ovaries
   C. fallopian tubes
   D. Graafian follicles

6. The area between the vagina and the anus is called the _____.
   A. cervix
   B. perimetrium
   C. perineum
   D. areola

7. A combination of physical and emotional symptoms that appear prior to the start of the menstrual flow and stop with its onset is _____.
   A. menopause
   B. menses
   C. toxic shock syndrome
   D. premenstrual syndrome

8. _____ is a hormone that allows for milk expulsion and the onset of labor.
   A. Oxytocin
   B. Progesterone
   C. Prolactin
   D. Testosterone

9. The muscular area located between the cervix and the vulva is called the _____.
   A. perineum
   B. vagina
   C. uterus
   D. fallopian tube

10. The _____ is a tube leading from the bladder through the penis via which semen is ejaculated.
   A. seminal vesicles
   B. seminiferous tubules
   C. ureter
   D. urethra

11. The organ that provides nourishment and oxygen to the fetus during pregnancy is called the _____.
   A. uterus
   B. placenta
   C. umbilical cord
   D. cervix

12. Sperm are produced at a rate of _____ per day.
   A. 100,000
   B. 500,000
   C. 300 million
   D. 500 million

13. Primary sex characteristics in a male include all of the following EXCEPT _____.
   A. growth of pubic, facial, and underarm hair
   B. growth of the penis and scrotum
   C. growth and activity of internal reproductive structures
   D. all of the above are primary sex characteristics

14. The _____ produce(s) a mucuslike fluid that provides nutrition and energy for the mobile sperm. This fluid accounts for 60% of the semen volume.
   A. epididymis
   B. seminiferous tubules
   C. seminal vesicles
   D. vas deferens

15. A human gestation period is usually _____ from the time of fertilization.
   A. 266 days
   B. 4 weeks
   C. three trimesters
   D. all of the above

16. An Apgar score of less than _____ indicates a newborn needs medical attention.
   A. 2
   B. 5
   C. 7
   D. 9

17. Proscar is an example of a(n) _____.
    A. HRT
    B. contraceptive
    C. ovulation stimulant
    D. treatment for menopause

18. The name of the blood test for prostatic hypertrophy is _____.
    A. VDRL
    B. PSA
    C. FTA
    D. ABS

19. A painless lump in the testicle may indicate which one of the following?
    A. Prostatitis
    B. Prostatic cancer
    C. Testicular cancer
    D. Epididymis

20. Which one of the following conditions can be caused by a bacterial infection?
    A. Benign prostatic hyperplasia
    B. Testicular cancer
    C. Endometriosis
    D. None of the above

21. A _____ is an imaging procedure that uses contrast media to visualize the uterus and fallopian tubes.
    A. Hysterosalpingography
    B. Mammography
    C. Colposcopy
    D. Cervicography

22. An imagining procedure using high-frequency sound waves to view the pelvic area is _____.
    A. colposcopy
    B. ultrasonography
    C. mammography
    D. cervicography

23. _____ is the displacement of the uterus into the vagina.
    A. Candidiasis
    B. Fibrocystic disease of the uterus
    C. Prolapsed uterus
    D. Toxic shock syndrome

24. _____ is(are) fluid-filled sacs that form on or near the ovaries.
    A. Ovarian cysts
    B. Endometriosis
    C. Fibroids
    D. None of the above

25. _____ is the premature separation of the placenta from the uterine wall, either partially or completely.
    A. Toxemia
    B. Ectopic pregnancy
    C. Placenta previa
    D. Placenta abruptio

Sentence Completion

Complete each sentence or statement.

1. _____ occurs when one or both testes do not descend and remain in the abdomen.

2. Circumcision is a procedure that removes the fold of skin at the end of the penis called the

   _____.

3. At ovulation, the egg is expelled from the _____ and is swept into the fallopian tube.

4. The _____ is known as the neck of the uterus.

5. _____ transport milk to the nipple.

6. The embryo reaches the uterus, around the _____ day.

7. Movement of the fetus occurs around the _____ month.

8. One minute after birth, a newborn is evaluated using a system called a(n) _____.

9. _____ occurs when the fertilized egg implants outside the uterus, usually in the fallopian

   tubes.

10. _____ is a sexually transmitted disease with symptoms that include purulent vaginal

   discharge, genital pain, and dysuria.

Short Answers

1. Trace the pathway that sperm follow through the five major structures of the male reproductive system, beginning with the testes and ending with the urethra.

2. Explain the purpose of semen.

3. List, identify, and describe the seven parts of the female reproductive system.

4. Explain the purpose of dialysis, and list two types.

CRITICAL THINKING

1. A newborn at 1 minute after birth presents with a heart rate below 100, respiratory rate that is slow and irregular, muscle tone that is limp, reflex of grimace, and pale in color. What is the infant's Apgar score? At 3 minutes, the heart rate was over 100, the respiratory rate was slow and irregular, muscle tone showed reflex of extremities, reflex withdrew foot, and his body was pink, but the extremities were blue. What is the infant's 3-minute score?

2. Kelly is a 22-year-old female patient. Kelly started menstruation at the age of 14 and has been sexually active for the past 3 years. She is being seen today with a chief complaint of vaginal itching. Upon examination the physician detects a foul-smelling, green frothy discharge, and after receiving laboratory test results, he diagnosis the condition as *Trichomonas* and prescribes an antibiotic. The physician asks you to talk with Kelly about her sexual partners, because this condition requires that all sexual partners be treated with an antibiotic. Left untreated, this condition can lead to sterility. The physician would also like for you to discuss safe sex practices and contraception with Kelly.
   Use your text, your institution's resource reference library, and/or the internet to address this issue as needed.

INTERNET RESEARCH

Keyword: (Use the name of the condition or disease you select to write about).

Select one condition or disease from Table 18-2, 18-4, 18-5, or 18-6 or other related condition or disease. Write a two-paragraph report regarding the condition or disease you selected, listing the etiology, signs and symptoms, diagnosis, therapy, and interventions. Cite your source. (You may not use the information on the tables exclusively for your report.) Be prepared to give a 2-minute oral presentation should your instructor assign you to do so.

WHAT WOULD YOU DO?

If you have accomplished the objectives in this chapter, you will be able to make better choices as a medical assistant. Take a look at this situation and decide what you would do.

Valerie has called her gynecologist for her annual Pap smear. The receptionist wanted to be sure that Valerie did not make her appointment during the time of her menses. Her menarche was at age 14. She has taken oral contraceptives in the past. She is now approaching age 50 and has excessive bleeding with each menstrual period. Her LMP was a week ago, and she is to have the Pap smear with her physical examination today. The medical assistant asks Valerie if she performs monthly BSEs. Dr. Jones started ordering a mammogram for Valerie on a yearly basis at age 35 because of a family history of fibrocystic disease of the breasts. Valerie asks Dr. Jones about taking HRT, because she seems to be approaching menopause and has PMS with each menstrual period. Dr. Jones replies that she will discuss this with Valerie after the Pap smear report has been returned. Do you understand why the various aspects of Valerie's appointment were handled the way they were?

1. **Why is it important that Valerie not make her appointment for her Pap smear during the time of menses?**

   _____

   _____

   _____

2. **What are the five stages of the menstrual cycle?**

_____

_____

_____

_____

3. **What is menarche? Are menstrual periods regular immediately following menarche?**

_____

_____

_____

4. **What is HRT? What classifications of medications are given for HRT? For oral contraception?**

_____

_____

_____

_____

_____

_____

5. **What is a BSE, and why is this important to be done approximately 1 week after menses?**

_____

_____

_____

_____

6. **What is fibrocystic disease of the breast? Why are mammograms and BSEs important for someone with this condition?**

_____

_____

_____

7. What is PMS?

_____

_____

8. What are the signs of menopause?

_____

_____

_____

_____

APPLICATION OF SKILLS

1. Label the diagrams.

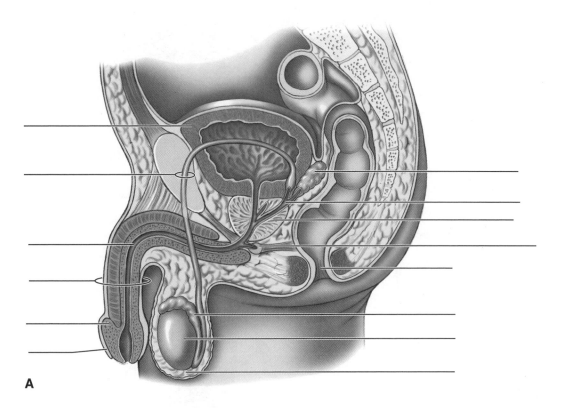

A

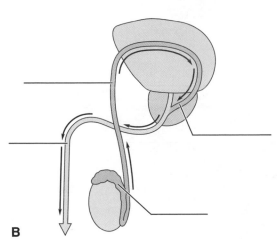

B

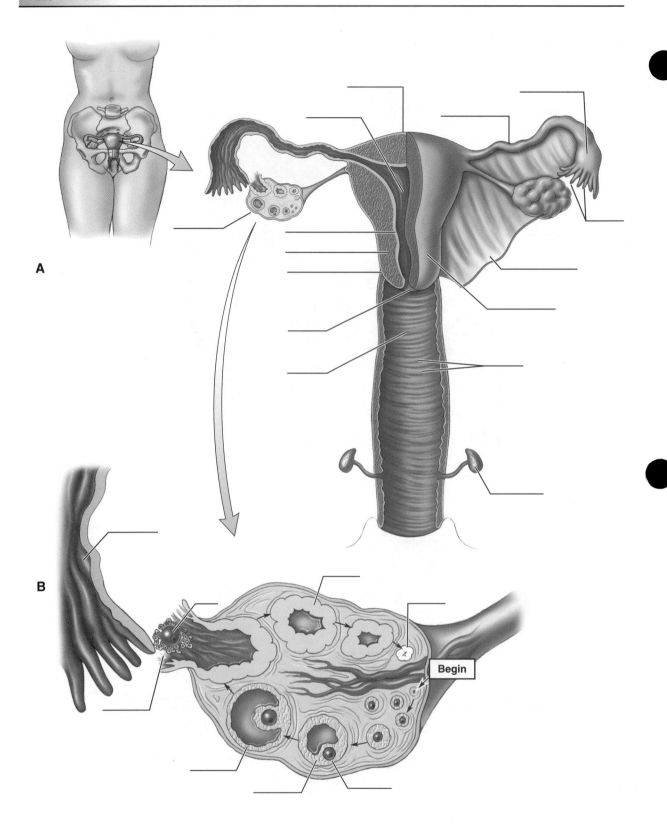

A

B

2. Define the following abbreviations.
   - BPH _____
   - GU _____
   - TUR _____
   - BCP _____
   - BSE _____
   - D&C _____
   - FBD _____
   - FSH _____
   - GYN _____
   - HRT _____
   - IUD _____
   - LH _____
   - LMP _____
   - OB _____
   - PMS _____
   - GC _____
   - PID _____
   - STD _____
   - VDRL _____

CHAPTER QUIZ

Multiple Choice

Identify the letter of the choice that best completes the statement or answers the question.

1. _____ are reproductive cells—eggs and sperm.
   A. Ovaries
   B. Testes
   C. Gonads
   D. Gametes

2. The _____ is where seminal vesicles and the vas deferens come together.
   A. seminiferous tubules
   B. bulbourethral gland
   C. ejaculatory duct
   D. urethra

3. The _____ is the organ that receives the egg.
   A. vagina
   B. uterus
   C. fallopian tube
   D. Graafian follicle

4. _____ is the hormone that prepares the uterus for the implantation of the fertilized egg and promotes female sex characteristics.
   A. Estrogen
   B. Testosterone
   C. Progesterone
   D. Oxytocin

5. The _____ connect(s) the ovaries to the uterus.
   A. ureters
   B. fallopian tubes
   C. Graafian follicles
   D. perineum

6. _____ occurs when the attachment of the placenta implants in the lower portion of the uterus and partially or completely covers the cervix.
   A. Ectopic pregnancy
   B. Placenta abruptio
   C. Placenta previa
   D. Endometriosis

7. The serous layer of the uterus is the called the _____.
   A. perimetrium
   B. endometrium
   C. myometrium
   D. osometrium

8. _____ is a fungal yeast infection of the vagina.
   A. *Trichomonas*
   B. Syphilis
   C. Human papilloma virus
   D. Candidiasis

9. The muscular area located between the cervix and vulva is called the _____.
   A. labia majora
   B. vagina
   C. uterus
   D. perineum

10. _____ is the medical term for "undescended or hidden testes."
    A. Epididymis
    B. Prostatitis
    C. Cryptorchidism
    D. None of the above

11. The hormone responsible for the stimulation of milk production is _____.
    A. estrogen
    B. oxytocin
    C. progesterone
    D. prolactin

12. _____ is the cessation of the menstrual cycle.
    A. Menarche
    B. Menses
    C. Menstruation
    D. Menopause

13. The hormone that increases during pregnancy and provides for pregnancy test results is _____.
    A. estrogen
    B. human chorionic gonadotropin
    C. testosterone
    D. prolactin

14. The hormone that releases progesterone and estrogen to thicken the uterine wall for pregnancy is the
    _____.
    A. corpus luteum
    B. luteinizing hormone
    C. Graafian follicle
    D. human chorionic gonadotropin

15. The _____ is where sperm is stored.
    A. vas deferens
    B. seminal vesicles
    C. scrotum
    D. epididymis

16. Gestation including the beginning day of the LMP is _____.
    A. 266 days
    B. 280 days
    C. 324 days
    D. none of the above

17. When fertilization occurs, the fusion of the sperm and egg forms a(n) _____.
    A. zygote
    B. fetus
    C. embryo
    D. infant

18. During parturition, crowning occurs and the fetus is expelled in stage _____.
    A. One
    B. Two
    C. Three
    D. Four

19. An Apgar score of less than _____ indicates a newborn needs medical attention.
    A. 9
    B. 8.5
    C. 8
    D. 7

20. The abbreviation of an intrauterine device for contraception is _____.
    A. CVD
    B. DUI
    C. IUD
    D. PID

CHAPTER NINETEEN

Endocrine System

VOCABULARY REVIEW

Matching: Match each term with the correct definition.

A. endocrine gland

B. exocrine gland

C. hormone

D. target organ

E. sella turcica

F. calcium tetany

G. adrenal cortex

H. steroid

I. adrenal medulla

J. islet of Langerhans

K. feedback

L. endocrinologist

M. anorexia

N. goiter

O. fasting blood sugar (FBS)

P. glucose tolerance test (GTT)

Q. hormone level test

R. radioactive iodine (RAI) uptake scan

S. thyroid function tests (TFTs)

_____ 1. Occurs when insufficient ADH is released from the posterior pituitary

_____ 2. Pancreas cells that produce the hormone insulin and cause secretion of the hormone glucagon

_____ 3. Blood test that indicates the amount of glucose present after a period of fasting

_____ 4. Main disease of the insulin-producing pancreas

_____ 5. Glands whose secretion reaches the epithelial surface, usually through a duct

_____ 6. Blood test measuring the body's ability to break down glucose

_____ 7. Specialist who treats diseases resulting from dysfunction of the endocrine system

_____ 8. Underproduction of thyroid glands in childhood causing a low metabolic rate, slow growth, and mental retardation

_____ 9. Secretes epinephrine and norepinephrine

_____ 10. Glands that secrete through a duct

_____ 11. Continuous muscle spasms caused by an abnormal level of calcium in the blood

_____ 12. Process that allows the body to stay in homeostasis

T. acromegaly

U. diabetes insipidus

V. cretinism

W. Graves disease

X. Addison disease

Y. diabetes mellitus

_____ 13. Lack of appetite

_____ 14. Organic compound derived from fats

_____ 15. Blood test measuring the amounts of ADH, cortisol, growth, and parathyroid hormones

_____ 16. Internal secretion by a gland or an organ that serves to regulate a body function

_____ 17. Results in adults when there is an over-production of thyroid hormone

_____ 18. Enlargement of thyroid gland not due to a tumor

_____ 19. Outer portion of the adrenal gland that secretes steroids

_____ 20. Contains receptors that cause it to react to certain hormones

_____ 21. Results from a deficiency of adrenocor-tical hormones

_____ 22. Blood test assessing T_3, T_4, and calcitonin

_____ 23. Depression in the sphenoid bone in the cranial cavity; holds the pituitary gland

_____ 24. Occurs in an adult when an excessive amount of growth hormone is secreted

_____ 25. Detects the thyroid's ability to concentrate and retain iodine

THEORY RECALL

True/False

Indicate whether the sentence or statement is true or false.

_____ 1. Hormones are secreted directly into the bloodsteam by glands that are referred to as ductless glands.

_____ 2. Sweat glands, sebaceous glands, and mammary glands are all part of the endocrine system.

_____ 3. The pineal gland is approximately the size of a pea and is held in the sella turcica.

_____ 4. Mineralocorticoids control sodium, potassium, and water balance, mainly through action on the kidneys.

_____ 5. The thyroid secretes five hormones.

Multiple Choice

Identify the letter of the choice that best completes the statement or answers the question.

1. The hormone responsible for contractions of the uterus during labor is _____.
   A. oxytocin
   B. ADH
   C. HCG
   D. aldosterone

2. The gland located in the neck on both sides of the trachea and larynx is _____.
   A. pituitary
   B. pineal
   C. thyroid
   D. none of the above

3. The gland located above the kidneys that help to control the body's metabolic rate is _____.
   A. prostate gland
   B. thymus
   C. pineal
   D. adrenal

4. The hormone _____ is secreted by the thymus.
   A. norepinephrine
   B. thymosin
   C. insulin
   D. melatonin

5. _____ is an increase of potassium in the blood.
   A. Hypocalcemia
   B. Hyperkalemia
   C. Hypernatremia
   D. Exophthalmia

6. _____ is a deficiency of glucose in the blood.
   A. Hypocalcemia
   B. Hyponatremia
   C. Hyperkalemia
   D. Hypoglycemia

7. _____ is the undergrowth of bone and body tissue in children.
   A. Graves disease
   B. Dwarfism
   C. Gigantism
   D. Cushing syndrome

8. _____ results from underactive thyroid secretion in adults.
   A. Exophthalmos
   B. Goiter
   C. Myxedema
   D. Addison disease

9. _____ is the hormone that responds to natural light and plays a role in sleep.
   A. Epinephrine
   B. Aldosterone
   C. Glucocorticoid
   D. Melatonin

10. _____ is the hormone that breaks down glucose into glycogen.
    A. Prostaglandin
    B. Insulin
    C. Thymosin
    D. Glucagon

11. There are _____ parathyroid glands.
    A. 3
    B. 4
    C. 5
    D. none of the above

12. The islets of Langerhans are scattered throughout the _____ and play a key role in the production of hormones used to regulate blood sugar.
    A. kidneys
    B. pancreas
    C. brain
    D. spleen

13. The pineal gland is a small cone-shaped organ in the brain that secretes _____.
    A. melatonin
    B. insulin
    C. prostaglandins
    D. none of the above

14. A(n) _____ feedback effect occurs when the gland is stimulated to increase hormone secretion instead of turning it off.
    A. equilateral
    B. bilateral
    C. positive
    D. negative

15. The combining form for "pituitary gland" is _____.
    A. adren/o
    B. crin/o
    C. hypophys/o
    D. natr/o

16. Which one of the following is the abbreviation for triiodothyronine?
    A. Trid
    B. T_3
    C. T_4
    D. none of the above

17. An example of a corticosteroid is _____.
    A. Amaryl
    B. Pitocin
    C. Deltasone
    D. Tapazole

18. A nondiabetic range for A1c is _____.
    A. 4% to 6%
    B. 6% to 7%
    C. 7% to 8%
    D. 8% to 10%

19. Which one of the following is NOT a warning sign of type 1 diabetes?
    A. Weight loss
    B. Unexplained irritability
    C. Nausea and vomiting
    D. Excessive hunger

20. The _____ is responsible for water reabsorption in the kidneys.
    A. anterior lobe of the pituitary gland
    B. posterior lobe of the pituitary gland
    C. adrenal cortex
    D. adrenal medulla

21. The hormone _____ stimulates growth and hormone activity of the testes and ovaries.
    A. ACTH
    B. MSH
    C. ADH
    D. FSH

22. The hormone _____ helps in carbohydrate metabolism and is active during stress.
    A. cortisol
    B. prolactin
    C. estrogen
    D. glucagon

23. _____ increases heart rate and blood pressure and is active during times of stress.
    A. Thyroxin
    B. Epinephrine
    C. Thyroid-stimulating hormone
    D. Norepinephrine

24. The medical term for "excessive urination" is _____.
    A. polyphagia
    B. polydipsia
    C. polyphagia
    D. polyuria

25. _____ is a test used for to evaluate bone density, hypoparathyroidism, and the size of the adrenal gland.
    A. CT scan
    B. MRI
    C. Radiography
    D. Ultrasonography

Sentence Completion

Complete each sentence or statement.

1. The _____ is known as the master gland.

2. _____ are steroid hormones produced by the adrenal cortex.

3. _____ is abnormal hairiness, especially in women.

4. _____ is a blood test that measures the body's ability to break down a concentrated glucose solution.

5. An enlargement of the thyroid gland caused by inadequate thyroid synthesis is called a(n) _____.

6. Signs and symptoms of _____ include a swollen face, enlargement of the lips, and a swollen and protruding tongue.

7. Signs and symptoms of _____ include elevated blood levels of HGH. Radiographs may show a pituitary tumor.

8. _____ is caused by the impaired ability of the thyroid gland to produce T_4.

9. When the target cells cannot take up sufficient quantities of insulin, it is referred to as _____.

10. Overproduction of the hormone cortisol may cause _____.

Short Answers

1. Explain the two main functions of the endocrine system.

   _____

   _____

2. Compare and contrast endocrine and exocrine glands.

_____

_____

_____

_____

3. Identify and locate the seven major endocrine glands.

_____

_____

_____

_____

_____

_____

_____

4. Name two organs that secrete hormones, and explain what hormone is secreted by each.

_____

_____

_____

_____

CRITICAL THINKING

1. Joanna is a 25-year-old mother of two. Joanna has recently been diagnosed with IDDM. Explain to Joanna what is IDDM and how it is monitored and treated.

2. Simon is a 19-year-old man who has been treated for gigantism. Explain the etiology, signs and symptoms, therapy, and interventions.
    Use your text, your institution's resource reference library, and/or the Internet to address the above as needed.

INTERNET RESEARCH

Keyword: (Use the name of the condition or disease you select to write about).

Select one condition or disease from Table 19-1 or other related condition or disease. Write a two-paragraph report regarding the condition or disease you selected, listing the etiology, signs and symptoms, diagnosis, therapy, and interventions. Cite your source. (You may not use the information on the tables exclusively for your report.) Be prepared to give a 2-minute oral presentation should your instructor assign you to do so.

WHAT WOULD YOU DO?

If you have accomplished the objectives in this chapter, you will be able to make better choices as a medical assistant. Take another look at this situation and decide what you would do.

Juliette, age 4, cannot get enough water to drink and has to void frequently. Her mother says that Juliette eats all the time, but she is losing weight. She is also lethargic. At times, her mother thinks that Juliette's breath has a fruity odor, although she does not chew fruit-flavored gum or eat fruit-flavored candy. After Dr. Jay checks Juliette, she tells her mother that she is concerned that Juliette has diabetes mellitus. Dr. Jay wants to do further testing as quickly as possible. She orders a fasting blood sugar test, which comes back with an elevated value. She follows this with a glucose tolerance test. When the glucose tolerance test result is abnormally high, Dr. Jay prescribes insulin for Juliette.

1. **What type of diabetes mellitus would you expect Juliette to have at age 4?**

   _____

2. **What is the difference between IDDM and NIDDM?**

   _____

   _____

   _____

3. **Are the symptoms listed for Juliette typical of those found for persons with diabetes?**

   _____

   _____

   _____

4. **What are the medical terms for "being hungry all the time," "having excessive thirst," and "having to void often"?**

   _____

5. **What other specific treatment will be needed to keep Juliette's blood sugar level lowered?**

_____

_____

_____

6. **What is the term for an "elevated blood sugar level"? What is the term for "sugar in the urine"?**

_____

_____

7. **What is a fasting glucose test? What is a glucose tolerance test?**

_____

_____

_____

8. **Diabetes insipidus has many of the same symptoms as diabetes mellitus. What symptoms are the same?**

_____

_____

_____

9. **What glands and hormones are associated with diabetes insipidus?**

_____

_____

_____

_____

10. **What is positive feedback? What is negative feedback? Why are these important in the endocrine system?**

_____

_____

_____

_____

_____

APPLICATION OF SKILLS

1. Label the diagrams.

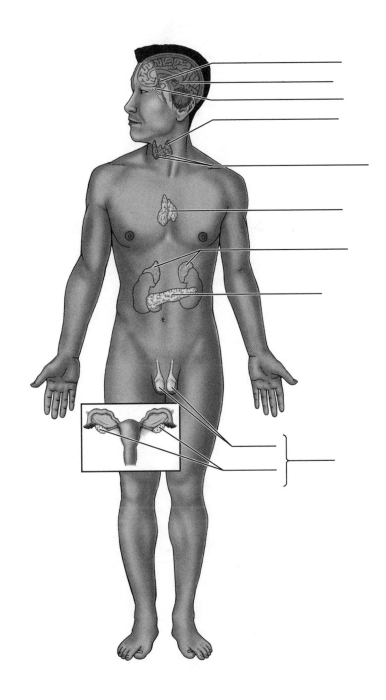

2. Define the following abbreviations.
   - ACTH _____
   - ADH _____
   - DM _____
   - FBS _____
   - GH _____
   - GTT _____
   - IDDM _____
   - NIDDM _____
   - T_3 _____
   - T_4 _____
   - TSH _____

CHAPTER QUIZ

Multiple Choice

Identify the letter of the choice that best completes the statement or answers the question.

1. The _____ gland(s) is(are) known as the master gland.
   A. pineal
   B. adrenal
   C. pituitary
   D. thyroid

2. The _____ gland(s) is(are) located above the kidneys.
   A. adrenal
   B. thymus
   C. parathyroid
   D. pineal

3. _____ is(are) hormone(s) responsible for the regulation of blood pressure, pain threshold, inflammation, and blood clotting.
   A. Antidiuretics
   B. Corticosteroids
   C. Prostaglandins
   D. Insulin

4. _____ is an increase of glucose in the blood.
   A. Hypoglycemia
   B. Hyperglycemia
   C. Hypercalcemia
   D. Hypokalemia

5. _____ is an increase of sodium in the blood.
   A. Hypercalcemia
   B. Hyperglycemia
   C. Hypokalemia
   D. Hypernatremia

6. _____ is a blood test measuring the amounts of ADH, cortisol, and growth and parathyroid hormones.
   A. A1c
   B. FBS
   C. Hormone level test
   D. Thyroid function test

7. _____ results in adults when there is an overproduction of thyroid hormone.
   A. Graves disease
   B. Cushing syndrome
   C. Diabetes mellitus
   D. Cretinism

8. _____ glands are whose secretion reaches the epithelial surface usually through a duct.
   A. Endocrine
   B. Exocrine
   C. Both endocrine and exocrine
   D. Neither endocrine nor exocrine

9. _____ is a type of corticosteroid.
   A. Pitocin
   B. Amaryl
   C. Deltasone
   D. Synthyroid

10. Which one of the following is a warning sign of diabetes type 1?
   A. Blurred vision
   B. Slow healing
   C. Numbness and tingling of the hands and feet
   D. None of the above

11. Which one of the following is a hormone produced by the thyroid gland?
   A. GH
   B. Calcitonin
   C. Parathormone
   D. Aldosterone

12. The adrenal medulla secretes which one of the following hormones?
   A. Testosterone
   B. Aldosterone
   C. Epinephrine
   D. Insulin

13. _____ is a lack of appetite.
   A. Exophthalmia
   B. Hirsutism
   C. Hypokalemia
   D. Anorexia

14. The medical term for "excessive thirst" is _____.
   A. polydipsia
   B. polyphagia
   C. polyuria
   D. none of the above

15. A(n) _____ is used to check for change in the size of soft tissue such as the pituitary, pancreas, and hypothalamus.
   A. CT scan
   B. MRI
   C. radiograph
   D. ultrasound

16. _____ is a blood test ordered to assess the amount of T_3, T_4, and calcitonin circulating in the blood.
   A. FBS
   B. GTT
   C. TFTs
   D. None of the above

17. _____ occurs in an adult when an excessive amount of growth hormone is secreted. The bones and soft tissue of the hands, feet, and face experience overgrowth.
   A. Dwarfism
   B. Gigantism
   C. Cretinism
   D. Acromegaly

18. The intervention for cretinism is _____.
   A. emotional support
   B. lifetime hormone replacement therapy
   C. encouraging patient to follow diet, reduce stress, and avoid infections
   D. encouraging patient to follow prescribed therapy for his or her lifetime

19. Clinical presentation of a "moon face," "buffalo hump," and obesity of trunk is indicative of _____.
   A. diabetes mellitus
   B. Cushing syndrome
   C. diabetes insipidus
   D. Addison disease

20. _____ is described as an enlargement of the thyroid gland caused by inadequate thyroid synthesis.
   A. Goiter
   B. Acromegaly
   C. Addison disease
   D. Cushing syndrome

CHAPTER TWENTY

Integumentary System

VOCABULARY REVIEW

Matching: Match each term with the correct definition.

A. dermatologist

B. turgor

C. dermis

D. keratin

E. melanin

F. whorls

G. sebaceous glands

H. sudoriferous glands

I. nails

J. cyst

K. polyp

L. benign

M. malignant melanoma

N. abrasion

O. contusion

P. laceration

Q. rule of nines

R. abscess

S. cicatrix

_____ 1. Black, asymmetrical lesion with uneven borders that grows faster than normal moles

_____ 2. Sweat glands; maintain body temperature

_____ 3. Contagious epithelial growths caused by a virus

_____ 4. Localized collection of pus that occurs on the skin or any body tissue

_____ 5. Specialist in the treatment of diseases and conditions of the skin

_____ 6. Abscess that occurs around a hair follicle

_____ 7. Not malignant

_____ 8. Ridges that fit snugly over the papillae on top of the dermis; coils or spirals that form fingerprints

_____ 9. Parasitic skin disorder caused by lice

_____ 10. Scar formation

_____ 11. Stalklike growth extending out from the mucous membrane

_____ 12. Pressure sore; bedsore

_____ 13. Waterproof protein that toughens the skin

T. decubitus ulcer

U. furuncle

V. pruritus

W. vitiligo

X. herpes simplex

Y. pediculosis

Z. verrucae

_____ 14. Growths of hard keratin that protect the ends of the fingers and toes

_____ 15. Blood vessels rupture and blood seeps into the tissue

_____ 16. Viral infection of the skin characterized by "cold sores" and "fever blisters"

_____ 17. Oil glands; release oil that lubricates the skin and hair

_____ 18. Severe itching

_____ 19. Jagged cuts; tissue edges are irregular

_____ 20. Thick-walled sac that contains fluid or semisolid material

_____ 21. Normal tension in the skin

_____ 22. Loss of pigment in the skin; milk-white patches

_____ 23. Epidermis is scraped off

_____ 24. Layer of skin that lies beneath the epidermis

_____ 25. System for evaluating the burns on a patient's total body surface area

_____ 26. Dark pigment that provides color to the skin and protects against the sun's ultra-violet rays

THEORY RECALL

True/False

Indicate whether the sentence or statement is true or false.

_____ 1. The skin is composed of the dermis, epidermis, and subcutaneous layer.

_____ 2. The epidermis is the deepest layer of the skin.

_____ 3. The dermis is thicker than the epidermis and lies beneath it.

_____ 4. A macule is a split or crack in the skin.

_____ 5. An incision is a smooth cut into the skin.

Multiple Choice

Identify the letter of the choice that best completes the statement or answers the question.

1. _____ is the most common inflammation of the skin; accompanied by papules, vesicles, and crusts.
   A. Furuncle
   B. Keloid
   C. Eczema
   D. Urticaria

2. Xylocaine is an example of a(n) _____ that blocks pain at the site where it is administered.
   A. anti-inflammatory
   B. analgesic
   C. antiviral
   D. none of the above

3. Salicylic acid is a(n) _____ medication used to remove warts.
   A. keratolytic
   B. antiviral
   C. corticosteroid
   D. antiinfective

4. _____ is a microscopic examination of skin lesions to screen for herpes virus.
   A. Wood's light examination
   B. Blood antibody titer
   C. Tzanck test
   D. Skin biopsy

5. Signs and symptoms of _____ include red, itchy rash with bull's eye appearance; joint pain and malaise.
   A. impetigo
   B. Lyme disease
   C. scleroderma
   D. scabies

6. _____ is a skin infection caused by fungus; classified according to body region.
   A. Lyme disease
   B. Scabies
   C. Tinea
   D. Pediculosis

7. A narrow band of epidermis at the base and sides of the nail is called the _____.
   A. nail bed
   B. lunula
   C. nail root
   D. cuticle

8. The medical term for "baldness" is _____.
   A. alopecia
   B. cicatrix
   C. onychomycosis
   D. none of the above

9. _____ is a parasitic skin disorder caused by lice.
   A. Onychomycosis
   B. Pediculosis
   C. Scabies
   D. Tinea

10. _____ are large abscesses that involve connecting furuncles.
    A. Cicatrix
    B. Melanoma
    C. Polyps
    D. Carbuncles

11. A sac or tube that anchors and contains an individual hair is called the _____.
    A. shaft
    B. follicle
    C. root
    D. none of the above

12. The medical term for a "precancerous growth of the skin" is _____.
    A. polyp
    B. vesicle
    C. actinic keratosis
    D. comedo

13. The skin layer that is mainly composed of adipose tissue and loose connective tissue is the _____.
    A. subcutaneous
    B. dermis
    C. epidermis
    D. both B and C

14. The medical term for a "flat discolored area of the skin" is _____.
    A. papule
    B. lesion
    C. wheal
    D. macule

15. Which degree of burn is reddened blistering of the dermis and epidermis layers of the skin?
    A. First
    B. Second
    C. Third
    D. Fourth

16. The medical term for "removal of surface epidermis by scratching, burning, or abrasion" is _____.
    A. erosion
    B. ichthyosis
    C. excoriation
    D. none of the above

17. An idiopathic hereditary dermatitis with dry, scaly, silver patches, usually on both arms, legs, and the scalp, is called _____.
    A. psoriasis
    B. eczema
    C. urticaria
    D. scleroderma

18. The medical term for an "erosion of the skin" (bedsore) is _____.
    A. lesion
    B. pustule
    C. polyp
    D. decubitus ulcer

19. Phase 1 on the healing process is known as the _____ phase.
    A. inflammation
    B. granulation
    C. maturation
    D. none of the above

20. A(n)_____ is an overgrowth of fibrous tissue at the site of scar tissue.
    A. ulcer
    B. polyp
    C. keloid
    D. furuncle

21. Benadryl is an example of a(n) _____ medication.
    A. antipruritic
    B. antiviral
    C. antifungal
    D. anesthetic

22. _____ is an infection of the skin and subcutaneous tissue caused by bacteria.
    A. Psoriasis
    B. Cellulitis
    C. Pediculosis
    D. Impetigo

23. In the condition of _____, the skin hardens and becomes leathery. Organs may also be affected by decreasing in size, and joints may swell and be painful.
    A. Lyme disease
    B. psoriasis
    C. scleroderma
    D. scabies

24. The combining form for "skin" is _____.
    A. albino/o
    B. diaphor/o
    C. histi/o
    D. dermat/o

25. The maturation phase of healing is phase _____.
    A. 1
    B. 2
    C. 3
    D. 4

Sentence Completion

Complete each sentence or statement.

1. A person unable to form melanin will have very white skin with no pigmentation and is referred to

   as a(n) _____ .

2. A(n) _____ is the duct opening that provides a pathway for fluid to leave the body.

3. The _____ is a white half-moon shape at the base of the nail.

4. Oil glands release _____ .

5. A clear blister is called a _____ .

6. A(n) _____ is a thick-walled sac that contains fluid or semisolid material.

7. _____ are skin cancers that appear as firm papules with ulcerations.

8. The abbreviation for "ointment" is _____ .

9. The abbreviation for "biopsy" is _____ .

10. The term for "scalelike" is _____ .

Short Answers

1. List the three main functions of the skin.

   _____

   _____

   _____

2. Identify the three layers of the skin and describe the structure and function of each.

_____

_____

_____

_____

_____

_____

_____

3. List and briefly describe nine common skin lesions.

_____

_____

_____

_____

_____

_____

_____

_____

4. Name two organs that secrete hormones and explain what hormone is secreted by each.

_____

_____

_____

_____

CRITICAL THINKING

1. Mrs. Kimerfield called the office this afternoon because her 8-year-old daughter Melanie brought a note home from school informing Mrs. Kimerfield that several of Melanie's classmates have head lice and that there is the potential that Melanie may also have it. Explain to Mrs. Kimerfield what to look for and how to treat it.

2. Identify the following types of fungal infections, by stating their location and a typical treatment of each.

- Tinea corporis _____

- Tinea pedis _____

- Tinea unguium _____

- Tinea cruris _____

- Tinea faciei _____

- Tinea capitis _____

Use your text, your institution's resource reference library, and/or the Internet to address the above as needed.

INTERNET RESEARCH

Keyword: (Use the name of the condition or disease you select to write about).

Select one condition or disease from Table 20-4 or other related condition or disease. Write a two-paragraph report regarding the condition or disease you selected, listing the etiology, signs and symptoms, diagnosis, therapy, and interventions. Cite your source. (You may not use the information on the tables exclusively for your report.) Be prepared to give a 2-minute oral presentation should your instructor assign you to do so.

WHAT WOULD YOU DO?

If you have accomplished the objectives in this chapter, you will be able to make better choices as a medical assistant. Take another look at this situation and decide what you would do.

Marilyn was taking a shower 2 weeks ago and found a large black mole on her shoulder. At first she wanted to ignore it, but after talking with her friend, she decided that she should see her family practice physician. This physician sent her to Dr. Nelson, a dermatologist, who diagnosed her lesion as a possible malignant melanoma. Dr. Nelson asked if she had any pruritus, a fissure, or crusting of the lesion. As Dr. Nelson examined Marilyn's shoulder, he noticed petechiae, ecchymosis, and purpura. When asked about these findings, Marilyn told the physician that the mole had itched and she had scratched the area in her sleep. On her leg was a furuncle that was inflamed and hot and appeared to have a pus formation. Upon completing the physical examination, Dr. Nelson noticed that Marilyn had the tendency to keloid formation based on the appearance of her old appendectomy scar. Marilyn had quite a few questions for the medical assistant about the meaning of some of the terms used by Dr. Nelson. Marilyn left the dermatologist's office with surgery scheduled for removal of the melanoma 2 days later.

1. **What is the etiology of a malignant melanoma?**

   _____

   _____

2. **How do the signs of a malignant melanoma differ from those of a benign lesion?**

   _____

   _____

   _____

3. What is pruritus? Fissure? Crusting?

_____

_____

_____

_____

4. What are petechiae? What is ecchymosis? Purpura?

_____

_____

_____

_____

5. What is the difference between a furuncle and a carbuncle?

_____

_____

_____

_____

6. Why would the physician be concerned that Marilyn had a history of keloids?

_____

_____

_____

_____

7. What are the stages of the healing process that you could expect Marilyn to have following surgery?

_____

_____

_____

_____

8. **What is a closed wound? Give two examples.**

_____

_____

_____

_____

9. **What is an open wound? Give two examples.**

_____

_____

_____

_____

APPLICATION OF SKILLS

Label the diagrams.

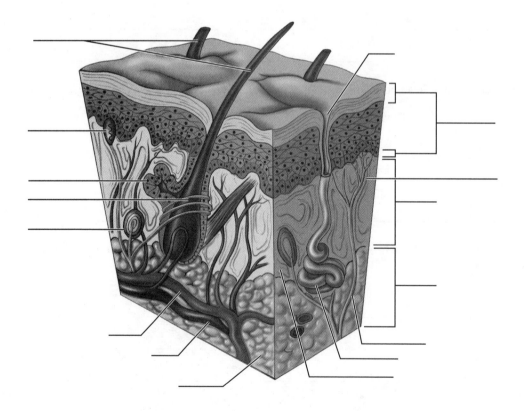

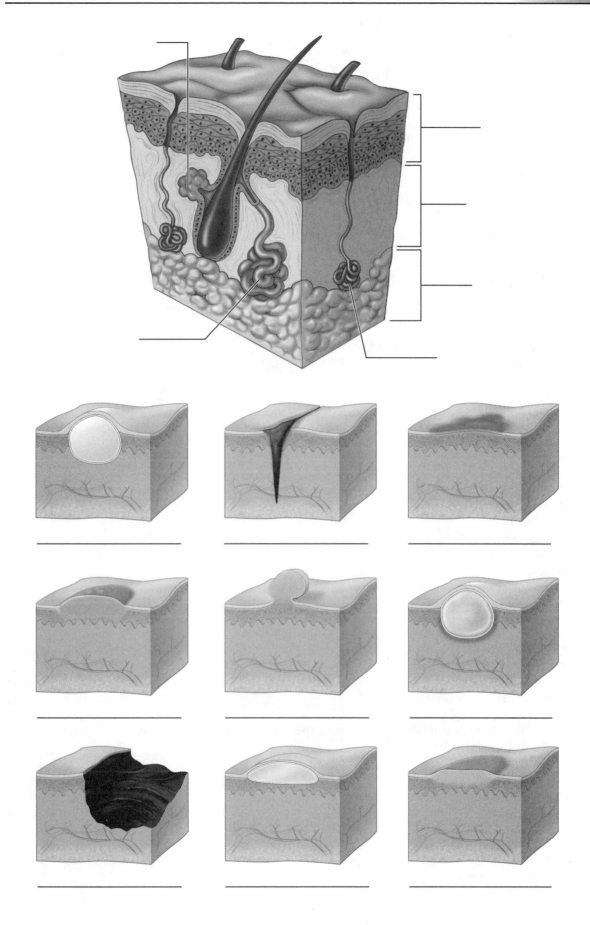

CHAPTER QUIZ

Multiple Choice

Identify the letter of the choice that best completes the statement or answers the question.

1. A(n) _____ has jagged cuts and tissue edges that are irregular.
   A. laceration
   B. incision
   C. abrasion
   D. contusion

2. _____ is an idiopathic, chronic systemic disease of the skin in which the skin hardens and become leathery.
   A. Impetigo
   B. Scleroderma
   C. Cellulitis
   D. Psoriasis

3. A(n) _____ is a split or crack in the skin.
   A. purpura
   B. contusion
   C. fissure
   D. onychomycosis

4. _____ are flat, pinpoint red spots.
   A. Ichthyosis
   B. Purpura
   C. Urticaria
   D. Petechiae

5. The deepest layer of skin is the _____.
   A. subcutaneous tissue
   B. epidermis
   C. dermis
   D. none of the above

6. A(n) _____ is an abscess that occurs around a hair follicle.
   A. carbuncle
   B. ulcer
   C. furuncle
   D. excoriation

7. _____ are oil glands that release oil that lubricates the skin and hair.
   A. Sudoriferous glands
   B. Sebaceous glands
   C. Lymph glands
   D. Adenoids

8. The _____ is Phase 2 of the healing process; collagen forms.
   A. inflammatory phase
   B. maturation phase
   C. granulation phase
   D. none of the above

9. _____ is the normal tension of skin.
   A. Turgor
   B. Rigor
   C. Flaccidity
   D. Cicatrix

10. A(n) _____ is a malignant skin lesion that is raised, with blood vessels around the edges.
    A. squamous cell carcinoma
    B. basal cell carcinoma
    C. malignant melanoma
    D. actinic keratosis

11. _____ is a skin disorder caused by itch mites.
    A. Lyme disease
    B. Pediculosis
    C. Scabies
    D. Tinea cruris

12. A patient with _____ exhibits blisters on the lips, inside of the mouth, and occasionally the nose.
    A. pediculosis
    B. verrucae
    C. tinea corporis
    D. herpes simplex

13. The combining form for "tissue" is _____.
    A. kerat/o
    B. histi/o
    C. hidr/o
    D. onych/o

14. Ung is the abbreviation for _____.
    A. "ointment"
    B. "nail border"
    C. "urgent"
    D. none of the above

15. Tetracycline is an example of a medication used for treating _____.
    A. fungi
    B. acne
    C. lice
    D. psoriasis

16. Zovirax is an example of a medication used for treating _____.
    A. scabies
    B. herpes simplex
    C. athletes foot
    D. burns

17. A Wood's light examination is used to detect _____.
    A. fungal skin infections
    B. reaction of the body to allergens
    C. viral infections
    D. bacterial infections

18. A burn patient's total body surface area is evaluated according to the _____ to determine the extent and/or severity of the burn.
    A. core body temperature
    B. full-thickness measurement
    C. rule of nines
    D. total body weight

19. The medical term for "ringworm" is _____.
    A. tinea capitis
    B. tinea corporis
    C. tinea faciei
    D. tinea pedis

20. The medical term for a "pore that is blocked, usually with sebum and bacteria" is _____.
    A. polyp
    B. furuncle
    C. comedo
    D. fissure

CHAPTER TWENTY-ONE

The Medical Office

VOCABULARY REVIEW

Matching: Match each term with the correct definition.

A. Americans With Disabilities Act (ADA)

B. breach of confidentiality

C. Health Insurance Portability and Accountability Act (HIPAA) of 1996

D. agenda

E. fax machine (facsimile)

F. itinerary

G. notebook computer

H. personal digital assistants (PDAs)

I. postage meter

J. preventive maintenance

K. facilities management

L. policy manual

M. procedures manual

N. backordered

O. capital goods

P. disposable goods

Q. inventory records

R. invoice

_____ 1. Document received with an order that lists the items ordered and itemizes those sent and those to arrive at a later date

_____ 2. Status of being out of stock; items that will be shipped at a later date

_____ 3. Office equipment that scans document, translates the information to electronic impulses, and transmits an exact copy of the original document from one location to another through a telephone line

_____ 4. Pocket-sized computer used for appointments, telephone numbers, notes, and other information used on a daily basis

_____ 5. Break in a patient's right to privacy

_____ 6. Entity that sells supplies, equipment, and services

_____ 7. Expendable or consumable supplies that are used and then discarded

_____ 8. Equipment that is reusable but less expensive and durable than capital equipment

_____ 9. Travel document that describes the overall trip and indicates what is scheduled to happen each day

_____ 10. Form prepared by the vendor describing the products sold by item number, quantity, and the price; used for paying the vendor

S. lead time

T. noncapital goods

U. order quantity

V. packing slip

W. purchase order

X. reorder point

Y. safety stock

Z. vendor

AA. warranty card

_____ 11. Provides for accessible routes and fixtures for use by the disabled

_____ 12. Regular servicing meant to prevent the breakdown of equipment

_____ 13. Card that accompanies a purchased item that provides protection for the buyer against defective parts for 90 days

_____ 14. Time it takes to receive an order once placed

_____ 15. Document used to order supplies; contains the name, address, and telephone number of a vendor and the quantity, price, and description of the items ordered

_____ 16. Document that includes the length of the meeting, topics to be covered, their order, and the person responsible for each

_____ 17. Maintaining the atmosphere and physical environment of an office

_____ 18. Optimal quantity of a supply to be ordered at one time

_____ 19. Manual containing specific instructions on how procedures are to be performed

_____ 20. Small, portable computer that can be carried easily

_____ 21. Documentation of physical assets and information that includes item description, date of purchase, price, and where purchased. Equipment serial numbers and service agreements are also recorded

_____ 22. Extra items on hand to avoid running out of stock (back-up supply)

_____ 23. Automated stamp machine

_____ 24. Mandates patient rights by providing guidelines for health care providers and insurance carriers to maintain confidentiality

_____ 25. Goods that are durable and are expected to last a few years; expensive

_____ 26. Minimum quantity of a supply to be available before a new order is placed

_____ 27. Manual that explains the day-to-day operations of the medical office and provides general information that affects all employees

THEORY RECALL

True/False

Indicate whether the sentence or statement is true or false.

_____ 1. A supply order should only be paid from a statement.

_____ 2. A professional cleaning staff typically cleans the office every night and arranges the reception area.

_____ 3. HIPAA provides federal regulations that require all public buildings be accessible to everyone.

_____ 4. A dedicated telephone line permits faxes to be sent and received 24 hours a day.

_____ 5. When leasing equipment, the office owns the equipment.

Multiple Choice

Identify the letter of the choice that best completes the statement or answers the question.

1. Tongue blades, syringes, and printer paper are all examples of _____ goods.
   A. disposable
   B. noncapital
   C. capital
   D. none of the above

2. The _____ is the optimal quantity of a supply to be ordered at one time.
   A. reorder point
   B. safety stock
   C. order quantity
   D. lead time

3. When an order is received, a(n) _____ is included in the package.
   A. purchase order
   B. packing slip
   C. invoice
   D. statement

4. Which one of the following is the first step in organizing a meeting?
   A. Prepare an agenda.
   B. Select a location and a meeting room.
   C. Send reminder notices to all participants.
   D. Assemble materials needed for the meeting.

5. Which one of the following is NOT needed to make travel arrangements for the physician?
   A. Dates of travel
   B. Number of people traveling
   C. Hotel reservations
   D. Favorite food

6. A _____ explains the day-to-day operations of the medical office.
   A. policy manual
   B. guidebook
   C. procedure manual
   D. none of the above

7. When a medical office is closed and unavailable to handle incoming calls, which one of the following is the most efficient method routinely used?
   A. Answering service
   B. Answering machine
   C. Forwarding all calls to the physician's home phone
   D. Both A and B are equally efficient

8. Maintenance of a procedure manual requires that _____.
   A. the physician's attorneys approve it
   B. the physician sends a memo once a year to remind everyone there is a procedure manual.
   C. all employees are required to date and initial that they have read the manual.
   D. none of the above

9. Which one of the following is NOT considered a medical office marketing tool?
   A. Brochure
   B. Web page
   C. Press release
   D. All of the above are marketing tools

10. Leasing is essentially _____ equipment for the office.
    A. buying
    B. renting
    C. both A and B
    D. neither A and B

11. Inventory records are used in maintaining an adequate supply for use in the office, for _____ purposes, and in case of fire or theft.
    A. depreciation
    B. capitation
    C. entrepreneurship
    D. none of the above

12. The first step in preparing a fax for transmission after gathering supplies and equipment is to _____.
    A. copy the patient's file
    B. check the file for a release of information
    C. prepare a coversheet
    D. photocopy the materials to be faxed on yellow paper for better transmission

13. _____ items are usually expensive and are expected to be permanent or at least last several years.
    A. Disposable
    B. Noncapital
    C. Capital
    D. None of the above

14. The *best* color of ink to use on a faxed document is _____.
    A. blue
    B. red
    C. black
    D. purple

15. If a fax is marked "for physician only," what should the medical assistant do?
    A. Do not accept the fax.
    B. Hand it directly to the physician.
    C. Give it to the office manager for his or her decision.
    D. Annotate it and then give to the physician.

16. When maintaining office equipment a file should be created for _____ or type of equipment.
    A. vendor
    B. medical assistant
    C. physician
    D. none of the above

17. To meet the minimum standards of the ADA, a wheelchair ramp longer than _____ feet must have two railings.
    A. 6
    B. 8
    C. 10
    D. 12

18. Internal restrooms must be _____ inches wide to be in compliance with the ADA.
    A. 24
    B. 32
    C. 36
    D. 42

19. Which one of the following is NOT a legal concern regarding fax machines and HIPAA regulations?
    A. Confidentiality–authorization signed
    B. Amount of information being sent
    C. Location of fax machine
    D. All of the above are legal concerns

20. A(n) _____ is a document that includes the length of a meeting, topics to be covered, their order, and the person responsible for each.
    A. itinerary
    B. agenda
    C. HIPAA mandate
    D. none of the above

Sentence Completion

Complete each sentence or statement.

1. When ordering supplies, a(n) _____ is typically initiated to keep track of what was ordered and when.

2. A(n) _____ describes an overall trip and indicates what is scheduled to happen each day.

3. You may want to create a(n) _____ to remind you that maintenance is routinely required on your office equipment.

4. A(n) _____ is a break in a patient's right to privacy.

5. A pocket-sized computer used for appointments, telephone numbers, etc., is called a(n) _____.

6. A(n) _____ is an automated stamp machine.

7. _____ is the time it takes to receive an order.

8. An item that is _____ is temporarily out of stock and will be shipped at a later date.

9. _____ is the term used for maintaining the atmosphere and physical environment of an office.

10. A(n) _____ is a card that accompanies a purchased item that provides protection for the buyer against defective parts for 90 days.

Short Answers

1. Design a plan for a medical office reception area that reflects HIPAA and ADA regulations and incorporates the seven considerations for a reception area.

_____

_____

_____

_____

2. List six types of office equipment and explain how each is used in the medical office.

_____

_____

_____

_____

3. Explain why inventory records are kept.

_____

_____

_____

_____

4. List three factors to be considered when establishing an inventory control system.

_____

_____

_____

_____

CRITICAL THINKING

The physician has requested a 10-cc syringe be available in exam room 3 for an I&D of a sebaceous cyst. When you went to the storage room to obtain the syringe, the box was empty. After searching the exam rooms, you were able to locate one 10-cc syringe, which you took into the doctor. After the procedure, you check the inventory supply reorder form for 10-cc syringes. No one has requested that 10-cc syringes be ordered. The office is completely out of 10-cc syringes; what would you now do?

INTERNET RESEARCH

Keywords: Health Insurance Portability and Accountability Act/Americans With Disabilities Act

Choose one of the following topics to research: patient confidentiality as it applies to HIPAA guidelines or the accommodations required of a medical facility under ADA guidelines. Write a two-paragraph report supporting your topic. Cite your source. Be prepared to give a 2-minute oral presentation should your instructor assign you to do so.

WHAT WOULD YOU DO?

If you have accomplished the objectives in this chapter, you will be able to make better choices as a medical assistant. Take a look at this situation and decide what you would do.

Janine is a new member of the office staff. She has not had any training in the medical assisting field but has been working as a receptionist in a loan office. On her first day at work, Janine is assigned to work at the front desk with the receptionist. As the patients for the day come in, Janine asks many personal questions about each patient and then proceeds to tell the receptionist what she knows about the patient. When told to be sure the names of the patients have been obliterated from the sign-in sheet, she uses a yellow highlighter. As she answers the telephone, everyone in the office can hear her conversations. Janine immediately moves the large plants in the reception area around so one is partially blocking the doorway. A fax from a surgeon arrives for Dr. Lopez, and Janine lays it on the front counter next to the sign-in sheet until she has a chance to give it to Dr. Lopez. When asked to move the fax, Janine replies that it would definitely be easier if the fax was just placed next to the front window rather than in the back room so she would not have to walk so far. Also, Janine does not understand why this office needs a dedicated line for the fax machine. Why not just let the fax line be connected to the multiline telephone at the front desk?

Janine was asked to leave a week later after she refused to maintain the equipment. As the office personnel looked for the manuals for the new equipment that had been purchased, no manuals could be found and when she was contacted, Janine admitted discarding them.

What should Janine be told about why she was asked to leave her job at the medical office?

1. **In many ways, Janine has broken confidentiality in the medical office as required by HIPAA. Name three ways that are obvious.**

2. **What is HIPAA, and how does it affect patient care?**

3. **Why is a multiline phone system important in a medical office?**

4. What special features should be considered when deciding on a phone system for the medical office?

_____

_____

_____

_____

5. How is ADA important in the medical office? What are three of the design features that are important for patient safety?

_____

_____

_____

_____

6. How did Janine make Dr. Lopez's office dangerous for a person with a physical disability?

_____

_____

_____

_____

7. Why is it important to keep manuals that are sent with new equipment?

_____

_____

_____

_____

8. Would you want Janine to be a fellow employee in a medical office with you? Defend your answer.

_____

_____

_____

_____

APPLICATION OF SKILLS

Procedure Check-off Sheets (*) and assignments from MACC CD (**)

1. Perform Procedure 21-1: Prepare and Send a Fax.*

2. Perform Procedure 21-2: Maintain Office Equipment.*

3. Perform Procedure 21-3: Inventory Control and Ordering Supplies*
   A. MACC CD
   MACC/Professionalism/Operational functions/Establishing and maintaining a supply inventory and ordering system.**

4. Perform Procedure 21-4: Develop Marketing Tools to Increase Visibility of a Medical Practice in the Community.*

5. Perform Procedure 21-5: Gather Community Resources.*

Student Name _____ Date _____

PROCEDURE 21-1: PREPARE AND SEND A FAX

TASK: Correctly send information by facsimile (fax), maintaining confidentiality.

CONDITIONS: Given the proper equipment and supplies, the student will be required to prepare and send a fax.

EQUIPMENT AND SUPPLIES
- Cover sheet
- Document(s) to be faxed
- Pen
- Telephone/fax machine

STANDARDS: Complete the procedure within _____ minutes and achieve a minimum score of _____ %.

Time began _____   **Time ended** _____

Steps	Possible Points	First Attempt	Second Attempt
1. Gather equipment and supplies.	5		
2. Prepare a fax to send			
a. Obtain or create a document to be faxed.	10		
b. Check file for release of information.	10		
c. Obtain the demographic information for the intended recipient.	5		
d. Create a company cover sheet template.	10		
e. Complete the cover sheet by filling in the required information.	10		
f. Prepare the document.	5		
3. Send a fax.			
a. Place the cover sheet and document in the fax machine as required by the manufacturer.	10		
b. Dial the telephone fax number of the recipient.	10		
c. Press start.	5		
d. When the document is completely through the machine, press the button if required or wait to receive a transmittal report.	10		
e. Remove the document from the machine and attach the transmittal report to the document.	10		
Total Points Possible	100		

Comments: Total Points Earned _____ Divided by _____ Total Possible Points= _____ % Score

*Instructor's Signature*_____

Student Name _____ Date _____

PROCEDURE 21-2: MAINTAIN OFFICE EQUIPMENT

TASK: Create an office procedure for maintaining office equipment.

CONDITIONS: Given the proper equipment and supplies, the student will be required to create a maintenance log for standard medical office equipment.

EQUIPMENT AND SUPPLIES
- List of office equipment to include all administrative and medical equipment, such as
  - Computer(s)
  - Telephone system
  - Transcription machine
  - Fax machine
  - Photocopy machine
  - Postage meter
  - Printer
  - Electrocardiograph machine
  - Glucometer
  - Cholesterol machine
  - Electronic thermometer(s)
  - Sigmoidoscope
  - Ultrasound equipment
  - X-ray equipment
- File folder(s)
- Medical equipment and office supply catalogs
- Computer – spreadsheet and word processing software or sheet provided by instructor for completion.
- Pen or pencil

STANDARDS: Complete the procedure within _____ minutes and achieve a minimum score of _____ %.

Time began _____   Time ended _____

Steps	Possible Points	First Attempt	Second Attempt
1. Inventory and then create a separate list for administrative and clinical equipment used in the facility. (Use classroom equipment.)	20		
2. Identify the vendor for each item.	10		
3. Create a file folder for each piece or type of equipment by vendor, type of equipment as determined by instructor.	10		
4. Create a maintenance log for each piece of equipment. Attach maintenance log on the left inside cover of the file folder.	10		
a. Print the name of the piece of equipment in the top right hand corner.	10		
b. List the manufacturer, identification number, date of purchase, and purchase price directly below the name.	10		
5. Physically inspect each piece of equipment.	10		
a. Ensure that each piece of equipment is in proper working order and is calibrated as mandated by the manufacturer.	10		
b. Look for frayed cords, broken parts, and improper functioning. Note on the maintenance log the date and the status of the equipment.	10		

Total Points Possible   100

Comments: Total Points Earned _____ Divided by _____ Total Possible Points = _____ % Score

Instructor's Signature _____

Student Name _____ Date _____

PROCEDURE 21-3: INVENTORY CONTROL AND ORDERING SUPPLIES

TASK: Create an inventory system for expendable supplies used in the doctor's office or clinic.

CONDITIONS: Given the proper equipment and supplies, role-play with a student or instructor the proper method of performing inventory control and ordering supplies.

EQUIPMENT AND SUPPLIES
- MACC CD/computer
- Supply list
- File box
- Supply inventory order cards – 3 × 5 or 5 × 7 index cards
- Blank file box divider cards
- Pen or pencil

STANDARDS: Complete the procedure within _____ minutes and achieve a minimum score of _____ %.

Time began _____   Time ended _____

Steps	Possible Points	First Attempt	Second Attempt
1. Create a list of all disposable supplies used in the facility.	10		
a. Separate the list into administrative and clinical supplies.	10		
b. Identify the vendor for each item.	10		
2. Create a divider card for each vendor.	5		
3. File the completed vendor divider cards.	5		
4. Create an inventory card for each disposable supply item on the supply list.	10		
5. Enter the unit price.	5		
6. Establish the reorder point.	5		
7. Inventory all items on the inventory list.	10		
8. Write the current number on hand next to the item on the supply list.	10		
9. Compare the quantity on hand to the reorder point on the inventory control card.	10		
10. Locate the inventory control card for each item that is highlighted.	5		
11. Order supplies.			
a. When an order has been placed, indicate the date ordered on the inventory card, amount ordered, and unit price.	5		
12. When the order is received, indicate the date and quantity received.	5		
13. Re-file the cards when the complete order has been received and the information is recorded.	5		
14. Restock the items.			
a. Place new items on the shelf behind the currently stocked supplies.	5		

Total Points Possible   115

Comments: Total Points Earned _____ Divided by _____ Total Possible Points = _____ % Score

Instructor's Signature _____

Student Name _____ Date _____

PROCEDURE 21-4: DEVELOP MARKETING TOOLS TO INCREASE VISIBILITY OF A MEDICAL PRACTICE IN THE COMMUNITY

TASK: Compile a list of marketing tools that can be used to increase a medical practice's visibility in the community.

CONDITIONS: Given the proper equipment and supplies, the student will be required to gather marketing resources within his or her community in preparation of creating marketing tools to increase a medical practice's visibility in the community.

EQUIPMENT AND SUPPLIES
- Telephone
- Telephone book
- Computer
- Internet
- Pen or pencil

STANDARDS: Complete the procedure within _____ minutes and achieve a minimum score of _____ %.

Time began _____   Time ended _____

Steps	Possible Points	First Attempt	Second Attempt
1. Research and gather information from your community to create marketing tools for promoting the medical practice.			
a. Gather examples of brochures and local newsletters and research Web pages from other medical practices or medical associations in your area.	20		
b. Contact the local newspaper for information on their guidelines for press releases.	15		
c. Locate and create a list of seminars or classes offered to medical professionals in your area for a 1-month period of time.	15		
d. Contact local or state telephone directory companies for information on advertising in their publications.	15		
2. Compile a specific list of the various marketing tools.	15		
3. Create a "Marketing" folder from the information gathered. Add information to the folder as you collect it.	10		
4. Turn in to the instructor gathered materials and folder.	10		

Total Points Possible   100

Comments: Total Points Earned _____ Divided by _____ Total Possible Points = _____ % Score

Instructor's Signature _____

Student Name _____ **Date** _____

PROCEDURE 21-5: GATHER COMMUNITY RESOURCES

TASK: Gather information from your local phone book, library, and newspaper or search the Internet and then create a reference document/brochure to increase a medical practice's visibility in the community and provide information to patients.

CONDITIONS: Given the proper equipment and supplies, the student will be required to gather community marketing information within their community and create a marketing tool/brochure to increase a medical practice's visibility in the community and provide information to patients.

EQUIPMENT AND SUPPLIES
- Local telephone book
- Local/state newspaper
- Internet access
- Computer – spreadsheet and word processing software
- Pen or pencil

STANDARDS: Complete the procedure within _____ minutes and achieve a minimum score of _____ %.

Time began _____   **Time ended** _____

Steps	Possible Points	First Attempt	Second Attempt
1. Research the resources available in your area using the local phone book, local/state newspaper, local library, or Internet: a minimum of five resources must be contacted.	25		
2. Create a list for each resource available that includes a telephone number, address, contact person, hours of operation, and what types of services each agency provides.	10		
3. Key the information gathered into a document either using a word processing software program or a spreadsheet software program. Double check your information for accuracy. Print a hard copy and save an electronic file on the computer.	15		
4. Create an informational marketing tool/brochure using the information gathered above as outlined by your instructor.	25		

Total Points Possible   75

Comments: Total Points Earned _____ Divided by _____ Total Possible Points = _____ % Score

Instructor's Signature _____

CHAPTER QUIZ

Multiple Choice

Identify the letter of the choice that best completes the statement or answers the question.

1. _____ mandates patient rights by providing guidelines for health care providers and insurance carriers.
   A. HIPAA
   B. ADA
   C. AMA
   D. State government

2. A(n) _____ is a piece of office equipment that scans a document, translates the information, and transmits an exact copy of the original over telephone lines.
   A. E-mail
   B. postage meter
   C. fax machine
   D. personal digital assistant

3. A document that includes the length of a meeting, topics to be covered, their order, and the person responsible for each is called a(n)_____.
   A. itinerary
   B. agenda
   C. minutes
   D. memo

4. _____ goods are durable and expensive and are expected to last a few years.
   A. Expendable
   B. Noncapital
   C. Capital
   D. None of the above

5. A(n) _____ is(are) documentation of physical assets and information that includes item description, date of purchase, and price.
   A. invoice
   B. inventory records
   C. packaging slip
   D. purchase order

6. _____ is the concept of maintaining the atmosphere of the physical environment of an office.
   A. Backordering
   B. Safety stocking
   C. Facilities management
   D. Preventative maintenance

7. Which one of the following is the first step in organizing a meeting?
   A. Assemble materials needed for the meeting.
   B. Send reminder notices to all participants.
   C. Select a location and a meeting room.
   D. Prepare an agenda.

8. A(n) _____ contains specific instructions on how tasks are to be performed.
   A. policy manual
   B. procedure manual
   C. guidebook
   D. none of the above

9. Which one of the following is NOT needed to make travel arrangements for the physician?
   A. Dates of travel
   B. Mode of transportation
   C. Hotel reservations
   D. Allergies

10. _____ occurs when a sign-in sheet is used that requests the patient to identify the reason for their visit.
    A. Fraud
    B. Malfeasance
    C. Breach of contract
    D. Breach of confidentiality

11. Which one of the following is NOT a function of a medical office reception area?
    A. Provides a place to greet patients upon their arrival
    B. Provides an area for patients to wait for provider
    C. Allows intake of patient information
    D. All are functions

12. To provide a comfortable reception area for patients, the temperature should not be above _____° F.
    A. 64
    B. 68
    C. 70
    D. 73

13. Only artificial plants or flowers should be used in the patient waiting area.
    A. True
    B. False

14. A typical multiline telephone system has _____ buttons.
    A. 3
    B. 6
    C. 9
    D. none of the above

15. The _____ feature on the telephone calls the last number dialed.
    A. call forwarding
    B. conference calling
    C. privacy
    D. repeat call

16. The _____ calling feature on a telephone system allows the physician to have a three-way conversation with consulting physicians and patient's families.
    A. conference
    B. dedicated
    C. call forwarding
    D. caller ID

17. A(n) _____ is a business entity that handles patient calls during hours the medical practice is closed.
    A. voice mail
    B. answering service
    C. pager
    D. answering machine

18. _____ is the science of adjusting the work environment so that injuries will be prevented.
    A. Osteopathy
    B. Chiropractics
    C. Ergonomics
    D. None of the above

19. Mail that has been metered in the office takes longer to reach its destination.
    A. True
    B. False

20. Leased equipment cannot be sold because it is not owned by the practice.
    A. True
    B. False

CHAPTER **TWENTY-TWO**

Medical Office Communication

VOCABULARY REVIEW

Matching: Match each term with the correct definition.

A. autopsy report

B. certified mail

C. cluster scheduling

D. consultation report

E. discharge summary

F. double booking

G. established patient

H. full-block format

I. history and physical (H&P) report

J. matrix

K. medical practice information booklet

L. modified-block format

M. modified-wave scheduling

N. new patient

O. open-hour scheduling

P. operative report

Q. progress notes

R. registered mail

_____ 1. Appointment scheduling technique that schedules more than one patient during the same appointment time period

_____ 2. Appointment scheduling technique based on the theory that each patient visit will not require the allotted time

_____ 3. Special mail-handling method used when the contents have a declared monetary value

_____ 4. Appointment scheduling technique that groups several appointments for similar types of examination; also called categorization scheduling

_____ 5. Appointment scheduling technique that divides an hour block into average-appointment time slots

_____ 6. Booklet or brochure that provides non-medical information for patients about standard office policies

_____ 7. Letter format in which all lines are flush with the left margin, except the first line of new paragraph, date, closing, and signature (which are centered)

_____ 8. Medical report that lists a surgical procedure performed, any pathologic specimens, the findings, and the medical personnel involved

_____ 9. Appointment scheduling technique that provides a definite time period for the patient to be seen

S. time-specified scheduling

T. wave scheduling

_____ 10. Letter format that has all lines flush with the left margin

_____ 11. Medical report written by a specialist who sees a patient for a primary physician and then returns care to the primary physician

_____ 12. Appointment scheduling technique that allows patients to be seen without an appointment

_____ 13. Medical report that provides details about the cause of a person's illness and death through both internal and external examination findings

_____ 14. Written findings of a patient's condition

_____ 15. Patient who has not received professional services from the physician or the medical office in the past 3 years

_____ 16. Medical report that provides a comprehensive review of a patient's hospital stay

_____ 17. Patient who has received professional services from the physician or the medical office in the past 3 years

_____ 18. Format used to mark off or reserve time in a schedule

_____ 19. Special mail-handling method used to prove an item was mailed and received

_____ 20. Medical report that consists of a patient's subjective and objective data

THEORY RECALL

True/False

Indicate whether the sentence or statement is true or false.

_____ 1. The HIPAA privacy rule allows for incidental disclosure of patient information as long as appropriate safeguards and rules are in place and followed.

_____ 2. Cluster scheduling is similar to wave scheduling, but instead of more than one patient being scheduled at the beginning of the hour, two patients are scheduled to see the physician at the same time.

_____ 3. A patient should be notified if they will be required to wait more than 20 minutes for the physician.

_____ 4. Mail should be arranged in order of importance and placed on the physician's desk.

_____ 5. The subject line of a business letter should be typed four lines below the salutation.

Multiple Choice

Identify the letter of the choice that best completes the statement or answers the question.

1. What is the purpose of the medical information booklet/brochure?
   A. Provides answers to nonmedical questions
   B. Outlines a treatment plan
   C. Provides the patient with a wound care instruction sheet
   D. None of the above

2. A medical assistant's/receptionist's voice should be _____ when answering the telephone.
   A. high pitched and loud
   B. expressive but pleasant
   C. low pitched and monotone
   D. none of the above

3. Of the following supplies, _____ is NOT necessary to answer the telephone efficiently?
   A. patient's chart
   B. message pad or notebook
   C. pen/pencil
   D. appointment book

4. Of the following, which ending of a telephone conversation is most appropriate?
   A. Bye bye
   B. Talk to ya later
   C. Ciao
   D. Thank you for calling, Ms. Jones

5. When speaking with a caller, a medical assistant should NEVER _____.
   A. identify himself or herself
   B. use slang terms
   C. ask questions
   D. listen attentively

6. When placing a caller on hold, the medical assistant should _____.
   A. ask the caller if they mind being on hold for a moment and then wait for response
   B. say, "Just a minute," and put the caller on hold
   C. say, "I'm putting you on hold," and then push the hold button
   D. none of the above

7. Which one of the following is NOT a common type of call a medical assistant would receive on a routine basis?
   A. Emergency
   B. Payment or account balance information request
   C. Appointment
   D. Sales/telemarketing

8. Which one of the following would NOT be an acceptable outgoing telephone call a medical assistant would make as part of a routine day?
   A. Call to mother about dinner plans
   B. Call to make outpatient appointments
   C. Call to change or confirm a patient's appointment
   D. All of the above are calls a medical assistant would routinely make

9. Which medical office professional would professionally handle an incoming call regarding a patient who has been poisoned?
   A. Physician
   B. Medical assistant
   C. Medical administrative assistant
   D. Pharmaceutical sales representative

10. If another physician calls the office to speak to the physician, you should _____.
    A. take a message and send the message to the physician
    B. transfer the call to the clinical medical assistant
    C. transfer the call immediately to the physician in most circumstances
    D. none of the above

11. When an outside laboratory calls with lab results, you should _____.
    A. transfer the call to the physician
    B. transfer the call to the individual requested by the lab
    C. transfer the call to the business office manager
    D. take a message and return the call later

12. If a patient "no-shows" an appointment, the medical assistant should _____.
    A. erase the patient's name so another patient can be scheduled
    B. write in ink next to the patient's name that the appointment was a no-show and document the occurrence in the patient's chart
    C. do nothing
    D. never schedule the patient for another appointment

13. The appointment book is a legal document; therefore, the medical assistant must use only _____ to write in the appointment book.
    A. green ink
    B. red ink
    C. black ink
    D. pencil

14. When a new patient calls the office for an appointment, you will need all of the following information EXCEPT _____.
    A. name
    B. address
    C. employer's name
    D. purpose of the visit

15. _____ gives each patient an appointment for a definite period of time.
    A. Wave scheduling
    B. Open-hour scheduling
    C. Cluster scheduling
    D. None of the above

16. Practices that schedule half of their patients on the hour and the other patients on the half-hour are using _____ scheduling.
    A. wave
    B. modified-wave
    C. cluster
    D. none of the above

17. _____ mail includes all sealed or unsealed letters up to and including 11 ounces.
    A. First class
    B. Second class
    C. Third class
    D. Fourth class

18. Which class of mail is used to send journals and magazines?
    A. First class
    B. Second class
    C. Third class
    D. Fourth class

19. When mailing an item that has a declared monetary value and is being sent first class, it is sent as _____ mail.
    A. certified
    B. insured
    C. registered
    D. restricted

20. Which one of the following describes how to correctly fold a letter for a size #10 envelope?
    A. Fold the letter in thirds face-up.
    B. Fold the letter in half and then into thirds face-down.
    C. Fold the letter in half face-up.
    D. Do not fold the letter.

21. Which one of the following does NOT apply when addressing an envelope?
    A. Use single spacing and block format.
    B. Use correct punctuation.
    C. Use the two-letter abbreviation for states.
    D. Use only capital letters to start words throughout the address.

22. When using letterhead, the _____ contains the name and address with Zip code to whom the letter is written.
    A. salutation
    B. enclosure notation
    C. inside address
    D. copy notation

23. The _____ notation lists all of the people receiving the letter in addition to the addressee.
    A. enclosure
    B. copy
    C. reference
    D. salutation

24. Immediately following a surgical procedure, a(n) _____ is dictated by the surgeon about the procedure.
    A. H&P report
    B. consultation report
    C. pathology report
    D. operative report

25. A(n) _____ is a final progress note about a patient who is leaving the hospital.
    A. radiology report
    B. H&P report
    C. discharge summary
    D. pathology summary

26. A(n) _____ includes the preliminary diagnosis for a patient's cause of death.
    A. H&P report
    B. discharge summary
    C. progress note
    D. autopsy report

Sentence Completion

Complete each sentence or statement.

1. Using _____ allows the medical assistant to indicate the reason for an appointment without writing out the reason using complete words and sentences.

2. A(n) _____ is any patient who has been seen in the past 3 years by the physician or provider in the practice.

3. A(n) _____ helps patients remember their next appointment and can be given to the patient at the end of their current appointment.

4. A second method of reminding a patient about their appointment is to give them a(n) _____.

5. The _____ is a great resource for familiarization of postal laws, regulations, and procedures.

6. Letters marked _____ are separated from other mail and delivered unopened to the person to whom they are addressed.

7. When you need to call a person or company in a different state, it is important to know in which _____ the person or company is located.

8. Most offices establish a _____ or develop some other format to block off time that is not to be used in patient scheduling.

9. In _____ scheduling, several appointments for similar types of examinations are grouped.

10. Before sending any written or keyed correspondence, you must _____ it to be certain the document is free of errors.

11. A(n) _____ is written for employees within the medical office setting to provide details about an upcoming event or meeting or to relay office policy decisions.

12. A(n) _____ is an article for a journal or other publication.

13. A(n) _____ is a person who listens to recorded dictation and converts it into a written document.

Short Answers

1. List the seven types of information documented when taking a telephone message.

_____

_____

_____

_____

_____

_____

_____

2. Why is it important to know the reason for a patient's office visit when making an appointment over the telephone?

_____

_____

_____

_____

3. Briefly describe the process of putting a caller on hold if more than one line is ringing.

_____

_____

_____

_____

4. List three pieces of information needed when scheduling an appointment for an established patient.

_____

_____

_____

5. Explain how to accommodate a patient who is habitually late for appointments.

_____

_____

_____

_____

6. List and describe the steps involved in preparing outgoing mail.

_____

_____

_____

_____

7. List the basic guidelines for effective written correspondence.

_____

_____

_____

_____

_____

8. List two complimentary closings in each of the following categories.

   Great respect: _____

   Formal: _____

   Less formal: _____

   Friendly: _____

CRITICAL THINKING

It has been an incredibly busy Monday and the telephones have not stopped ringing. You currently have six callers on hold. Prioritize each caller by using a scale of 1 to 6, with 1 being the most important call to handle and 6 being the least important call to handle, and then write a brief summary of how each of the following callers should be handled.

_____ a. Dr. Jacobs is on line 1 and is waiting to speak to the physician.
_____ b. Hartley is on line 2 and would like to make an appointment for next month.
_____ c. Sara Raphael is on line 3 and would like her prescription of Vicodin refilled as she is still in a lot of pain. This is her third refill request.
_____ d. Porter is on line 4 and is calling to discuss his wife's pregnancy test results.
_____ e. Caria Thopher is on line 5 with a personal call for the clinical medical assistant Grace.
_____ f. The laboratory is on line 6 and would like to give someone test results.

INTERNET RESEARCH

Keywords: Telephone Etiquette, Medical Appointment Scheduling.

Choose one of the following topics to research: Telephone etiquette; various methods of medical appointment scheduling. Write a two-paragraph report supporting your topic. Cite your source. Be prepared to give a 2-minute oral presentation should your instructor assign you to do so.

WHAT WOULD YOU DO?

If you have accomplished the objectives in this chapter, you will be able to make better choices as a medical assistant. Take a look at this situation and decide what you would do.

Tara is a new medical assistant at a physician's office. Dr. Vickers has hired her to answer the phone and to greet patients as they arrive, as well as to assist with making appointments as needed. On a particularly busy day, the phone is ringing with two lines already on hold, and a new patient arrives at the reception desk. Steve, the physician's assistant, asks Tara to make an appointment for another patient to see Dr. Vickers as soon as possible. Since the office makes appointments in a modified wave, Steve tells the patient to wait to be seen because Tara has found an opening in about a half-hour. In all the confusion Tara does not return to the patients who are on hold for several minutes, and one of the calls is an emergency. Furthermore, Tara is short-tempered with the new patient who has arrived at the office. Tara's frustration about the busy schedule she is expected to keep shows, and the new patient states that she is not sure that she has chosen the best physician's office for her medical care.

What effect will Tara's frustration have on this medical office? How would you have handled the situation differently?

1. Why is the role of the receptionist so important in putting a patient at ease?

   _____

   _____

2. When answering the phone, what are the voice qualities that are important in making a good impression?

   _____

   _____

3. What are the guidelines necessary in answering multiline calls?

   _____

   _____

   _____

   _____

4. What information should be obtained from a patient when making appointments?

   _____

   _____

   _____

   _____

5. Why is a patient information booklet important for a new patient?

   _____

   _____

   _____

   _____

6. What is modified-wave appointment scheduling? What are the problems with this type of scheduling?

   _____

   _____

   _____

   _____

7. How should Tara have handled the callers placed on hold?

_____

_____

_____

APPLICATION OF SKILLS

Procedure Check-off Sheets (*) and assignments from MACC CD (**)

1. Perform Procedure 22-1: Give Verbal Instructions on How to Locate the Medical Office.*

2. Perform Procedure 22-2: Create a Medical Practice Information Brochure.*

3. Perform Procedure 22-3: Answer a Multiline Telephone System.*
   A. MACC CD
   MACC/Administrative skills/General office duties/The telephone/Taking a telephone message.**
   Practice taking two telephone messages.

4. Perform Procedure 22-4: Prepare and Maintain an Appointment Book.*
   A. MACC CD
   MACC/Administrative skills/General office duties/Appointments/Preparing & maintaining the appointment book.**

5. Perform Procedure 22-5: Schedule a New Patient.*
   A. MACC CD
   MACC/Administrative skills/General office duties/Appointments/Scheduling a new patient**

6. Perform Procedure 22-6: Schedule Outpatient and Inpatient Appointments.*
   A. MACC CD
   MACC/Administrative skills/General office duties/Appointments/Scheduling an outpatient diagnostic test**
   B. MACC CD
   MACC/Administrative skills/General office duties/Appointment/Scheduling an inpatient admission and an inpatient surgical procedure**

7. Perform Procedure 22-7: Compose Business Correspondence.*
   A. MACC CD
   MACC/Professionalism/Communication/Proofreading written correspondence**

8. Perform Procedure 22-8: Compose a Memo.*

9. Perform Procedure 22-9: Transcribe a Machine-Dictated Document.*

Student Name _____ Date _____

PROCEDURE 22-1: GIVE VERBAL INSTRUCTIONS FOR LOCATING THE MEDICAL OFFICE

TASK: Provide verbal instructions to a caller on how to locate the medical office.
CONDITIONS: Given the proper equipment and supplies, the student will be required to give verbal instructions to a patient on how to locate the medical office.

EQUIPMENT AND SUPPLIES
- Telephone or telephone training system
- City map
- Pen or pencil
- Telephone/fax machine

STANDARDS: Complete the procedure within _____ minutes and achieve a minimum score of _____ %.

Time began _____   Time ended _____

Steps	Possible Points	First Attempt	Second Attempt
1. Gather equipment and supplies.	5		
2. Address the patient or caller in a polite and professional manner.	20		
3. Determine the place of origin for the patient.	10		
4. Determine the most direct route to the medical office, with alternate routes if possible. Provide the person with major cross streets or landmarks.	25		
5. Allow the caller sufficient time to write the directions.	10		
6. Provide the caller with the office's telephone number.	10		
7. Ask the caller if they have any questions.	10		
8. Politely end the call after answering any questions.	10		

Total Points Possible: 100

Comments: Total Points Earned _____ Divided by _____ Total Possible Points = _____ % Score

Instructor's Signature _____

Student Name _____ Date _____

PROCEDURE 22-2: CREATE A MEDICAL PRACTICE INFORMATION BROCHURE

TASK: Create a patient information booklet for a "mock" medical practice.
CONDITIONS: Given the proper equipment and supplies, the student will be required to create an informational brochure for his or her "mock" practice.

EQUIPMENT AND SUPPLIES
- Computer
- Software program that allows for brochure layouts
- Examples of local medical practice brochures and local medical office policies
- Pen or pencil

STANDARDS: Complete the procedure within _____ minutes and achieve a minimum score of _____ %.

Time began _____   **Time ended** _____

Steps	Possible Points	First Attempt	Second Attempt
1. Write and key a short paragraph describing each of the following topics and other information as needed.			
a. Description of the practice	10		
b. Physical location of facility	10		
c. Parking options	10		
d. Telephone numbers, e-mail addresses, and Web page	10		
e. Office hours	10		
f. Names and credentials of staff members	10		
g. Types of services	10		
h. Appointment scheduling and cancellation policies	10		
i. Payment options	10		
j. Prescription refill policy	10		
k. Types of accepted insurance	10		
l. Referral policy	10		
m. Release of records policy	10		
n. Emergency protocols	10		
o. Name of a contact person in the event the physician is unavailable	10		
p. Frequently asked questions	10		
q. Any special considerations	10		
2. Proofread the keyed paragraphs.	15		
3. Determine the layout of the brochure to provide ready access of information to patient. Include the following considerations:			
a. Visually pleasing	5		
b. Placement of logo	5		
c. Name, address, and telephone number of the practice prominently placed	5		

Steps	Possible Points	First Attempt	Second Attempt
4. Print the final version of the brochure. Submit to instructor.			

Total Points Possible: 100

Comments: Total Points Earned _____ Divided by _____ Total Possible Points = _____ % Score

Instructor's Signature _____

Student Name _____ Date _____

PROCEDURE 22-3: ANSWER A MULTILINE TELEPHONE SYSTEM

TASK: Answer a multiline telephone system in a professional manner, by responding to a request for action, placing a call on hold, transferring a call to another party, and accurately recording a message for action by another staff member or in a patient's medical record; either role-play or actual procedure.

CONDITIONS: Given the proper equipment and supplies, role-play with a student or instructor how to respond to a telephone requests for action, placing a call on hold, transferring a call to another party, and accurately recording a message for action by another staff member or in a patient's medical record.

EQUIPMENT AND SUPPLIES
- MACC CD/computer
- Telephone
- Appointment book
- Message pad
- Telephone emergency triage reference guide
- Physician referral sheet
- Pen or pencil
- Headset (optional)

STANDARDS: Complete the procedure within _____ minutes and achieve a minimum score of _____ %.

Time began _____   Time ended _____

Steps	Possible Points	First Attempt	Second Attempt
1. Answer the telephone by third ring using good telephone techniques. Speak distinctly with a pleasant tone, at a moderate rate, with sufficient volume.	50		
2. Greet with the appropriate time of day, identifying the office and yourself, verify the identity of the caller, and request the caller's telephone number.	10		
3. Provide the caller with the requested information or service concerning: 1) Appointments 2) Payments or account balance information 3) Physician referrals 4) Emergencies	40		
4. If you are unable to assist the caller, transfer the caller to the person who can assist by placing caller on hold and wait for a response. Transfer the call. If the caller does not want to hold, take a message.	10		
5. Multiple lines are ringing; use correct techniques for two ringing lines.	25		

Steps	Possible Points	First Attempt	Second Attempt
6. Take a message by collecting information for return of the call.	30		
7. Terminate the call in an appropriate manner.	25		

Total Points Possible: 200

Comments: Total Points Earned _____ Divided by _____ Total Possible Points = _____ % Score

Instructor's Signature _____

Student Name _____ **Date** _____

PROCEDURE 22-4: PREPARE AND MAINTAIN AN APPOINTMENT BOOK

TASK: Establish the matrix of an appointment book page and schedule a patient appointment.

CONDITIONS: Given the proper equipment and supplies, the student will be required to matrix an appointment book and schedule appointments.

EQUIPMENT AND SUPPLIES
- MACC CD/computer
- Appointment book
- Office policy for office hours and list of physician's availability
- Pencil

STANDARDS: Complete the procedure within _____ minutes and achieve a minimum score of _____ %.

Time began _____ **Time ended** _____

Steps	Possible Points	First Attempt	Second Attempt
1. Identify and mark the matrix according to office policy.	25		
2. Allow appointment times for emergency visits and unexpected needs.	10		
3. Schedule appointment(s) providing the needed information for appropriate patient care, for canceling appointments, and for efficient time management.	15		

Total Points Possible: 50

Comments: Total Points Earned _____ Divided by _____ Total Possible Points = _____ % Score

Instructor's Signature _____

Student Name _____ Date _____

PROCEDURE 22-5: SCHEDULE A NEW PATIENT

TASK: Schedule a new patient for an office visit.
CONDITIONS: Given the proper equipment and supplies, the student will be required to schedule a new
  patient appointment.

EQUIPMENT AND SUPPLIES
- MACC CD/computer
- Appointment book
- Telephone
- Pencil

STANDARDS: Complete the procedure within _____ minutes and achieve a minimum score of _____ %.

Time began _____   **Time ended** _____

Steps	Possible Points	First Attempt	Second Attempt
1. Obtain preliminary information necessary for scheduling an appropriate appointment.	10		
2. Obtain the patient's demographics information and chief compliant.	10		
3. Determine whether the patient was referred by another physician.	10		
4. Enter the appointment in the appointment book using information and alternatives for maintenance of appointment book.	10		
5. Obtain additional information at the time the appointment is made as per office policies or patient needs.	10		

Total Points Possible: 50

Comments: Total Points Earned _____ Divided by _____ Total Possible Points = _____ % Score

Instructor's Signature _____

Student Name _____ Date _____

PROCEDURE 22-6: SCHEDULE OUTPATIENT AND INPATIENT APPOINTMENTS

TASK: Schedule a patient for a physician-ordered test or procedure and admission, in both an outpatient and an inpatient setting or inpatient admission, with the time frame requested by the physician, confirm the appointment with the patient, and issue all required instructions

CONDITIONS: Given the proper equipment and supplies, the student will be required to schedule outpatient and inpatient appointments

EQUIPMENT AND SUPPLIES
- MACC CD/computer
- Physician's order for either an outpatient or an inpatient diagnostic test procedure or inpatient admission
- Patient chart
- Test preparation or preadmission instructions
- Telephone

STANDARDS: Complete the procedure within _____ minutes and achieve a minimum score of _____ %.

Time began _____   Time ended _____

Steps	Possible Points	First Attempt	Second Attempt
Outpatient			
1. Schedule appointment using an order for an outpatient diagnostic test(s) or procedure(s) and the expected time frame for results.	15		
2. Precertify the procedure(s) and/or test(s) with the patient's insurance company.	10		
3. Determine patient availability.	10		
4. Contact the facility and schedule the procedure(s) and/or test(s).	10		
5. Notify the patient of the arrangements.	10		
6. Conduct follow-up.	10		
Inpatient			
1. Schedule appointment using an order for an inpatient diagnostic test or procedure and the expected time frame for results.	15		
2. Precertify the procedure(s) and/or test(s) with the patient's insurance company.	10		
3. Determine patient availability.	10		
4. Contact the facility and schedule the procedure(s) and/or test(s).	10		
5. Notify the patient of the arrangements.	10		
6. Conduct follow-up.	10		
Inpatient			
1. Schedule hospital admission.	15		
2. Precertify the admission with the patient's insurance company.	10		
3. Determine patient availability.	10		

Steps	Possible Points	First Attempt	Second Attempt
4. Contact the facility and schedule the procedure(s) and/or test(s).	10		
5. Notify the patient of the arrangements.	10		
6. Conduct follow-up.	10		

Total Points Possible: 195

Comments: Total Points Earned _____ Divided by _____ Total Possible Points = _____ % Score

Instructor's Signature _____

Student Name _____ Date _____

PROCEDURE 22-7: COMPOSE BUSINESS CORRESPONDENCE

TASK: Compose, key, and proofread a business letter ready for mailing referring a patient to a specialist, using the guidelines of a common style.

CONDITIONS: Given the proper equipment and supplies, the student will be required to schedule compose, key, and proofread a business letter.

EQUIPMENT AND SUPPLIES
- MACC CD/Computer
- Word processor, computer with a printer, or typewriter
- Paper
- Letterhead stationery
- Telephone
- Pen/pencil

STANDARDS: Complete the procedure within _____ minutes and achieve a minimum score of _____ %.

Time began _____   Time ended _____

Steps	Possible Points	First Attempt	Second Attempt
1. Assemble all needed equipment and supplies.	5		
2. Prepare a rough draft of the letter.	25		
3. Proofread the letter and correct errors.	10		
4. Prepare the final draft of the letter and proofread for errors.	10		
5. Print a copy on letterhead and prepare document for signature by appropriate person.	10		
6. Prepare the correspondence for mailing.	20		
7. Add correct postage.	10		
8. Mail the letter.	10		

Total Points Possible: 100

Comments: Total Points Earned _____ Divided by _____ Total Possible Points = _____ % Score

Instructor's Signature _____

Student Name _____ Date _____

PROCEDURE 22-8: COMPOSE A MEMO

TASK: Compose, key, and proofread a memo.
CONDITIONS: Given the proper equipment and supplies, the student will be required to compose, key, and proofread a memo.

EQUIPMENT AND SUPPLIES
- Computer
- Paper
- Pen/pencil

STANDARDS: Complete the procedure within _____ minutes and achieve a minimum score of _____ %.

Time began _____   **Time ended** _____

Steps	Possible Points	First Attempt	Second Attempt
1. Assemble all needed equipment and supplies.	5		
2. Create a memo form, using the guidelines presented in the chapter.	15		
3. Fill in the required data.	10		
4. Ensure the format is correct.	10		
5. Distribute the memo to the proper recipients.	10		

Total Points Possible: 50

Comments: Total Points Earned _____ Divided by _____ Total Possible Points = _____ % Score

Instructor's Signature _____

Student Name _____ Date _____

PROCEDURE 22-9: TRANSCRIBE A MACHINE-DICTATED DOCUMENT

TASK: Transcribe a machine-dictated document, in the correct format and error free.
CONDITIONS: Given the proper equipment and supplies, the student will be required to transcribe, key, and proofread a machine-dictated document.

EQUIPMENT AND SUPPLIES
- Computer
- Transcription machine with foot pedal and headset
- Word processing software, computer with a printer, or typewriter
- Reference materials (English and medical dictionaries)
- Paper
- Pen/pencil
- Cassette tape with dictated materials

STANDARDS: Complete the procedure within _____ minutes and achieve a minimum score of _____ %.

Time began _____   Time ended _____

Steps	Possible Points	First Attempt	Second Attempt
1. Assemble all equipment and supplies.	5		
2. Turn on computer and transcription equipment.	5		
3. Adjust the volume and speed control to comfortable levels.	5		
4. Listen to the dictated report and key the document using the appropriate format.	25		
5. Proofread and edit the document using proofreading marks and reference materials.	25		
6. Make corrections.	5		
7. Print the document.	5		
8. Rewind the tape back to the beginning.	5		
9. Turn off equipment.	5		
10. Remove the cassette from the transcriber.	5		
11. Submit the original document, the proofread document, and the final draft to your instructor.	5		

Total Points Possible: 50

Comments: Total Points Earned _____ Divided by _____ Total Possible Points = _____ % Score

Instructor's Signature _____

CHAPTER QUIZ

Multiple Choice

Identify the letter of the choice that best completes the statement or answers the question.

1. A patient who has not been seen in the medical office for _____ is considered a new patient.
   A. 6 months
   B. 12 months
   C. 3 years
   D. 5 years

2. A letter that has all lines flush with the left margin, except for the first line of a new paragraph and date, closing, and signature lines, is in _____ format.
   A. modified-block
   B. full-block
   C. abstract
   D. manuscript

3. A _____ is a document used for formal publication.
   A. matrix
   B. memo
   C. progress notes
   D. manuscript

4. The importance of a triage manual is which one of the following?
   A. Helps the receptionist screen incoming calls and determine the level of urgency
   B. Provides the receptionist with information about the practice's policies and services
   C. Provides a list of routine questions to ask a patient scheduling an appointment
   D. None of the above

5. Which one of the following is not a piece of information you need to obtain when taking a telephone message?
   A. Caller's name
   B. Caller's telephone number
   C. Callers date of birth
   D. Caller's message

6. In which one of the following types of schedules does every patient have an appointment for a definite time?
   A. Wave scheduling
   B. Time-specified scheduling
   C. Modified-wave scheduling
   D. Cluster scheduling

7. _____ is used for interoffice communication.
   A. Manuscript
   B. Formal business letter
   C. Memo
   D. Journal

8. _____ help(s) the medical assistant see what needs to be corrected before sending out correspondence.
   A. Proofreader marks
   B. Dictionary
   C. Spell-check
   D. All of the above

9. _____ reports are initiated by the medical office before treatment begins.
   A. Radiology
   B. Consultation
   C. Discharge summary
   D. History and physical

10. _____ describes the surgical procedure and includes pathologic specimens, results, and personnel involved.
    A. H&P
    B. OP report
    C. Autopsy
    D. Discharge summary

11. _____ requires that someone listens to recorded information and produces the information in a written document.
    A. Dictation
    B. Proofreading
    C. Shorthand
    D. Transcription

12. _____ mail is used when it is necessary to prove that a letter was delivered.
    A. Registered
    B. Certified
    C. Express
    D. Overnight

13. _____ is(are) special services offered by both the U.S. Postal Service and Western Union.
    A. Air mail
    B. Telegram
    C. Mailgrams
    D. Express mail

14. If a patient calls the office with a question about an insurance payment, the _____ would typically handle the call.
    A. Physician
    B. Clinical medical assistant
    C. Administrative medical assistant
    D. None of the above

15. The abbreviation used on the appointment book for a complete physical exam is which one of the following?
    A. CPE
    B. CPX
    C. CPR
    D. None of the above

16. The abbreviation S/R noted in the appointment book means the patient is being seen for _____.
    A. Surgery
    B. Superficial reattachment
    C. Suture removal
    D. Sinus/respiratory disorder

17. Scheduling where more than one patient is booked for the same time slot on the schedule is called
    _____.
    A. cluster scheduling
    B. double booking
    C. modified-wave scheduling
    D. open-hour booking

18. Your physician just called the office; she is going to be 2 hours late to see patients this morning due to
    an emergency with a patient at the hospital. Which one of the following is the best way to handle this
    situation?
    A. Call the scheduled patients, explain the situation, and offer to reschedule their appointment.
    B. Call the scheduled patients and explain the situation and that it would be best if they could arrive
       at their scheduled time, as it will be a first-come first-serve basis when the physician arrives.
    C. Inform the patients of the delay, and ask them to wait patiently and offer them a beverage.
    D. None of the above

19. When scheduling a patient for a hospital admission, you must have a written order from the physician.
    A. True
    B. False

20. If the physician receives a letter marked "Personal," you should open it immediately, annotate it, and
    place on the physician's desk.
    A. True
    B. False

CHAPTER TWENTY-THREE

Medical Records and Chart Documentation

VOCABULARY REVIEW

Matching: Match each term with the correct definition.

A. acronym

B. active file

C. aging labels

D. caption

E. coding

F. conditioning

G. cross-reference

H. database

I. electronic medical record

J. filing

K. indexing

L. key unit

M. numeric filing

N. out guides

O. problem-oriented medical record

P. progress notes

Q. purge

R. SOAP

_____ 1. Patient medical records kept in a computer file; also called "paperless chart"

_____ 2. Data concerning a patient's medical care and its results

_____ 3. Method of filing that organizes records by their final digits

_____ 4. Words that describe the contents, name, or subject matter on a label

_____ 5. Method of arranging files using numbers

_____ 6. To clean out, as with excessive data in patient files

_____ 7. Type of chart format that divides each patient problem into subjective data, objective data, assessment, and plan for treatment

_____ 8. Process of removing staples and paper clips and mending a document before filing

_____ 9. Information source and storage

_____ 10. Separators that replace a file folder when it is removed from the file cabinet; contains a notation of the date and the name of who signed out the file

_____ 11. Arranging documents in a particular order for filing ease

S. sorting

T. terminal-digit filing

———— 12. Process of underlining a keyword to indicate how a document should be filed

———— 13. Word formed from the first letter of several words

———— 14. Chart format that is arranged according to a patient's health complaint

———— 15. First unit to be filed

———— 16. Notification system showing a file stored in more than one place

———— 17. Records of current patient

———— 18. Process of determining how a record will be filed

———— 19. Labels on a chart that identify the year

———— 20. Process of putting documents in a folder

THEORY RECALL

True/False

Indicate whether the sentence or statement is true or false.

———— 1. Medical records provide evidence of patient assessments, interventions, and communications

———— 2. Progress notes are a list of the current medications taken by the patient.

———— 3. SOAP formatting is extremely advantageous when more than one physician is treating the patient, because all information pertaining to a specific problem can be located in a concise format.

———— 4. The proper method of correcting errors in a medical record is to use correction fluid and reenter the correct information.

———— 5. The caption on a file label is used to identify the contents of the file.

Multiple Choice

Identify the letter of the choice that best completes the statement or answers the question.

1. The _____ process is the determination of how a record will be filed.
   A. indexing
   B. sorting
   C. annotating
   D. none of the above

2. In alphabetical filing, a _____ name is used as the key indexing unit.
    A. first
    B. middle
    C. last
    D. any of the above

3. Which of the following names would be filed before Mary Lynn Sommers?
    A. Mary Anne Winters
    B. M. Sorenson
    C. Mary Samuels
    D. Miriam Sommers

4. Which of the following names would be filed first?
    A. John Johnston
    B. Johnny Johnsten
    C. J. Jackson
    D. Jeremiah Jacobson

5. Which one of the following would be filed first?
    A. Professor Elijah Carlson
    B. President Eldon Anderson
    C. Congressman Elliason
    D. General George Franklin

6. _____ filing organizes a number by the final digits of the number.
    A. End-numeric
    B. Alpha-numeric
    C. First-digit
    D. None of the above

7. A file is "_____" when a checkmark is placed on the document indicating it should be filed.
    A. conditioned
    B. indexed
    C. sorted
    D. released

8. Inactive files are the files of a patient who has not visited the practice in _____.
    A. a time span set by the practice
    B. 1 year
    C. 3 years
    D. 7 years

9. A _____ is a reminder aid that organizes events by date.
    A. database file
    B. tickler file
    C. giggle file
    D. reminder file

10. Which one of the following files is NOT a standard form included in a patient record?
    A. Health history
    B. Consent to treatment
    C. Birth certificate
    D. Consent to disclose health information

11. If an established patient sees the physician for (a) _____, a new file must be made because the patient's complete health information would not be made available to an employer.
    A. pregnancy
    B. home-related injury
    C. work-related injury
    D. natural disaster

12. _____ regulations require providers to issue a written statement to each patient telling them about how the patient's health information may be used.
    A. HIPAA
    B. OSHA
    C. CLIA
    D. State

13. When initiating a file for a new patient, the first step in the procedure is to _____.
    A. create a file label
    B. attach alphabetic, color-coded labels
    C. attach an encounter form
    D. obtain and review a patient information form

14. If two patients have the exact same name, which of the following would determine which patient's file is filed first?
    A. Address
    B. Date of birth
    C. Social Security number
    D. The patient who has seen the physician more frequently

15. A _____ medical record is arranged according to the patient's health complaint.
    A. CCPH
    B. POMR
    C. SOAP
    D. none of the above

16. "My ankle hurts" is which one of the following types of information?
    A. Subjective
    B. Objective
    C. Assessment
    D. Plan

17. Which one of the following is "objective information"?
    A. There is swelling and bruising of the ankle and foot.
    B. The foot is hot to the touch.
    C. When the patient is walking to the exam room, you notice it is painful for the patient to put weight on the foot.
    D. All of the above is objective information.

18. All entries in a patient's record should begin with the _____.
    A. patient's name
    B. date of the encounter
    C. physician's signature
    D. none of the above

19. When choosing a filing system, the practice needs to consider all of the following EXCEPT _____.
    A. available space
    B. potential volume of patients
    C. available budget
    D. what is aesthetically pleasing

20. _____ has established rules to assist in efficient alphabetic filing.
    A. ARMA
    B. AAMA
    C. AHIMA
    D. None of the above

21. Which one of the following is a disadvantage to numeric filing?
    A. Expansion is unlimited.
    B. It is more confidential.
    C. It is easy to misfile.
    D. It is easy to remove inactive files.

22. The filing system that has stationary shelves and a door cover that slides up and back into a cabinet and can hold approximately 1000 records is a _____ file cabinet.
    A. vertical
    B. drawer
    C. lateral, open-shelf
    D. lateral, drawer

23. As computerization becomes increasingly sophisticated in medical offices, the use of electronic medical records is growing in popularity and will soon become the industry standard. Which one of the following is NOT an advantage of this type of system?
    A. All entries are legible.
    B. The record can be accessed by multiple practitioners at the same time.
    C. There is an inability to secure all records and maintain confidentiality.
    D. Printouts are easily retrieved.

24. _____ are dividers of a different size and color than a file folder. They should always be used when a file is removed from the storage system.
    A. Manila envelopes
    B. Out guides
    C. Book markers
    D. File labels

25. The _____ filing method uses letters of the alphabet to determine how files are arranged.
    A. Mendoza
    B. Alphabetical
    C. Numerical
    D. Indexing

Sentence Completion

Complete each sentence or statement.

1. _____ is the acronym for the Association of Records Mangers and Administrators.

2. Professional titles, general titles, and professional numeric and seniority suffixes are always indexed _____.

3. _____, articles, conjunctions, and symbols are considered separate indexing units.

4. In the _____ filing method, patient files are given numbers and arranged in numeric sequence.

5. Because patient addresses may change frequently, most medical offices use the patient's date of birth or _____ rather than the address when two patient names are identical.

6. Numbers expressed in digit form are indexed before alphabetic letters or words and _____ are filed before Roman numerals.

7. The files filed using the _____ filing method are more likely to be misfiled, and they must be constantly updated and maintained.

8. _____ filing is the most common form of numeric filing.

9. _____ a file prior to being filed ensures the file is in good condition because all staples and paper clips are removed and any torn edges are mended.

10. If the medical office does not have a computerized reminder system, it is an excellent idea for the medical assistant to create a(n) _____ about upcoming events such as license renewal, payments, and call-backs.

Short Answers

1. List the three steps for correcting an entry error in the patient's medical record.

   _____

   _____

   _____

2. State the three considerations for selecting a filing system.

   _____

   _____

   _____

3. Discuss the advantages and disadvantages of numeric filing.

   _____

   _____

   _____

   _____

4. Discuss the advantages and disadvantages of alphabetic filing.

   _____

   _____

   _____

   _____

5. List six supplies typically used with a filing system.

   _____

   _____

   _____

6. Explain the need to purge files regularly in a medical practice.

   _____

   _____

   _____

CRITICAL THINKING

Mr. Meredith called the office this morning inquiring about the status of lab results for his wife, Sharon. Sharon was seen last Friday in the office, and the lab results came in this morning. The lab reports have been filed in her patient file and are in a stack of files on Dr. Henry's desk for review. Describe how you would handle this call.

INTERNET RESEARCH

Keyword: Alphanumeric Filing Systems, Terminal Digit Filing Systems

Choose one of the following topics to research: Alphanumeric filing systems and terminal digit filing systems. Write a two-paragraph report supporting your topic. Cite your source. Be prepared to give a 2-minute oral presentation should your instructor assign you to do so.

WHAT WOULD YOU DO?

If you have accomplished the objectives in this chapter, you will be able to make better choices as a medical assistant. Take a look at this situation and decide what you would do.

Deanna is a new administrative medical-assisting extern at Dr. Juanea's office. Shirley, the office manager, asks Deanna to prepare a file for a new patient who will be seen tomorrow in the office. Shirley tells Deanna to be sure that she has color-coded the file folder and that the necessary forms have been included inside. In this office, the medical records are problem oriented, and all records are SOAP format; both are new concepts to Deanna, who was taught to prepare source-oriented records. After Deanna has prepared the new patient's file, Shirley asks her to pull the necessary records for tomorrow's appointments from the lateral open-shelf file cabinet containing patient records filed in alphabetic order. As she pulls the records, Deanna is to annotate the patient list for tomorrow's schedule. With the assistance of Shirley, Deanna will also purge the inactive patient records.

Would you be able to perform these tasks?

1. **Why is the medical record necessary? What are its uses?**

   _____

   _____

   _____

   _____

2. **What is meant by "color-coding" a patient file?**

   _____

   _____

3. What forms should Deanna be sure are in the new record?

_____

_____

_____

4. What is meant by "problem-oriented" medical records?

_____

_____

5. What does SOAP mean?

_____

_____

_____

6. What is a "source-oriented" patient record?

_____

_____

7. What are the advantages of open-shelf filing? What are the disadvantages?

_____

_____

_____

_____

8. Why is alphabetic filing advantageous? What are the disadvantages?

_____

_____

_____

_____

9. What will Deanna do to "annotate" a patient list?

_____

_____

_____

10. What is "purging" a file or a record? Why should patient records be purged on a regular basis?

_____

_____

_____

_____

APPLICATION OF SKILLS

Procedure Check-off Sheets (*) and assignments from MACC CD (**)

1. Perform Procedure 23-1: Pull Patient Records.*

2. Perform Procedure 23-2: Register a New Patient.*

3. Perform Procedure 23-3: Initiate a Patient File for a New Patient Using Color-Coded Tabs.*
   A. MACC CD MACC/Administrative skills/General office duties/The medical record/Initiating a medical file for a new patient**
      Set up and organize a medical file for a new patient that contains the personal data necessary for a complete record and any other information required by the medical office.
   B. MACC CD
      MACC/General office duties/The medical record/Color coding patient charts**

4. Perform Procedure 23-4: Add Supplementary Items to an Established Patient File.*
   A. MACC CD
      MACC/Administrative skills/General office duties/The medical record/Adding supplementary items to established patient file**
      Add supplemental documents and progress notes to patient files, observing standard steps in filing, while creating an orderly file that will facilitate ready reference to any item of information.

5. Perform Procedure 23-5: Maintain Confidentiality of Patients and Their Medical Records.*
   A. MACC CD
      MACC/Administrative skills/General office duties/The medical record/Preparing a record release form**

6. Perform Procedure 23-6: File Medical Records Using the Alphabetic System.*
   A. MACC CD
      MACC/Administrative skills/General office duties/The medical record/Filing medical records using the alphabetical system**
      Correctly file a set of patient charts, using an established alphabetical filing system.

7. Perform Procedure 23-7: File Medical Records Using the Numeric System.*
   A. MACC CD
      MACC/Administrative skills/General office duties/The medical record/Filing medical charts using the numeric system**
      Correctly file a set of patient charts, using an established numeric filing system.

Student Name _____ Date _____

PROCEDURE 23-1: PULL PATIENT RECORDS

TASK: Before the start of the business day, pull patient charts for daily appointment schedule.

CONDITIONS: Given the proper equipment and supplies, the student will be required to role-play with another student or an instructor the proper method for pulling patient records based on a full day's appointment schedule (10 to 12 patient files requested of 30 to 50 files).

EQUIPMENT AND SUPPLIES
- Computer
- Appointment book, appointment list
- Pen/pencil
- Tape
- Stapler
- Two-hole punch
- Patient files

STANDARDS: Complete the procedure within _____ minutes and achieve a minimum score of _____ %.

Time began _____   **Time ended** _____

Steps	Possible Points	First Attempt	Second Attempt
1. Assemble all equipment and supplies.	5		
2. Locate and review the day's schedule.	5		
3. Generate the daily appointment list (type, photocopy, or print from the computer).	5		
4. Identify the full name of each scheduled patient.	5		
5. Obtain the patient's records from the filing system; place a checkmark next to each patient's name on the appointment book as each record is obtained.	10		
6. Review each record for completeness.	5		
7. Annotate the appointment list with any special considerations.	5		
8. Arrange all records sequentially by appointment time.	5		
9. Place the records in a specified location that is out of view from unauthorized persons.	5		

Total Points Possible: 50

Comments: Total Points Earned _____ Divided by _____ Total Possible Points = _____ % Score

Instructor's Signature _____

Student Name _____ Date _____

PROCEDURE 23-2: REGISTER A NEW PATIENT

TASK: Complete a registration form for a new patient, obtaining all required information for credit and insurance claims.

CONDITIONS: Given the proper equipment and supplies, the student will be required to complete a new patient registration form by role-playing with another student or an instructor.

EQUIPMENT AND SUPPLIES
- Computer
- Registration form
- Pen
- Clipboard
- Private conference area

STANDARDS: Complete the procedure within _____ minutes and achieve a minimum score of _____ %.

Time began _____   Time ended _____

Steps	Possible Points	First Attempt	Second Attempt
1. Assemble all equipment and supplies.	5		
2. Establish a new patient status.	5		
3. Obtain and document the required information. (When role-playing this procedure, information obtained can be fictitious.)	25		
4. Review the entire form for completeness, make corrections as required.	15		

Total Points Possible: 50

Comments: Total Points Earned _____ Divided by _____ Total Possible Points = _____ % Score

Instructor's Signature _____

PROCEDURE 23-3: INITIATE A PATIENT FILE FOR A NEW PATIENT USING COLOR-CODED TABS

TASK: Set up and organize a file that contains the personal data necessary for a complete record and other information required by the medical office for a new patient. This should be completed using a color-coded filing system.

CONDITIONS: Given the proper equipment and supplies, the student will be required to initiate a patient file for a new patient using color-coded tabs.

EQUIPMENT AND SUPPLIES
- MACC CD/computer
- End-cut file
- A-Z color-coded tabs (self-adhesive)
- Blank file label (self-adhesive)
- Color-coded year label (annual age dating label)
- Medical alert or other label types as appropriate
- Forms:
  - Patient information
  - Assignment of benefits
  - Waiver
  - Treatment authorizations
  - Referral slips
  - Health history
  - Hospital discharge summaries
  - Surgery reports
  - Progress notes
  - Visit log
  - Prescription flow sheet
  - Laboratory reports
  - Diagnostic reports
  - Consultation reports
  - Miscellaneous correspondence

STANDARDS: Complete the procedure within _____ minutes and achieve a minimum score of _____ %.

Time began _____   **Time ended _____**

Steps	Possible Points	First Attempt	Second Attempt
1. Assemble all equipment and supplies.	5		
2. Obtain and review a completed patient information form.	10		
3. Place the completed and reviewed form on the left inside cover of the file, using the method preferred by the medical facility.	10		
4. Place progress note form and prescription flow sheet on the inside right cover of the file with the progress note form on top. File additional forms in reverse chronological order, meaning the most recent on top.	10		
5. Create a file label.	10		
6. Attach the file label in the center of the file tab.	10		
7. Attach alphabetic, color-coded labels.	10		
8. Attach the current year "aging" label above the first-name initial tab.	5		
9. Compile the file. Place the appropriate patient information, health history, and other forms in the patient file.	10		

Steps	Possible Points	First Attempt	Second Attempt
10. Attach a "Medical Alert" label on the front of the file.	5		
11. Prepare a ledger card or enter the patient information into a computerized management program.	10		
12. Attach an encounter form (super bill) to the outside of the patient's file.	5		

Total Points Possible: 100

Comments: Total Points Earned _____ Divided by _____ Total Possible Points = _____ % Score

Instructor's Signature _____

Student Name _____ Date _____

PROCEDURE 23-4: ADD SUPPLEMENTARY ITEMS TO AN ESTABLISHED PATIENT FILE

TASK: Add supplemental documents and progress notes to patient files, observing standard steps in filing while creating an orderly file that facilitates ready reference to any information.

CONDITIONS: Given the proper equipment and supplies, the student will be required to add supplementary items to an established patient file.

EQUIPMENT AND SUPPLIES
- MACC CD/computer
- Patient file
- Assorted documents (provided by instructor)
- Stapler
- Clear tape
- Two-hole punch
- Alphanumeric sorter

STANDARDS: Complete the procedure within _____ minutes and achieve a minimum score of _____ %.

Time began _____   Time ended _____

Steps	Possible Points	First Attempt	Second Attempt
1. Assemble all equipment and supplies.	5		
2. Retrieve the appropriate file from the file storage area.	5		
3. Condition the document.	5		
4. Release the document.	5		
5. Index and code the document.	10		
6. Sort for filing.	5		
7. File each document according to categories into the established patient's file, with the most recent document on top.	10		
8. Return file to the storage area.	5		

Total Points Possible: 50

Comments: Total Points Earned _____ Divided by _____ Total Possible Points = _____ % Score

Instructor's Signature _____

Student Name _____ Date _____

PROCEDURE 23-5: MAINTAIN CONFIDENTIALITY OF PATIENT INFORMATION AND THEIR MEDICAL RECORDS

TASK: Explain through role-playing how to maintain confidentiality of patient information and their medical records.

CONDITIONS: Given the proper equipment and supplies, the student will be required to explain how to maintain confidentiality of patient information and their medical records.

EQUIPMENT AND SUPPLIES
- MACC CD/computer
- Authorization form for "Release of Medical Records"
- HIPAA release form

STANDARDS: Complete the procedure within _____ minutes and achieve a minimum score of _____ %.

Time began _____   Time ended _____

Steps	Possible Points	First Attempt	Second Attempt
1. Assemble all supplies and equipment.	5		
2. Select a partner to be a patient as you assume the role of the administrative medical assistant.	5		
3. Explain to the "patient" through role-playing how the integrity of confidences shared in the office is maintained regarding the following medical office types	15		
a. Attorney is calling the office to gain information about a patient.	5		
b. Release of information about a minor	5		
c. Advertising and media	5		
d. Computerized medical records	5		
4. Explain to the "patient" through role-playing how confidences shared in the office are maintained regarding the following specialty topics.	15		
a. Child abuse	5		
b. Sexually transmitted diseases	5		
c. Sexual assault	5		
d. Mental health	5		
e. AIDS and HIV	5		
f. Substance abuse	5		
5. Explain to the "patient" through role-playing how the following situations regarding confidentiality issues are handled in the medical office.	15		
a. Subpoenaed medical records	5		
b. HIPAA guidelines	5		
c. Areas of mandated disclosure by state and federal regulations	5		
6. Explain to the "patient" through role-playing the "Patient's Bill of Rights."	15		

7. Explain to the "patient" through role-playing how
to complete an authorization form for release
of medical records   15

Total Points Possible: 150

Comments: Total Points Earned _____ Divided by _____ Total Possible Points = _____ % Score

Instructor's Signature _____

Student Name _____ Date _____

PROCEDURE 23-6: FILE MEDICAL RECORDS USING THE ALPHABETIC SYSTEM

TASK: Correctly file a set of patient records using an established alphabetic filing system.

CONDITIONS: Given the proper equipment and supplies, the student will be required to file medical charts using the alphabetic system.

EQUIPMENT AND SUPPLIES
- MACC CD/computer
- Patient files
- Alphanumeric sorter

STANDARDS: Complete the procedure within _____ minutes and achieve a minimum score of _____ %.

Time began _____   **Time ended** _____

Steps	Possible Points	First Attempt	Second Attempt
1. Assemble all supplies and equipment.	5		
2. Retrieve the appropriate patient files from the file storage area.	15		
3. Use an out guide.	10		
4. Complete documentation as appropriate.	15		
5. Add any supplemental forms or records generated according to office procedures.	15		
6. Sort the files alphabetically, using a "desktop sorter" if possible.	15		
7. Remove the files from the sorter and return the files to the storage area, correctly filing them alphabetically into the appropriate sequence.	15		
8. Remove out guide.	10		

Total Points Possible: 100

Comments: Total Points Earned _____ Divided by _____ Total Possible Points = _____ % Score

Instructor's Signature _____

Student Name _____ **Date** _____

PROCEDURE 23-7: FILE MEDICAL RECORDS USING THE NUMERIC SYSTEM

TASK: Correctly file a set of patient charts, using an established numeric filing system.

CONDITIONS: Given the proper equipment and supplies, the student will be required to file medical charts using a numeric system.

EQUIPMENT AND SUPPLIES
- MACC CD/computer
- Patient files
- Numeric sorter

STANDARDS: Complete the procedure within _____ minutes and achieve a minimum score of _____ %.

Time began _____   **Time ended** _____

Steps	Possible Points	First Attempt	Second Attempt
1. Assemble all supplies and equipment.	5		
2. Retrieve the proper numeric code from the appropriate system file.	15		
3. Use an out guide.	10		
4. Complete documentation as appropriate.	15		
5. Add any supplemental forms or records generated according to office procedures.	15		
6. Sort the files numerically, using a "desktop sorter" if possible.	15		
7. Remove the files from the sorter and return the files to the storage area, correctly filing them into the appropriate numeric sequence.	15		
8. Remove out guide.	10		

Total Points Possible: 100

Comments: Total Points Earned _____ Divided by _____ Total Possible Points = _____ % Score

Instructor's Signature _____

CHAPTER QUIZ

Multiple Choice

Identify the letter of the choice that best completes the statement or answers the question.

1. _____ is a method of arranging files using straight numbers.
   A. Alphabetical filing
   B. Numerical filing
   C. Terminal digit filing
   D. Problem-oriented filing

2. _____ is the process of determining how a record will be filed.
   A. Conditioning
   B. Indexing
   C. Coding
   D. Purging

3. Word(s) that describe the content's name or subject matter on a label is called _____.
   A. acronym
   B. key unit
   C. cross-reference
   D. caption

4. _____ is a chart format that uses dividers to separate the different types of patient information.
   A. Problem-oriented medical record format
   B. Electronic medical record format
   C. Source-oriented format
   D. None of the above

5. A type of chart format that divides each patient problem into subjective data, objective data, assessment, and plan for treatment is _____.
   A. SOAP
   B. POMR
   C. SOBP
   D. WRI

6. A _____ is entered into the patient's record and is used to update the status of the patient's health. These are added to the patient's chart each time the patient visits the office.
   A. problem list
   B. tickler file
   C. progress note
   D. caption

7. The physician owns the medical record, but the patient owns the information.
   A. True
   B. False

8. When might a medical assistant use a patient's date of birth as an indexing unit for filing?
   A. Never
   B. When two patients have the same name and same address
   C. When two patients have the same name but different addresses
   D. When a patient does not have a permanent address

9. Which one of the following names would be filed first?
   A. Lolita Gonzales
   B. Edward Green III
   C. Cleo Gonzales Esq.
   D. Juanita Esperanza

10. Which one of the following names would be filed second?
    A. Lolita Gonzales
    B. Edward Green III
    C. Cleo Gonzales Esq.
    D. Juanita Esperanza

11. Which one of the following names would be filed first?
    A. Aurelia Hunter
    B. Laura Hinkleman
    C. Sister Mary Catherine
    D. Kimberly Edades

12. Which one of the following names would be filed first?
    A. Timothy O'Shea
    B. Simon Samuelson
    C. Kelly Sherwin
    D. Belinda deLarue

13. Professional titles and professional, numeric, and seniority suffixes are always indexed _____.
    A. first
    B. second
    C. last
    D. does not matter

14. Which one of the following is a charting "DON'T"?
    A. Chart anything you did not see or do.
    B. Use black ink because it is easier to photocopy.
    C. Verify the name on the file before charting.
    D. All of the above are Don'ts.

15. Which one of the following is NOT part of the decision when selecting a filing system?
    A. Selection of supplies
    B. Types of storage equipment
    C. Available space
    D. All of the above would be considered when selecting a filing system.

16. In which filing system are records more protected in case of fire?
    A. Lateral-open shelf
    B. Vertical-drawer
    C. Rotary
    D. Lateral-drawer

17. _____ filing is most commonly used in small to medium-sized offices.
    A. Alphabetical
    B. Numerical
    C. Terminal-digit
    D. Geographical

18. Which one of the following is a disadvantage of direct filing?
    A. The correct spelling of the name must be known to find a folder.
    B. Alphabetical filing is the easiest system to learn.
    C. Only one sorting is required.
    D. None of the above

19. All punctuation is disregarded when indexing personal and business names.
    A. True
    B. False

20. When filing, the first name of the patient is considered the key unit.
    A. True
    B. False

CHAPTER TWENTY-FOUR

Financial Management

VOCABULARY REVIEW

Matching: Match each term with the correct definition.

A. accounting

B. accounts receivable

C. aging report

D. asset

E. balance sheet

F. credit

G. daysheet

H. debit

I. deposit

J. employee's withholding allowance certificate

K. endorse

L. exemption

M. financial statements

N. gross wages

O. income statement

P. liability

Q. net income

R. nonsufficient funds

_____ 1. Amount of money not able to be collected

_____ 2. Amount remaining after liabilities are subtracted from assets

_____ 3. Writing a check using future date, so check can be deposited only after date on check

_____ 4. State of a checkbook and a bank statement being in balance

_____ 5. To sign or place a signature on the back of a check that transfers the rights of ownership of funds

_____ 6. Report that shows how long debt has gone unpaid

_____ 7. Reports that indicate the financial condition of a business

_____ 8. Money placed in an account of a financial institution

_____ 9. Form that each new employee fills out to declare exemption from tax withholdings for earnings

_____ 10. Recording system using a specially designed document device for the increased efficiency of recording daily transactions; also called one-write system

S. one-write system

T. owner's equity

U. payable

V. payroll

W. pegboard system

X. postdated

Y. reconciled

Z. statement of owner's equity

AA. T-account

BB. third-party check

CC. transaction

DD. write-off

_____ 11. Total amount of money earned by employee before deductions are taken

_____ 12. Financial activity of a business

_____ 13. Indication that the payer did not have adequate funds in the bank to cover the amount of a check written

_____ 14. Numerical language of business that describes its activities

_____ 15. Record of patient transactions showing an amount due

_____ 16. Reports showing the results of income and expenses over time

_____ 17. Another name for pegboard system

_____ 18. Amount owed: debt

_____ 19. Employees' salaries, wages, bonuses, net pay, and deductions

_____ 20. Amount representing a payment: recorded on the right side of an accounting sheet

_____ 21. Amount of money earned that is not taxable

_____ 22. Resulting figure when income is greater than expenditures

_____ 23. Anything of value owned by a business that can be used to acquire other items

_____ 24. Amount representing a charge or debt owed: recorded on the left side of a T-account

_____ 25. Representing liability; accounts payable are money and funds owed to someone else

_____ 26. Check signed over to another party, who is not the original payee

_____ 27. Report on the financial condition of a business on a certain date

_____ 28. Journal for recording the day's activities

_____ 29. Tool used to analyze the effect of a transaction on an account

_____ 30. Report that shows changes in the owner's financial interest over time

THEORY RECALL

True/False

Indicate whether the sentence or statement is true or false.

_____ 1. A write-off is done when a portion or the entire amount of the charges cannot be collected.

_____ 2. The statement-receipt is a charge form that lists the ICD-9 and CPT codes most frequently used in the medical practice.

_____ 3. Checks marked paid in full should not be accepted unless the amount covers the entire current balance.

_____ 4. Bookkeeping is the basic process of recording the financial activities of the business.

_____ 5. The income statement reports the changes in the owner's financial interest during a reporting period and gives an explanation on why the investment has changed.

Multiple Choice

Identify the letter of the choice that best completes the statement or answers the question.

1. The legislation requiring a disclosure statement informing a patient of a procedure's total cost, including finance charges, which is required when a patient will make more than four payments, is called _____.
   A. Federal Insurance Contributions Act
   B. Federal Truth in Lending Act
   C. Federal Employees' Compensation Act
   D. Federal Unemployment Act

2. A(n) _____ is when money is prepared and sent to a financial institution to be placed in an account.
   A. deposit
   B. ABA number
   C. endorsement
   D. debit

3. _____ are sometimes given to other health care professionals and their families.
   A. Adjustments
   B. Professional discounts
   C. Write-offs
   D. Exemptions

4. Payroll is the financial record of employees' _____.
   A. salaries
   B. wages
   C. deductions
   D. all of the above

5. A(n) _____ is the amount of an individual's earnings that is exempt from income taxes based on the number of dependents.
   A. deduction
   B. exemption
   C. withholding
   D. none of the above

6. The total earnings paid to an employee after payroll taxes and other deductions have been taken is called _____.
   A. salary
   B. net pay
   C. wages
   D. all of the above

7. The legislation that provides funds to support retirement benefits, dependents of retired workers, and disability benefits is called _____.
   A. Federal Insurance Contribution Act
   B. Federal Unemployment Tax Act
   C. Federal Employees' Compensation Act
   D. none of the above

8. _____ acts as a journal for recording the day's activities.
   A. Daysheet
   B. Pegboard
   C. Ledger card
   D. Payroll register

9. _____ contains demographics about the patient as well as important billing information.
   A. Daysheet
   B. Pegboard
   C. Ledger card
   D. None of the above

10. _____ is a fixed fee that is paid by the patient at each office visit.
    A. Co-insurance
    B. Co-payment
    C. Restrictive endorsement
    D. None of the above

11. A(n) _____ shows the results of income and expenses over time, usually a month or year.
    A. balance sheet
    B. financial statement
    C. income statement
    D. accounts payable statement

12. A(n) _____ are reports that tell the owner the fiscal condition of the practice.
    A. balance sheet
    B. financial statement
    C. income sheet
    D. none of the above

13. A(n) _____ fund is an amount of cash kept on hand that is used for making small payments for incidental supplies.
    A. gross wages
    B. owner's equity
    C. petty cash
    D. none of the above

14. _____ is a document indicating the activity in an account.
    A. Statement-receipt
    B. Statement of ownership
    C. Statement
    D. Superbill

15. The _____ is also known as the Wage and Hour Law.
    A. Social Security law
    B. Federal Labor Standards Act
    C. Tax Payment Act
    D. Federal Unemployment Act

16. The _____ requires employers to not only withhold income tax and then pay it to the IRS but also keep accurate records of the names, addresses, and SS number of person(s) employed.
    A. Social Security law
    B. Federal Labor Standards Act
    C. Tax Payment Act
    D. Federal Unemployment Act

17. Federal law requires _____ to be deducted from the employee's gross pay.
    A. Social Security tax
    B. Medicare tax
    C. Federal income tax
    D. All of the above

18. _____ is(are) part of the accounting equation.
    A. Assets
    B. Liabilities
    C. Owner's equity
    D. All of the above

19. In T-accounts, the left side is also known as a(n) _____.
    A. asset
    B. credit
    C. debit
    D. equity

20. _____ is the listing of a physician's charges for service.
    A. Balance sheet
    B. Fee schedule
    C. Ledger cards
    D. None of the above

Sentence Completion

Complete each sentence or statement.

1. _____ is considered the "language" of business.

2. _____ reports the financial condition of a medical practice on a given date.

3. When a patient does not have enough money in his or her bank account, it will be returned

   for _____.

4. _____ is a person owing a debit.

5. _____ is also known as a superbill.

6. The resulting figure when income is greater than expenditures is called _____.

7. _____ is a paper showing the date, amount of transaction, what was purchased, and who

   purchased the item.

8. _____ is the listing of all cash and checks to be deposited to a certain account of a

   business's financial institution.

9. The amount remaining after the liabilities are subtracted from the assets is called _____.

10. A(n) _____ is an amount that is added or subtracted from the physician's fee, changing

    the patient's account balance.

Short Answers

1. List and explain the three important accounting principles.

   _____

   _____

   _____

   _____

   _____

2. Explain the two major purposes for using the pegboard system.

_____

_____

_____

_____

3. List the five verifications you must make in order to accept a check.

_____

_____

_____

4. Explain in detail the four types of endorsements.

_____

_____

_____

_____

_____

_____

5. Explain the four types of billing cycles.

_____

_____

_____

_____

_____

_____

CRITICAL THINKING

You started working for Dr. Palmer 2 weeks ago as the administrative medical assistant. Dr. Palmer asked you this morning to create a list of all the patients with an outstanding balance on their account, determine which accounts are overdue, and send collection letters to all patients with an outstanding account balance over 120 days. You determine that only one account, Marjory Kreswin, has an outstanding balance over 120 days past due. Draft a collection letter stating that she has 10 days to bring the balance current or you will be required to send her account to a collection agency.

INTERNET RESEARCH

Keyword: "Collection Regulations" in your state

Research the collection regulations in your state, and compose a list of 10 regulations. Cite your source. Be prepared to discuss your list of regulations with your classmates in an oral presentation should your instructor assign you to do so.

WHAT WOULD YOU DO?

If you have accomplished the objectives in this chapter, you will be able to make better choices as a medical assistant. Take a look at this situation and decide what you would do.

Meredith is the office manager for a private physician. She is responsible for the financial management of the office. She is the person who tracks the assets and liabilities for the accountant and interprets "owner equity" so that the physician will know the net value of the practice. As part of her job description Meredith also disburses petty cash. She makes sure that the vouchers, with receipts attached, and the cash on hand balance at the end of each workday. As each patient leaves the office, the payments for office visits are collected. The goal is to collect whatever is necessary from patients (co-payment, coinsurance) on the day of service. If patient receivables are current, outstanding insurance claims become the main focus for accounts receivable. Another one of Meredith's duties is to approve or disapprove of professional discounts and write-offs as fee adjustments. Finally, she generates collection letters and telephone calls for overdue and delinquent accounts.

Would you be able to perform these responsibilities in the medical office?

1. **What are assets? What are liabilities?**

   _____

   _____

   _____

   _____

2. **Why is it important for a physician to be aware of the owner equity before spending money for new equipment?**

   _____

   _____

   _____

   _____

3. What is petty cash, and how is it used by the medical office?

_____

_____

_____

4. Why is it important for Meredith to complete a petty cash voucher each time that money is removed from the petty cash fund?

_____

_____

_____

5. Why is it important to keep accounts receivable at a low level?

_____

_____

_____

6. What are professional discounts?

_____

_____

_____

7. What is a write-off?

_____

_____

_____

8. How should a collection phone call be handled?

_____

_____

_____

APPLICATION OF SKILLS

Procedure Check-off Sheets (*) and assignments from MACC CD (**)

1. Perform Procedure 24-1: Manage an Account for Petty Cash.*
   A. MACC CD
   MACC/Administrative skills/Financial management/Accounts receivable and payable/Accounting for petty cash**
   Establish a petty cash fund, maintain an accurate record of expenditures, and replenish the fund as necessary.

2. Perform Procedure 24-2: Post Service Charges and Payments Using a Pegboard System.*
   A. MACC CD
   MACC/Administrative skills/Financial management/Accounts receivable and payable/Posting service charges and payments using a pegboard**
   Post service charges and payments using a pegboard.

3. Perform Procedure 24-3: Record Adjustments and Credits.*
   A. MACC CD MACC/Administrative skills/Financial management/Accounts receivable and payable/Posting service charges and payments using a pegboard** (continued from Procedure 24-2 screens 18-55)

4. Perform Procedure 24-4: Prepare a Bank Deposit.*
   A. MACC CD
   MACC/Administrative skills/Financial management/Banking/Preparing a bank deposit**
   Correctly prepare a bank deposit for the day's receipts and complete appropriate office records related to the deposit.

5. Perform Procedure 24-5: Reconcile a Bank Statement.*
   A. MACC CD
   MACC/Administrative skills/Financial management/Banking/Reconciling a bank statement**
   Correctly reconcile a bank statement with the checking account.

6. Perform Procedure 24-6: Explain Professional Fees Before Services Are Provided.*

7. Perform Procedure 24-7: Establish Payment Arrangements on a Patient Account.*

8. Perform Procedure 24-8: Explain a Statement of Account.*
   A. MACC CD
   MACC/Administrative skills/Financial management/Billing and collection/Explaining professional fees**
   Explain the physician's fees so that the patient understands his or her obligations.

9. Perform Procedure 24-9: Prepare Billing Statements and Collecting Past-Due Accounts.*
   A. MACC CD
   MACC/Administrative skills/Financial management/Billing and collections/Preparing monthly billing statements**
   Process monthly statements and evaluate accounts for collection procedures.

Student Name _____ Date _____

PROCEDURE 24-1: MANAGE AN ACCOUNT FOR PETTY CASH

TASK: Establish a petty cash fund, maintain an accurate record of expenditures, and replenish the fund as necessary.

CONDITIONS: Given the proper equipment and supplies, the student will be required to file establish a petty cash fund, maintain an accurate record of expenditures, and replenish the fund as necessary.

EQUIPMENT AND SUPPLIES
- MACC CD/computer
- Petty cash box or envelope
- Petty cash expense record
- Petty cash vouchers with receipts or list of petty cash expenditures
- Two blank checks
- Calculator
- Pen or pencil

STANDARDS: Complete the procedure within _____ minutes and achieve a minimum score of _____ %.

Time began _____   Time ended _____

Steps	Possible Points	First Attempt	Second Attempt
1. Assemble all supplies and equipment.	5		
2. Establish the amount needed in the petty cash fund.	5		
3. Write a check for the determined amount, and put the cash in the petty cash box or envelope.	10		
4. Record the beginning balance to the petty cash record.	5		
5. Prepare a petty cash voucher for each amount withdrawn from the fund, and attach a sales receipt or an explanation of the payment.	10		
6. Enter each expense in the petty cash expense record, allocating them to the correct disbursement categories. Calculate the new balance remaining in the fund.	10		
7. When the fund balance has reached the established minimum, count the remaining currency in the petty cash box.	10		
8. Total all vouchers in the petty cash box.	10		
9. Add the voucher total to the amount in the petty cash fund. This should equal the original amount of the petty cash fund.	5		
10. Prepare a check for "cash" for the amount that was used from the fund for incidental expenses. Enter the check number on the petty cash expense record.	10		
11. Cash the check and add the replacement cash to the cash box.	5		

Steps	Possible Points	First Attempt	Second Attempt
12. Record the amount added to the fund on the expense record.	5		
13. Bring the balance forward.	10		

Total Points Possible   100

Comments: Total Points Earned _____ Divided by _____ Total Possible Points = _____ % Score

Instructor's Signature _____

Student Name _____   **Date** _____

PROCEDURE 24-2: POST SERVICE CHARGES AND PAYMENTS USING A PEGBOARD SYSTEM

TASK: Post service charges and payments using a pegboard.
CONDITIONS: Given the proper equipment and supplies, the student will be required to file post service charges and payments using a pegboard system.

EQUIPMENT AND SUPPLIES
- MACC CD/computer
- Pegboard
- Calculator
- Daysheet (daily journal)
- Receipt-charge slip
- Ledger cards
- Previous day's balance
- List of patients and services
- Fee schedule
- Pen or pencil

STANDARDS: Complete the procedure within _____ minutes and achieve a minimum score of _____ %.

Time began _____   **Time ended** _____

Steps	Possible Points	First Attempt	Second Attempt
1. Assemble all supplies and equipment.	5		
2. Prepare the pegboard for today's activities.	15		
3. Date the daysheet and carry forward appropriate balances.	10		
4. Obtain the ledger cards for patients scheduled for appointments.	10		
5. Prepare the ledger card and the charge slip as appropriate.	10		
6. Attach the charge slip to patient's chart and store ledger card as appropriate.	10		
7. Locate on the pegboard the receipt with the number that matches the number on the patient's charge slip.	10		
8. After professional visit, reinsert receipt-charge slip and the patient's ledger card to the daysheet and complete.	10		
9. Obtain payment and record the payment amount and the new balance.	10		
10. Remove the completed receipt from the pegboard and give the patient the receipt.	10		
11. Refile the ledger card.	10		
12. Check all columns of the daysheet using a pencil to verify totals are accurately recorded.	10		
13. At the end of the day, total the figures in each column, and add to prove sheet balances.	10		

Copyright © 2005 by Elsevier Inc.

Steps	Possible Points	First Attempt	Second Attempt
14. Add previous page totals and today's totals and prove balances of columns.	10		
15. Write in ink the proof totals on the bottom of the daysheet and add the total number of pages in the Sheet Number space at the top of the daysheet pages.	10		

Total Points Possible   150

Comments: Total Points Earned _____ Divided by _____ Total Possible Points = _____ % Score

Instructor's Signature _____

Student Name _____ Date _____

PROCEDURE 24-3: RECORD ADJUSTMENTS AND CREDITS USING A PEGBOARD SYSTEM

TASK: Record adjustments such as insurance payments, write-offs professional discounts, and nonsufficient funds (NSF) using pegboard.

CONDITIONS: Given the proper equipment and supplies, the student will be required to file record adjustments such as insurance payments, write-offs professional discounts and non-sufficient funds.

EQUIPMENT AND SUPPLIES
- MACC CD/computer
- Pegboard
- Calculator
- Daysheet (daily journal)
- Ledger cards
- Previous day's balance
- List of patients and services
- Fee schedule
- Pen/pencil

STANDARDS: Complete the procedure within _____ minutes and achieve a minimum score of _____ %.

Time began _____ **Time ended** _____

Steps	Possible Points	First Attempt	Second Attempt
Recording Adjustments			
1. Assemble all supplies and equipment.	5		
2. Obtain the patient's ledger card and align it on the daysheet.	10		
3. Complete ledger card as appropriate for a payment on account.	25		
4. Re-file the ledger card.	5		
5. Provide information for a refund if the patient's account has a credit balance showing the adjustment for the refund on the ledger card using the appropriate information.	15		
Recording Nonsufficient Funds			
1. Obtain the patient's ledger card and align it with the fist available empty row on the daysheet.	10		
2. Complete the ledger card as appropriate for recording an NSF check.	25		
3. Re-file the ledger card and prepare necessary documents for notification to patient.	5		
Total Points Possible	100		

Comments: Total Points Earned _____ Divided by _____ Total Possible Points = _____ % Score

Instructor's Signature _____

Student Name _____ Date _____

PROCEDURE 24-4: PREPARE A BANK DEPOSIT

TASK: Correctly prepare a bank deposit for the day's receipts and complete appropriate office records related to the deposit.

CONDITIONS: Given the proper equipment and supplies, the student will be required to prepare a bank deposit.

EQUIPMENT AND SUPPLIES
- MACC CD/computer
- Currency
- Checks for deposit
- Deposit slip
- Endorsement stamp (optional)
- Deposit envelope
- Pen or pencil

STANDARDS: Complete the procedure within _____ minutes and achieve a minimum score of _____ %.

Time began _____   Time ended _____

Steps	Possible Points	First Attempt	Second Attempt
1. Assemble all supplies and equipment.	5		
2. Organize currency.	5		
3. Count currency, then record amount on the bank deposit slip as appropriate.	10		
4. Prepare the checks for deposit.	15		
5. Complete the deposit slip, documenting each check appropriately.	15		
6. Total the amount of deposit, entering the total as appropriate.	5		
7. Record the appropriate amount of the deposit in the office checkbook.	10		
8. Photocopy the front and back of the deposit slip if duplicate deposit slip was not available.	5		
9. Place the currency, checks, and completed deposit slip in appropriate place for deposit.	5		

Total Points Possible   75

Comments: Total Points Earned _____ Divided by _____ Total Possible Points = _____ % Score

Instructor's Signature _____

Student Name _____ Date _____

PROCEDURE 24-5: RECONCILE A BANK STATEMENT

TASK: Reconcile a bank statement.

CONDITIONS: Given the proper equipment and supplies, the student will be required to reconcile a bank statement.

EQUIPMENT AND SUPPLIES
- MACC CD/computer
- Ending balance of previous statement
- Current bank statement
- Canceled checks for current month
- Checkbook stubs
- Calculator
- Pen or pencil

STANDARDS: Complete the procedure within _____ minutes and achieve a minimum score of _____ %.

Time began _____   Time ended _____

Steps	Possible Points	First Attempt	Second Attempt
1. Assemble all supplies and equipment.	5		
2. Compare the closing balance of the previous statement with the beginning balance of the current statement.	10		
3. Compare the checks written with the items on the statement using appropriate means to verify checks have cleared the bank.	20		
4. List and total the outstanding checks.	10		
5. Complete the bank statement reconciliation worksheet on the back of the bank statement, or apply the bank statement reconciliation formula.	10		
6. Reconcile deposits, including any positive adjustments made by bank.	10		
7. Add outstanding deposits to the bank statement reconciliation formula.	10		
8. Calculate the corrected bank statement balance.	10		
9. Adjust the checkbook balance by subtracting any bank charges that appear on the bank statement.	10		
10. If the checkbook balance and the statement balance do not agree, check the appropriate figures and make adjustments as necessary.	5		

Total Points Possible   100

Comments: Total Points Earned _____ Divided by _____ Total Possible Points = _____ % Score

Instructor's Signature _____

Student Name _____ Date _____

PROCEDURE 24-6: EXPLAIN PROFESSIONAL FEES BEFORE SERVICES ARE PROVIDED

TASK: Explain professional fees to the patient to provide understanding of his or her obligations before receiving services.

CONDITIONS: Given the proper equipment and supplies, the student will role-play with another student or an instructor how to explain professional fees to the patient.

EQUIPMENT AND SUPPLIES
- Physician's fee schedule
- Surgical cost estimate
- Estimate of medical expenses form
- Private area for discussion

STANDARDS: Complete the procedure within _____ minutes and achieve a minimum score of _____ %.

Time began _____   Time ended _____

Steps	Possible Points	First Attempt	Second Attempt
1. Assemble all supplies and equipment.	5		
2. Provide privacy for discussion.	5		
3. Display a professional attitude.	10		
4. Provide an estimate of anticipated fees before services are provided.	10		
5. Determine whether the patient has specific concerns that may hinder payment.	10		
6. Make appropriate arrangements for further discussion between the physician (instructor) and patient (student) if further explanation is necessary.	10		

Total Points Possible   50

Comments: Total Points Earned _____ Divided by _____ Total Possible Points = _____ % Score

Instructor's Signature _____

Student Name _____ Date _____

PROCEDURE 24-7: ESTABLISH PAYMENT ARRANGEMENTS ON A PATIENT ACCOUNT

TASK: Establish a payment plan for paying for services on a large ("high-dollar") or overdue account.
CONDITIONS: Given the proper equipment and supplies, the student will role-play with another student or an instructor making payment arrangements on a patient account.

EQUIPMENT AND SUPPLIES
- Patient's billing statement (ledger card and account information)
- Calendar
- "Truth in Lending Form"
- Paper
- Pen
- Private area for discussion

STANDARDS: Complete the procedure within _____ minutes and achieve a minimum score of _____ %.

Time began _____ Time ended _____

Steps	Possible Points	First Attempt	Second Attempt
1. Assemble all supplies and equipment.	5		
2. Determine that all information on the billing statement is correct.	10		
3. Discuss payment arrangements accepted by the practice.	20		
4. Explain any finance charges that will accrue on the account (for the purposes of this activity, use a 2% finance charge).	10		
5. Determine date of first payment.	5		
6. Prepare the "Truth in Lending" statement.	15		
7. Have the person responsible for the account sign the form if the agreement requires more than four installments.	10		
8. Document the agreement by making notes to the ledger card in the appropriate place in patient chart.	15		
9. Copy the statement and provide copy to patient. Place original in patient record or other place as appropriate under office policy.	10		
Total Points Possible	100		

Comments: Total Points Earned _____ Divided by _____ Total Possible Points = _____ % Score

Instructor's Signature _____

Student Name _____ Date _____

PROCEDURE 24-8: EXPLAIN A STATEMENT OF ACCOUNT TO A PATIENT

TASK: Explain a statement of account to a patient to provide understanding of his or her obligations.
CONDITIONS: Given the proper equipment and supplies, the student will role-play with another student or an instructor the explanation of a statement of account to a patient.

EQUIPMENT AND SUPPLIES
• MACC CD/computer
• Patient statement
• Patient information form
• Encounter form(s)
• Physician's fee schedule
• Private area for discussion

STANDARDS: Complete the procedure within _____ minutes and achieve a minimum score of _____ %.

Time began _____   Time ended _____

Steps	Possible Points	First Attempt	Second Attempt
1. Assemble all supplies and equipment.	5		
2. Determine that the patient has the correct statement and discover what seems to be the problem.	5		
3. Examine the statement for any possible errors.	10		
4. Review with the patient each of the items that appears on the statement.	15		
5. If an error is located, correct it immediately and apologize to the patient.	5		
6. Address patient concerns hindering payment arrangements.	5		
7. If there was no error and your discussion does not resolve the patient's concerns, make arrangements for a discussion between the physician and patient to resolve the problem.	5		

Total Points Possible   50

Comments: Total Points Earned _____ Divided by _____ Total Possible Points = _____ % Score

Instructor's Signature _____

Student Name _____ **Date** _____

PROCEDURE 24-9: PREPARE BILLING STATEMENTS AND COLLECT PAST-DUE ACCOUNTS

TASK: Process monthly statements and evaluate accounts for collection procedures.

CONDITIONS: Given the proper equipment and supplies, the student will prepare statements for billing and process collection letter(s) for past-due accounts.

EQUIPMENT AND SUPPLIES
- MACC CD/computer
- Patient ledger card
- Patient information form
- Collection form letters
- Computer
- Stationary and envelopes
- Collection agency commission requirements
- Pen or pencil

STANDARDS: Complete the procedure within _____ minutes and achieve a minimum score of _____ %.

Time began _____   **Time ended** _____

Steps	Possible Points	First Attempt	Second Attempt
Preparing Billing Statements			
1. Assemble all supplies and equipment.	5		
2. Determine the billing schedule for the medical practice (provided by instructor).	5		
3. Determine the accounts with outstanding balances.	20		
4. Separate the accounts for routine billing and for past-due actions.	20		
Performing Routine Billing			
5. Prepare ledger cards for billing statements.	25		
6. Print out computer-generated statements as applicable.	25		
7. Prepare statements for mailing.	15		
Collecting Past-Due Accounts			
8. Obtain all patient ledger cards with past-due balances.	15		
9. Separate accounts according to the action required, according to length of aging of account.	15		

Steps	Possible Points	First Attempt	Second Attempt
10. Create the appropriate form letter for each account using company stationery, "mail" (turn in to the instructor) to the patient or turn accounts over to collection agency (instructor) as appropriate.	55		

Total Points Possible 200

Comments: Total Points Earned _____ Divided by _____ Total Possible Points = _____ % Score

Instructor's Signature _____

CHAPTER QUIZ

Multiple Choice

Identify the letter of the choice that best completes the statement or answers the question.

1. _____ is an amount owed by the medical practice.
   A. Asset
   B. Liability
   C. Owner's equity
   D. None of the above

2. _____ reports the changes in the owner's financial interest during a reporting period and why the interest has changed.
   A. Bank statement
   B. Financial statement
   C. Income statement
   D. Statement of owner's equity

3. _____ is a special device used to write the same information on several forms at one time.
   A. Daysheet
   B. Encounter form
   C. Pegboard
   D. None of the above

4. _____ is a charge form that lists the ICD-9 and CPT codes most frequently used in the medical practices.
   A. Receipt-charge slip
   B. Encounter form
   C. Superbill
   D. Both B and C

5. _____ is collected to support the federal health insurance program for people aged 65 and older.
   A. FUTA
   B. FICA
   C. Medicare tax
   D. SUTA

6. The Wage and Hour Law is also known as the Fair Labor Standards Act.
   A. True
   B. False

7. _____ records debit and credit activity of a patient in the practice.
   A. Financial statement
   B. Income statement
   C. Ledger card
   D. None of the above

8. _____ is a numbered form used to track petty cash withdrawals.
   A. Transaction
   B. Ledger
   C. Voucher
   D. all of the above

9. The pegboard system is also known as the one-write system.
   A. True
   B. False

10. An AR report that is beneficial to the financial success of the medical practice is called the _____ report.
    A. aging
    B. financial
    C. summary
    D. none of the above

11. _____ is a fixed percentage of a medical cost, paid by the patient.
    A. Co-pay
    B. Co-insurance
    C. Both A and B
    D. None of the above

12. _____ is(are) part of the accounting equation.
    A. Assets
    B. Liabilities
    C. Owner's equity
    D. All the above

13. _____ endorsement is a type of endorsement in which only a signature is listed on the back of the check.
    A. Blank
    B. Restrictive
    C. Qualified
    D. None of the above

14. The amount recorded on the right side of the T-account is called a debit.
    A. True
    B. False

15. _____ contains demographics about the patient as well as important billing information.
    A. Financial statement
    B. Ledger cards
    C. Encounter forms
    D. None of the above

16. When accepting a check for payment, you must verify _____.
    A. current address
    B. correct provider name
    C. affixed signature
    D. All of the above

17. The ABA number _____.
    A. helps to identify the payer's bank
    B. is located on the right corner of each check
    C. helps to identify the location of the bank
    D. all the above

18. Federal law requires _____ to be deducted from a person's gross pay.
    A. SUTA
    B. Medicare tax
    C. medical insurance premiums
    D. none of the above

19. Total earnings paid to an employee after payroll taxes and other deductions have been taken out is called gross pay.
    A. True
    B. False

20. Accounting is considered the language of business.
    A. True
    B. False

CHAPTER TWENTY-FIVE

Medical Coding

VOCABULARY REVIEW

Matching

Match each term with the correct definition.

A. acute

B. chief complaint

C. concurrent condition

D. contributory factors

E. diagnosis

F. eponym

G. established patient

H. guidelines

I. instructional terms

J. key components

K. main term

L. medical decision making

M. medical necessity

N. morbidity rate

O. new patient

P. pertinent past, family, and social history

Q. presenting problem

R. primary diagnosis

_____ 1. Condition considered as the patient's major health problem; used in outpatient coding

_____ 2. Occurring over the long term or recurring frequently

_____ 3. *ICD-9-CM* supplementary codes for factors influencing health status and reasons for contact with health services when a diagnosis needs further explanation or when the patient has no disease process for coding

_____ 4. Rules that determine items necessary to interpret and report procedures and services appropriately

_____ 5. Issues that affect a decision

_____ 6. Disease, condition, noun, synonym, or eponym that helps the coder find the correct code or range of codes in an index

_____ 7. *ICD-9-CM* supplementary codes for external causes of injury and poisoning

_____ 8. Person who has not received professional services from the physician, or another physician of the same practice, within the past 3 years

_____ 9. Three main factors taken into account when selecting a level of E/M service in *CPT* coding

S. referral

T. review of systems

U. secondary condition

V. subjective findings

W. E-codes

X. V-codes

Y. chronic

Z. coordination of care

AA. history of present illness

BB. modifier

CC. greatest specificity

DD. principal diagnosis

_____ 10. Transfer of a patient's care to another health care provider at the request of a member of the health care team

_____ 11. Occurring now; of short-term duration

_____ 12. Approach to managing a patient's care when a provider asks other health care providers to assist

_____ 13. Documentation that verifies a procedure is needed

_____ 14. Chronological description of the patient's present illness from the first sign or symptom to the present

_____ 15. Pertinent background information about a patient's family and the patient visiting a health care provider

_____ 16. Condition that occurs at the same time as the primary diagnosis and affects the patient's treatment or recovery from the primary condition

_____ 17. Rate of disease or illness or proportion of diseased persons in a given population or location

_____ 18. Condition the patient experiences at the same time as the primary diagnosis

_____ 19. Statement in the patient's own words describing the reason for the office visit; should be documented in the patient's words

_____ 20. Information provided by the patient and generally not measurable by health care professionals

_____ 21. Determination of the nature of a disease based on signs, symptoms, and laboratory findings

_____ 22. Symptoms, disease, or condition that is currently causing a problem and that is the reason for the patient visiting a health care provider

_____ 23. Person who has been treated by a member of the health care team in the past 3 years

_____ 24. How the physician looks at all the information gathered on examining and testing the patient and then factors this into a decision for a treatment plan

_____ 25. Inventory of body systems obtained through a series of questions seeking to identify signs and symptoms that the patient may be experiencing or has experienced

_____ 26. Words or phrases that have a special meaning to provide needed information

_____ 27. Person or persons for whom something has been named, or the name is so derived

_____ 28. Means by which the reporting physician can indicate a service or procedure performed has been altered by some specific circumstance, but its definition or code has not changed

_____ 29. Coding to the highest level of documentation available; not using only a three-digit code when a four- or five-digit code exists to better describe the disease or procedure

_____ 30. Diagnosis, determined after study, that was the cause for a patient's hospital admission; used only for inpatient coding

THEORY RECALL

True/False

Indicate whether the sentence or statement is true or false.

_____ 1. "Diagnosis" is defined as determining the nature of a disease based on signs, symptoms, and laboratory findings.

_____ 2. A primary diagnosis is the condition established to be chiefly responsible for triggering the admission of the patient to the hospital for treatment.

_____ 3. CPT stands for Current Procedural Terminology.

_____ 4. Chief complaint is a statement usually made by the patient in his or her own words that describes the reason for the visit.

_____ 5. The U.S National Center for Health Services is used to track mortality and morbidity rates.

Multiple Choice

Identify the letter of the choice that best completes the statement or answers the question.

1. Volume _____ of the *ICD-9-CM* is a numerical listing of the diseases and injury codes and consists of 17 chapters.
   A. 1
   B. 2
   C. 3
   D. 4

2. Volume _____ of the *ICD-9-CM* is included when it will be used specifically for hospital coding.
   A. 1
   B. 2
   C. 3
   D. 4

3. The first *CPT* manual appeared in _____.
   A. 1956
   B. 1966
   C. 1976
   D. none of the above

4. _____ is a key component in a determination of the level of E/M service to be selected.
   A. History
   B. Examination
   C. The difficulty of medical decision making
   D. All of the above

5. Volume _____ of the *ICD-9-CM* consists of an alphabetic listing of terms and codes.
   A. 1
   B. 2
   C. 3
   D. 4

6. _____ provide a classification of environmental events, circumstances, and conditions as the cause of injury, poisoning, and other adverse effects.
   A. E-codes
   B. V-codes
   C. *ICD-9*-codes
   D. *CPT*-codes

7. _____ owns and publishes the disease classification and releases an updated version of *ICD* about every 10 years.
   A. London Bills of Mortality
   B. World Health Organization
   C. Health Insurance Portability and Accountability
   D. None of the above

8. _____ is a type of examination.
   A. Comprehensive
   B. Detailed
   C. Problem focused
   D. All of the above

9. _____ is a type of medical decision making.
   A. High complexity
   B. Straightforward
   C. Moderate complexity
   D. All of the above

10. A medical record must include _____.
   A. the nature of the problem
   B. the appropriate amount of time spent with the patient
   C. both A and B
   D. none of the above

11. In _____, the U.S. Congress passed the Medical Catastrophic Coverage Act.
   A. 1937
   B. 1948
   C. 1988
   D. 2000

12. _____ is a disorder that is affecting the patient at the same time as the primary diagnosis but not necessarily affecting the prognosis of the primary condition.
   A. Concurrent condition
   B. Secondary condition
   C. Systemic condition
   D. None of the above

13. The _____ is used by hospitals and allows for up to four concurrent conditions, ranked in the order of severity.
   A. CMS 1500
   B. UB-92
   C. both A and B
   D. none of the above

14. Volume _____ codes of the *ICD-9-CM* represent the means for the hospital to receive reimbursement for their facility overhead.
   A. 1
   B. 2
   C. 3
   D. 4

15. Effective diagnostic and procedural coding requires _____.
   A. a good knowledge of terminology
   B. familiarity with the *ICD-9* and *CPT*
   C. discipline to read all explanations from medical records
   D. all of the above

Sentence Completion

Complete each sentence or statement.

1. The _____ code manual lists and describes codes for services and procedures.

2. _____ codes are temporary codes used for new technology, services, and procedure.

3. _____ requires the health care provider to render a service at the request of another health care professional, such as a second opinion.

4. The _____ is whatever symptoms, illness, or injury is causing the encounter.

5. _____ is death from a particular disease.

6. In *CPT*, Volume 1 all titles and codes are printed in _____.

7. _____ are groups of four-digit code numbers listed after three-digit categories.

8. _____ is information regarding past events.

9. _____ are additional information segments related to coding.

10. A(n) _____ is a patient who has not received any professional services from the physician, or another physician of the same practice, within the past 3 years.

Short Answers

1. List six agencies and organizations that use *ICD-9-CM* codes.

_____

_____

_____

2. Explain what "main term" means, and list four items represented by main terms in *ICD-9-CM* coding.

_____

_____

_____

_____

3. Explain the purpose of the *ICD-9-CM* system.

_____

_____

_____

4. Explain three factors that must be determined before the process of E/M coding begins

_____

_____

_____

_____

5. Explain what a "special report" should include.

_____

_____

_____

_____

CRITICAL THINKING

Dr. Peterson has asked you to update her podiatric clinic's superbill with new diagnostic and procedure codes. She handed you the following list and would like you to have it completed by the end of the day.

1. Locate the procedure codes for the following:
   a. Office Visits—New Patient
      1) Problem Focused   _____
      2) Expanded Focused   _____
      3) Detailed   _____
   b. Office Visits—Established Patient
      1) Problem Focused   _____
      2) Expanded Focus   _____
      3) Detailed   _____

c. Consultations
   1) Initial Visit   _____
   2) Expanded Focused   _____
   3) Detailed   _____
   4) Comprehensive   _____
   5) Second Opinion   _____
   6) Special Report   _____
d. Injections
   1) Tendon/Ligament   _____
   2) Small Joint/Bursae   _____
   3) Nerve Block   _____
   4) Intralesional Injection   _____
e. Casts and Splints
   1) Flexible Cast (unna)   _____
   2) Short Leg Walker   _____
   3) Impression Cast   _____
   4) Short Leg Cast   _____
   5) AirCast Pneumatic   _____
f. Supplies
   1) Foot Orthoses, Rigid   _____
   2) Sterile Tray, Major   _____
   3) Post-op Shoe   _____
   4) Medication   _____
g. Radiology
   1) Foot, 2 Views   _____
   2) Foot, 3 Views   _____
   3) Ankle, 2 Views   _____
   4) Ankle, 3 Views   _____
h. Surgery
   1) Abscess, Skin I&D   _____
   2) Aspiration, Cyst   _____
   3) Debride Infected Skin   _____
   4) Nail Avulsion   _____
   5) Nail/Matrix Excision   _____
   6) Remove Foreign Body Subq   _____

2. Locate the diagnostic codes for the following:
   a. Abscess Cellulitis   _____
   b. Abscess Plantar   _____
   c. Arthritis, Osteo   _____
   d. Gout   _____
   e. Bunion   _____
   f. Contusion   _____
   g. Cyst, Inclusion   _____
   h. Dermatitis, Contact   _____
   i. Diabetes Mellitus   _____
   j. Fibroma, Plantar   _____
   k. Fracture, Toe   _____
   l. Ganglion, Synovial   _____
   m. Hammer Toe   _____
   n. Lymphedema   _____
   o. Neuritis   _____
   p. Onychocryptosis   _____

q. Raynaud's Disease _____
r. Tarsal Tunnel Syndrome _____
s. Tendinitis Achilles _____
t. Tinea Pedis _____
u. Ulcer, Pressure _____
v. Varicose Veins _____
w. Verruca _____
x. Xerosis _____

INTERNET RESEARCH

Keywords: Diagnostic Coding, Procedural Coding

Choose one of the following topics to research: Diagnostic Coding guidelines or Procedural Coding guidelines. Cite your source. Be prepared to give a 2-minute oral presentation should your instructor assign you to do so.

WHAT WOULD YOU DO?

If you have accomplished the objectives in this chapter, you will be able to make better choices as a medical assistant. Take another look at this situation and decide what you would do.

Jenny, a medical assistant, is the insurance clerk in a large medical practice. She has been with the practice for 10 years and has gradually learned how to perform coding. She uses the *ICD-9-CM* codes and the *CPT-4* codes daily. Phyllis, a longtime patient, was seen today with a chief complaint of a sore throat, influenza, and a chronic cough. Phyllis has diabetes mellitus and hypertension as well as chronic obstructive pulmonary disease. The physician not only examined her respiratory tract and listened to her heart but checked her other body systems as well. He also reviewed her symptoms and took a past history as it related to her presenting symptoms. The medical decision making was more complex for Phyllis because many medications used for cough contain sugar.

When Phyllis left the office, Jenny immediately began the process of coding her visit. Would you be able to code this visit?

1. **Why is coding a medical visit so important, and what is actually being accomplished by coding?**

   _____

   _____

   _____

2. **What part of the medical visit is coded using *ICD-9-CM* codes?**

   _____

   _____

   _____

3. What part of the medical visit is coded using *CPT* codes?

_____

_____

4. What is a diagnosis?

_____

_____

5. What is the difference between Volume 1 and Volume 2 of the *ICD-9-CM* manual?

_____

_____

_____

6. What is a chief complaint? Which of the above symptoms is the chief complaint?

_____

_____

_____

7. What is the primary diagnosis above? Concurrent conditions? Secondary conditions?

_____

_____

_____

_____

_____

8. Why are words such as "probable," "suspected," and "rule out" not used with outpatient diagnosis coding?

_____

_____

_____

_____

_____

9. **How would you code the *CPT* E/M code pertaining to the history above? How would you use *CPT* codes for the medical decision making?**

_____

_____

_____

_____

_____

APPLICATION OF SKILLS

Procedure Check-off Sheets (*) and Assignments from MACC CD (**)

1. Perform Procedure 25-1 Diagnostic Coding.*
   A. MACC CD
      MACC/Administrative skills/Health insurance activities/Assigning ICD-9-CM codes**
      Assign the proper *ICD-9-CM* code based on medical documentation for auditing and billing purposes.

2. Perform Procedure 25-2 Procedural Coding.*
   A. MACC CD
      MACC/Administrative skills/Health insurance activities/Assigning CPT codes**
      Assign the proper *CPT* code based on medical documentation for auditing and billing purposes.

Student Name _____ Date _____

PROCEDURE 25-1: DIAGNOSTIC CODING

TASK: Assign the proper *International Classification of Diseases (ICD-9-CM)* code based on medical documentation to the highest degree of specificity.

CONDITIONS: Given the proper equipment and supplies, the student will assign the proper *ICD-9-CM* code based on medical documentation to the highest degree of specificity.

EQUIPMENT AND SUPPLIES
- MACC CD/computer
- Current *ICD-9-CM* codebook
- Medical dictionary
- Patient's medical records
- Pen or pencil

STANDARDS: Complete the procedure within _____ minutes and achieve a minimum score of _____ %.

Time began _____   Time ended _____

Steps	Possible Points	First Attempt	Second Attempt
1. Assemble all supplies and equipment.	5		
2. Identify the key term in the diagnostic statement.	10		
3. Locate the diagnosis in the Alphabetic Index (Volume 2, Section 1) of the *ICD-9-CM* codebook.	20		
4. Read and use footnotes, symbols, or instructions.	15		
5. Locate the diagnosis in the Tabular List (Volume 1).	10		
6. Read and use the inclusions and exclusions noted in the Tabular List.	10		
7. Assign the code to the highest degree of specificity appropriate.	20		
8. Document in the medical record.	10		
9. Ask yourself these final questions (NO points awarded for this section).	0		
a. Have you coded to the highest degree of specificity?			
b. When you transferred the code to the patient form and to subsequent records and forms, did you record the code accurately?			
c. Are there any secondary diagnoses or conditions addressed during the encounter that need to be coded?			

Total Points Possible: 100

Comments: Total Points Earned _____ Divided by _____ Total Possible Points = _____ % Score

Instructor's Signature _____

Student Name _____ Date _____

PROCEDURE 25-2: PROCEDURAL CODING

TASK: Assign the proper *Current Procedural Terminology* (CPT) code to the highest degree of specificity based on medical documentation for auditing and billing purposes.

CONDITIONS: Given the proper equipment and supplies, the student will assign the proper (CPT) code to the highest degree of specificity based on medical documentation for auditing and billing purposes.

EQUIPMENT AND SUPPLIES
- MACC CD/computer
- Current *CPT* codebook
- Medical dictionary
- Patient's medical records
- Pen or pencil

STANDARDS: Complete the procedure within _____ minutes and achieve a minimum score of _____ %.

Time began _____   **Time ended** _____

Steps	Possible Points	First Attempt	Second Attempt
1. Assemble all supplies and equipment.	5		
2. Read the introduction, guidelines, and notes of a current *CPT* codebook.	10		
3. Review all service and procedures performed on the day of the encounter; include all medications administered and trays and equipment used.	20		
4. Identify the main term in the procedure.	15		
5. Locate the main term in the alphabetical index. Review any subterms listed alphabetically under the main term.	10		
6. Verify the code sets in the tabular (numerical) list. Select the code with the greatest specificity.	10		
7. Determine if a modifier is required.	20		
8. Assign the code using all necessary steps for proper code determination.	10		
9. Ask yourself these final questions (NO points awarded for this section). a. Have you coded to the highest degree of specificity? b. When you transferred the code to the patient form and to subsequent records and forms, did you record the code accurately? c. Are there any secondary diagnoses or conditions addressed during the encounter that need to be coded?	0		

Total Points Possible: 100

Comments: Total Points Earned _____ Divided by _____ Total Possible Points = _____ % Score

*Instructor's Signature*_____

CHAPTER QUIZ

Multiple Choice

Identify the letter of the choice that best completes the statement or answers the question.

1. _____ are codes used for external causes of injury and poisoning.
   A. A
   B. E
   C. V
   D. J

2. Volume _____ is included in the *ICD-9 CM* manual only when it will be used specifically for hospital coding.
   A. 1
   B. 2
   C. 3
   D. none of the above

3. The first *CPT* book appeared in _____ as a result of an effort by the AMA to create a method of accurately and universally identifying all medical and surgical procedures and services.
   A. 1938
   B. 1945
   C. 1966
   D. 1978

4. The *ICD-9-CM* books are updated every _____ years.
   A. 5
   B. 7
   C. 10
   D. 12

5. The _____ is used by hospitals and allows for up to four concurrent conditions, ranked in the order of severity.
   A. CMS 1500
   B. UB-92
   C. both A and B
   D. none of the above

6. "Diagnosis" is defined as the determination of the nature of a disease based on signs, symptoms, and laboratory findings.
   A. True
   B. False

7. *ICD-9* Volume _____ consists of an alphabetic listing of terms and codes with special tables.
   A. 1
   B. 2
   C. 3
   D. 4

8. Effective diagnostic and procedural coding requires _____.
   A. a good knowledge of terminology
   B. familiarity with the *ICD-9-CM* and *CPT*
   C. discipline to read all explanations from medical records.
   D. all of the above

9. In 1948, the World Health Organization developed a publication that could be used to track morbidity rates.
   A. True
   B. False

10. In the *ICD-9-CM* Volume _____, all of the titles and codes are printed in bold.
    A. 1
    B. 2
    C. 3
    D. 4

11. Volume _____ of the *ICD-9-CM* is the numerical listings of disease and injury codes and consists of 17 chapters.
    A. 1
    B. 2
    C. 3
    D. 4

12. _____ is a key component in a determination of the level of E/M service to be selected.
    A. History
    B. Examination
    C. Difficulty of medical decision making
    D. All of the above

13. _____ codes are supplementary codes for factors influencing health status and reasons for contact with health services when a diagnosis needs further explanation or when the patient has no disease process for coding.
    A. E
    B. F
    C. J
    D. V

14. A primary diagnosis is the condition considered to be the patient's major health problem.
    A. True
    B. False

15. CPT stands for Current Procedure Terminology.
    A. True
    B. False

16. A medical record must include the _____.
    A. nature of the problem
    B. appropriate amount of time spent with the patient
    C. both A and B
    D. none of the above

17. The semicolon is critical when coding procedures.
    A. True
    B. False

18. _____ is NOT a type of examination.
    A. Comprehensive
    B. Detailed
    C. Problem focused
    D. Exhaustive

19. In *ICD-9-CM* coding, a main term represents a _____.
    A. disease
    B. condition
    C. noun
    D. all of the above

20. Chief complaint is a statement usually made by the patient in his or her own words that describes the reason for the visit.
    A. True
    B. False

CHAPTER TWENTY-SIX

Medical Insurance

VOCABULARY REVIEW

Matching

Match each term with the correct definition.

A. allowable charges

B. birthday rule

C. capitation

D. CHAMPVA

E. clearinghouse

F. CMS-1500

G. comprehensive plan

H. coordination of benefits

I. cost containment

J. curriculum vitae

K. explanation of benefits

L. fraud

M. gatekeeper

N. HCFA Common Procedure Coding System

O. HIPAA

P. health maintenance organization

Q. indemnity plan

R. major medical benefits

_____ 1. Person retired from the U.S. military services

_____ 2. Medical insurance plan that covers both basic and major medical costs

_____ 3. American Hospital Association 2003 update of "Patient's Bill of Rights"

_____ 4. Person or company involved in the physician-patient relationship but not part of implied contract

_____ 5. Amount of a professional service fee that an insurance company is willing to accept

_____ 6. Type of physician's resume listing education, in-service training, hospital affiliations, professional organizations, and any publications written

_____ 7. Insurance plan in which patients pay the provider and submit a claim form for reimbursement from their insurance company

_____ 8. Form sent by the insurance carrier to the patient and the medical practice that explains the amount of reimbursement or the reason for denial of a submitted claim

_____ 9. 10-digit lifetime identification number issued to health care providers by Medicare

S. managed care

T. national provider identification

U. nonparticipating provider

V. partial disability

W. patient care partnership

X. precertification

Y. preferred provider organization

Z. primary care physician

AA. release of information

BB. resource-based relative value scale

CC. third party

DD. TRICARE

EE. usual, customary, and reasonable

FF. veteran

_____ 10. Organization that receives electronic claim forms from medical providers and processes them for payment

_____ 11. Physician responsible for most of the ongoing care of a patient

_____ 12. Scale that uses a complex formula to determine Medicare fees based on geographical area expenses

_____ 13. Managed care plan that pays a predetermined amount to a provider over a set time regardless of the number of services rendered to their subscribers in the period

_____ 14. Civilian Health and Medical Program of the Department of Veterans Affairs; health benefits program that provides coverage to the spouse or widow(er) of a U.S military veteran

_____ 15. Primary care physician designated by an HMO to provide ongoing care to a patient and to authorize referrals to specialists when deemed necessary

_____ 16. Insurance rule that states the policy of the parent whose birthday is first in the calendar year holds the primary insurance for any dependent

_____ 17. Health insurance claims form, also known as the "universal" claim form that can be filled with all insurance companies; formally HCFA-1500

_____ 18. Standardized coding system that uses CPT, national, and local codes to process Medicare claims; used primarily for supplies, materials, injections, and certain procedures and services not defined in CPT

_____ 19. State in which a person can perform a portion of his or her job duties

_____ 20. Organization that provides comprehensive health care services for plan participants at a fixed rate

_____ 21. Health care system that provides a list of providers who have signed a contract with the insurance carrier to provide services to the insured

_____ 22. Comprehensive federal health care program for all active duty and retired U.S. military personnel and eligible family members; formally known as CHAMPUS

_____ 23. Insurance term stating that total reimbursement from primary and secondary insurance companies will not exceed the total cost of the charges

_____ 24. Intentional misrepresentation of medical facts as they relate to a claim for health care services

_____ 25. Insurance coverage beyond basic medical benefits used for expenses incurred by lengthy illness or serious injury

_____ 26. Physician who has not signed a contract with an insurance company to participate in health care for the insured

_____ 27. Referring to typically charged or prevailing fees for health care services in a geographical area

_____ 28. Term referring to methods used to control the rising cost of health care

_____ 29. Method used for determining in advance how much the patient's insurance policy will reimburse for a particular service or procedure

_____ 30. Federal legislation to improve health insurance availability for those who lose coverage

_____ 31. Network of health care services and benefits designed for a group of individuals who pay premiums to join the insurance plan

_____ 32. Authorization signed by the patient that gives the provider permission to disclose certain health information to the insurance carrier or other health care providers or pertinent parties (e.g., attorney) as deemed appropriate

THEORY RECALL

True/False

Indicate whether the sentence or statement is true or false.

_____ 1. A preferred provider organization is a health care delivery arrangement that offers insured individuals certain incentives if they choose health care providers from a list of those who are contracted with the PPO.

_____ 2. The Consolidated Omnibus Reconciliation Act (COBRA) was enacted in 1996 and requires employers with five or more employees to continue to offer coverage of their group health plan up to 18 months in the event of voluntary or involuntary termination of employment.

_____ 3. Disability income insurance is insurance that pays benefits to the policyholder if he or she becomes unable to work as a result of an illness or injury that is not related to work.

_____ 4. A medical savings account is only used for medical care with taxed dollars.

_____ 5. CMS-1500 is the name given to a universal claim form used to report outpatient services to all government programs.

Multiple Choice

Identify the letter of the choice that best completes the statement or answers the question.

1. _____ rules apply when a patient is covered by more than one insurance policy.
   A. Co-payment
   B. COB
   C. Co-insurance
   D. Managed care

2. _____ is(are) (a) reason(s) for dramatic increases in health care costs.
   A. Underpayment of premiums
   B. Overuse and misuse of medical supplies
   C. Not enough people wanting insurance
   D. Increase in the elderly population

3. _____ have policies in which major medical and basic benefits apply.
   A. Comprehensive plans
   B. Fee-for-service plans
   C. Managed care plans
   D. PPOs

4. _____ is a method of structuring fees.
   A. Usual, customary, and reasonable
   B. Capitation
   C. Relative value scale
   D. All of the above

5. _____ is a method of setting Medicare fees.
   A. RVU
   B. RBRVS
   C. RVS
   D. URC

6. The Medicare program was developed in _____, initially as a national health insurance for elderly people.
   A. 1932
   B. 1948
   C. 1959
   D. 1966

7. CHAMPVA is a health benefits program that provides coverage to the spouse or widower and to the children of veterans who _____.
   A. are rated permanently and totally disabled because of service-connected disability
   B. were rated permanently and totally disabled because of a service-connected condition at the time of death
   C. died during active duty and whose dependents are not otherwise eligible for TRICARE benefits
   D. all of the above

8. _____ is when an individual has loss of speech, loss of hearing in both ears, loss of sight in both eyes, or loss of the use of two limbs.
   A. Total disability
   B. Partial disability
   C. Residual disability
   D. Catastrophic disability

9. _____ is a secondary insurance policy for Medicare-eligible individuals.
   A. MediCal
   B. Medicaid
   C. MediGap
   D. Medi-Medi

10. _____ is a statement giving the health care provider permission to disclose certain health information to the patient's insurance carrier.
    A. ROI
    B. OCR
    C. FECA
    D. RVS

11. A(n) _____ has no errors or omissions and is the best defense against delays or rejections.
    A. clean claim
    B. electronic claim
    C. paper claim
    D. quick claim

12. _____ policy is an insurance policy purchased by a company for its employees or by a group representing similar professions.
    A. Individual
    B. Private
    C. Group
    D. Public

13. CMS is responsible for the operation of the Medicare program and for the selection of the regional insurance companies, called _____.
    A. fiscal intermediaries
    B. adjusters
    C. agents
    D. none of the above

14. The patient must be _____ years of age to qualify for Medicare, unless the person is disabled.
    A. 55
    B. 60
    C. 65
    D. 70

15. _____ covers nonmilitary employees of the federal government.
    A. FICA
    B. FECA
    C. HCFA
    D. SSDI

Sentence Completion

Complete each sentence or statement.

1. _____ is a term used to describe and measure the various health care services and encounters rendered in connection with a specific injury or period of illness.

2. _____ is an insurance contract purchased by individuals who are not eligible for group policies or who do not qualify for government-sponsored plans.

3. _____ is the method used for determining in advance how much the patient's insurance policy will reimburse or pay for a particular service or procedure.

4. _____ is an organization that receives claims from medical facilities, checks them for completeness and accuracy, and forwards them electronically to the proper carrier.

5. The primary care physician who can refer patients to specialists is also known as the _____.

6. A(n) _____ is the yearly amount the patient "must pay out of pocket" before the insurance will pay on any claims.

7. A(n) _____ is the monthly, quarterly, or annual payment for insurance coverage.

8. _____ is a state in which an individual is unable to perform the requirements of any
   employment.

9. _____ is an organized group of participating providers for an insurance plan; policies may
   have "in-network" or "out-of-network" benefits.

10. _____ is an agent; insurance company that processes Medicare claims.

Short Answers

1. Explain how insurance companies establish UCR fees.

   _____

   _____

   _____

2. Explain the two ways HMOs are organized.

   _____

   _____

   _____

3. Explain in detail the three parts of Medicare.

   _____

   _____

   _____

   _____

4. Explain the advantages of electronic claims over paper claims.

   _____

   _____

   _____

   _____

5. List those who are eligible for TRICARE.

_____

_____

_____

_____

_____

CRITICAL THINKING

You have a patient, Celeste, whose parents are getting divorced. Celeste's mother is the parent who typically brings Celeste to the doctor. On this visit, however, Celeste's father brings her in. He claims that Celeste's mother is responsible for paying her doctor bills. You personally know that her father is supposed to carry the insurance policy for Celeste. How would you handle this situation? Research on the Internet or using resources in your community to answer this question.

INTERNET RESEARCH

Keywords: Medicare, Medicaid, any third-party carrier such as Blue Cross/Blue Shield, Principal Mutual, etc.

Choose one of the following topics to research: Medicare guidelines for your state, Medicaid guidelines for your state, or any third-party carrier. Cite your source. Be prepared to give a 2-minute oral presentation should your instructor assign you to do so.

WHAT WOULD YOU DO?

If you have accomplished the objectives in this chapter, you will be able to make better choices as a medical assistant. Take another look at this situation and decide what you would do.

Dr. Jay has hired Maria as his insurance clerk. Maria's previous experience was with household liability claims and coverage. She has not had experience with the CMS-1500 or with coding of medical conditions. She is not aware that the claim begins with the appointment and patient registration, and ends with payment by the insurer. Jude Beck, a new patient of Dr. Jay, is seen in the office for what appears to be diabetes mellitus. An ECG, urinalysis, and blood test were done during the visit without checking with Mr. Beck's insurance first. In his notes Dr. Jay states that he must "rule out diabetes mellitus," so Maria codes this as the "primary diagnosis" and sends the claim without a final diagnosis. When the results of the lab work are received, Dr. Jay documents in the medical record that the final diagnoses are dehydration and hypertension with tachycardia. When the registration form was completed, Mr. Beck failed to check off which of his insurance companies is primary and which is secondary. In processing the claim, Maria sends it with a diagnosis of "diabetes mellitus" to one of the two insurance companies, which turns out to be the secondary insurer. The claim is denied because there is no EOB attached from the primary payer. Maria does not resubmit the claim to the company that is actually the primary carrier. Could you explain to Maria what went wrong and how the claim should have been handled?

1. Why is it important for the registration form to be completed accurately?

   _____

   _____

   _____

2. Why would the secondary insurance not pay for the claim before payment by the primary carrier?

   _____

   _____

   _____

3. What are the guidelines for coding a "rule out" diagnosis in the outpatient setting?

   _____

   _____

   _____

   _____

4. Why is preauthorization so important when dealing with insurance?

   _____

   _____

   _____

   _____

5. What is the implication for Mr. Beck of Maria not tracking the claims?

   _____

   _____

   _____

   _____

6. What is an "EOB"?

   _____

   _____

7. Why does the EOB of primary insurance need to be sent to the secondary insurance?

_____

_____

_____

8. Why is a "clean claim" so important in obtaining insurance payment?

_____

_____

_____

_____

APPLICATION OF SKILLS

Procedure Check-off Sheets (*) and Assignments from MACC CD (**)

1. Perform Procedure 26-1: Apply Managed Care Policies and Procedures.*
   A. MACC CD
      MACC/Administrative skills/Health insurance activities/Obtaining a managed care precertification**
      Obtain precertification from a patient's HMO for requested services or procedures.
   B. MACC CD
      MACC/Administrative skills/Health insurance activities/Obtaining a managed care referral**
      Obtain a referral from a patient's HMO for requested consultation or treatment.

2. Perform Procedure 26-2: Complete the CMS-1500 Claim Form.*
   A. MACC CD
      MACC/Administrative skills/Health insurance activities/Assigning _ICD-9-CM_ codes**
      Assign the proper _ICD-9-CM_ code based on medical documentation for auditing and billing purposes.
   B. MACC CD
      MACC/Administrative skills/Health insurance activities/Assigning CPT codes**
      Assign the proper CPT codes based on medical documentation for auditing and billing purposes.
   C. MACC CD
      MACC/Administrative skills/Health insurance activities/Completing and insurance claim form**
      Apply third-party guidelines to prepare an insurance claim.
      Complete an insurance claim form.
      Use physician's fee schedule to determine the charges.

Student Name _____ Date _____

PROCEDURE 26-1: APPLY MANAGED CARE POLICIES AND PROCEDURES

TASK: Obtain precertification from a patient's HMO for requested services or procedures. Obtain a referral from a patient's HMO for requested consultation or treatment.

CONDITIONS: Given the proper equipment and supplies, the student will role-play with another student or an instructor applying managed care policies and procedures.

EQUIPMENT AND SUPPLIES
- MACC CD/computer
- Photocopy of patient's insurance identification card
- Patient's information form
- Patient's encounter form
- Patient's medical record
- Precertification form
- Pen or pencil

STANDARDS: Complete the procedure within _____ minutes and achieve a minimum score of _____ %.

Time began _____   Time ended _____

Steps	Possible Points	First Attempt	Second Attempt
1. Assemble all supplies and equipment.	5		
2. Gather the documents and information necessary to obtain a managed care precertification.	5		
3. Review the records to be sure all information is available.	5		
4. Complete the precertification/referral form.	5		
5. Proofread the entire form to ensure it is accurate.	15		
6. Send the form to the insurance carrier for review and action (submit to the instructor).	5		
7. Wait for a response from the managed care organization (instructor returns paper).	5		
8. Process and place a copy of the completed form in the patient's file. Give the original to the patient (student).	5		

Total Points Possible: 50

Comments: Total Points Earned _____ Divided by _____ Total Possible Points = _____ % Score

Instructor's Signature _____

Student Name _____ Date _____

PROCEDURE 26-2: COMPLETE THE CMS-1500 CLAIM FORM

TASK: Apply third-party guidelines and use a physician's fee schedule to complete an insurance claim form.

CONDITIONS: Given the proper equipment and supplies, the student will role-play with another student or an instructor completing a CMS-1500 claim form.

EQUIPMENT AND SUPPLIES
- MACC CD/computer
- Photocopy of the patient's insurance identification card
- Patient's information form
- Patent's encounter form
- Patient's medical record
- Physician's fee schedule
- CMS-1500 insurance claim form
- Pen or pencil

STANDARDS: Complete the procedure within _____ minutes and achieve a minimum score of _____ %.

Time began _____   Time ended _____

Steps	Possible Points	First Attempt	Second Attempt
1. Assemble all supplies and equipment.	5		
2. Identify the patient's primary third-party payer, or the company or agency to which the claim will be submitted.	15		
3. Enter the name and address of the third-party payer in the top right corner of the insurance form using all-capital letters and no punctuation.	15		
4. Complete blocks 1–13 of the form.	50		
5. Complete the Physician/Supplier Section, blocks 14–33 of the CMS-1500 form.	100		
6. Review the claim for completion and corrections.	15		
7. Submit the claim (to instructor).	0		

Total Points Possible: 100

Comments: Total Points Earned _____ Divided by _____ Total Possible Points = _____ % Score

Instructor's Signature _____

CHAPTER QUIZ

Multiple Choice

Identify the letter of the choice that best completes the statement or answers the question.

1. _____ rules apply when a patient is covered by more than one insurance policy.
   A. Co-payment
   B. COB
   C. Co-insurance
   D. Managed care

2. Disability income insurance is insurance that pays benefits to the policyholder if he or she becomes unable to work as a result of an illness or injury that is not related to work
   A. True
   B. False

3. _____ program was developed in 1966, initially as a national health insurance for elderly people.
   A. Medicaid
   B. Workers' Compensation
   C. Blue Cross/Blue Shield
   D. Medicare

4. COBRA was enacted in 1985 and requires employers of _____ or more employees to continue to offer coverage in their group health care plan to former employees.
   A. 5
   B. 10
   C. 20
   D. 50

5. Medical savings accounts are only used to pay for medical care with pretax dollars.
   A. True
   B. False

6. CMS is responsible for the operation of the Medicare program and for selection of the regional insurance companies, called _____.
   A. fiscal intermediaries
   B. adjusters
   C. agents
   D. none of the above

7. _____ is one of the methods of structuring fees.
   A. Relative value scale
   B. Capitation
   C. Usual, customary, and reasonable
   D. All the above

8. A person who is not permanently disabled must be _____ years of age to qualify for Medicare.
   A. 55
   B. 60
   C. 65
   D. 68

9. _____ is a method of setting Medicare fees.
    A. RVU
    B. RBRVS
    C. RVS
    D. URC

10. A(n) _____ is an insurance policy purchased by a company for its employees.
    A. individual policy
    B. group policy
    C. private policy
    D. public policy

11. _____ has policies in which major medical and basic benefits apply.
    A. Comprehensive plan
    B. Fee-for-service plan
    C. Managed care plan
    D. PPO

12. When an individual has loss of speech, loss of hearing in both ears, loss of sight in both eyes, or loss of the use of two limbs, it is referred to as a _____ disability.
    A. total
    B. residual
    C. catastrophic
    D. partial

13. _____ covers nonmilitary employees of the federal government.
    A. FICA
    B. FECA
    C. FEMA
    D. FAMA

14. _____ is(are) (a) reason(s) for dramatic increases in health care costs.
    A. Overuse and misuse of medical supplies
    B. Not enough people wanting insurance
    C. Increase in the elderly population
    D. Not enough people wanting insurance

15. The CMS-1500 is the name given to a universal claim form use to report outpatient services to all government health programs.
    A. True
    B. False

16. _____ is a fixed fee that is paid by the patient at each visit.
    A. Co-payment
    B. Co-insurance
    C. Premium
    D. Allowable charge

17. _____ is a documented medical condition that is present in the patient before the insurance policy goes into effect.
    A. Precertification
    B. Preauthorization
    C. Preexisting condition
    D. None of the above

18. _____ is a term used to describe and measure the various health care services provided for a specific injury or period of illness.
    A. Medical necessity
    B. Episode of care
    C. Guidelines
    D. Comprehensive plan

19. A proof of education, training, and experience is termed a curriculum vitae.
    A. True
    B. False

20. CHAMPUS is a health care program for members of the U.S. military.
    A. True
    B. False

CHAPTER TWENTY-SEVEN

Computers in the Medical Office

VOCABULARY REVIEW

Matching

Match each term with the correct definition.

A. boot up

B. cold boot

C. default

D. floppy disk

E. hard drive

F. host

G. ink-jet printer

H. Internet service provider

I. menus

J. motherboard

K. network

L. password

M. peripherals

N. prompt

O. read-only memory

P. search engine

Q. software

R. spreadsheet

_____ 1. Productivity software that allows the computer user to work with facts and figures

_____ 2. Monitor that displays options that can be selected by touching them on the screen

_____ 3. List of commands or options, typically found on the top of the computer screen, that can be selected by the user

_____ 4. Computer system that scans and reads typewritten characters and converts them to digitized files

_____ 5. Term used to indicate that a computer system has been activated and is ready to use

_____ 6. External disk storage device that holds large amounts of data

_____ 7. Computers interconnected to exchange information

_____ 8. Main device in the computer used to store and retrieve information

_____ 9. External components attached to the computer, such as the speakers

_____ 10. Secondary storage device for computer data

S. touch screen

T. tutorial

U. URL

V. warm boot

W. wizard

X. zip drive

Y. database management

Z. optical character recognition

_____ 11. "Intelligence" of a computer; tells the computer what to do; computer program

_____ 12. Company that provides a "host" access to the Internet

_____ 13. Uniform resource locator; Internet address

_____ 14. Starting the computer when it has been in "off" mode

_____ 15. Printer that produces characters and graphics by imprinting ink onto paper

_____ 16. Productivity software application that helps the user do calculations by entering numbers and formulas in a grid of rows and columns

_____ 17. Circuit board that contains memory chips; power supply, and vital components for processing data in the computer

_____ 18. Sequence of screens that direct the user to produce test-based documents

_____ 19. Selection or option automatically chosen by most computer programs if not directed by the user to do otherwise

_____ 20. Term used when the computer system has been on and must be restarted because it "freezes up"

_____ 21. Special set of characters known only to the user and the person who assigned the characters; designed to secure and protect unauthorized entry to a computer

_____ 22. Stored data that can be read but not changed

_____ 23. Self-guided step by step learning process that teaches generic skills needed to use software

_____ 24. Message displayed by the computer to request information or to help the user proceed

_____ 25. Specialized program designed to find specific information on the Internet

_____ 26. Computer that is the main computer in a system of connected terminals

THEORY RECALL

True/False

Indicate whether the sentence or statement is true or false.

_____ 1. Messages are transmitted over the Internet when a URL is entered into the browser.

_____ 2. The "motherboard" is an external component attached to the computer.

_____ 3. A 3.5-inch floppy disk holds more information than a CD–ROM.

_____ 4. Wizards are a sequence of screens that directs users through multiple steps to help them accomplish a desired task.

_____ 5. Word processing is a system of entering and editing text that requires interaction between a person and a computer.

Multiple Choice

Identify the letter of the choice that best completes the statement or answers the question.

1. A computer's function is to _____ data.
   A. input
   B. generate
   C. store
   D. all of the above

2. The OCR computer system _____ and reads typewritten data.
   A. saves
   B. scans
   C. distributes
   D. replies

3. _____ is(are) a system of entering and editing text that requires interaction between a person and a computer.
   A. PDF processing
   B. Spreadsheet
   C. Word processing
   D. Search engines

4. Hardware located outside of the computer is called _____.
   A. adjuncts
   B. peripherals
   C. accessories
   D. random memory

5. Major priority is to protect the hard drive. It is necessary to run a backup tape _____.
   A. daily
   B. weekly
   C. monthly
   D. bimonthly

6. _____ contains memory chips, power supply, and vital components for processing.
   A. Keyboard
   B. Monitor
   C. Motherboard
   D. Modems

7. _____ are rated by the size and number of dots or pixels.
   A. Scanners
   B. Monitors
   C. Laser printers
   D. None of the above

8. _____ copy is also known as a printed copy.
   A. Soft
   B. Hard
   C. Warm
   D. Cold

9. Browsers and Websites contain _____ that allow a user to enter a topic or group of words into a text box to retrieve information or locate a Website.
   A. Web addresses
   B. ISP numbers
   C. domain names
   D. search engines

10. _____ software aids in manipulating numerical data for financial management, such as for setting up a budget.
    A. Word processing
    B. Spreadsheet
    C. Data fields
    D. None of the above

11. A _____ is a device that transfers data from one computer to another over telephone or cable lines.
    A. motherboard
    B. scanner
    C. modem
    D. sound card

12. A _____ is a combination of letters and numbers that serves to identify the person using the computer.
    A. browser
    B. password
    C. user ID
    D. privacy code

13. _____ is the sum total of managing all of the facets of running a medical practice.
    A. Database management
    B. Practice management
    C. Employee management
    D. Financial management

14. _____ is a special set of numbers or characters or a combination of numbers and characters known only to the user.
    A. Browser
    B. Password
    C. User ID
    D. Privacy code

15. The "reports" feature of any practice management program allows the medical practice to manage all of the following EXCEPT_____.
    A. cash flow
    B. budget
    C. patient schedules
    D. physician's personal finances

16. The _____ is the main device a computer uses to store and retrieve information.
    A. modem
    B. email
    C. hard drive
    D. soft drive

17. _____ contains instructions to the CPU on how to set itself up when the system is initially turned on.
    A. RAM
    B. ISP
    C. URL
    D. ROM

18. The _____ is the "brain" of the computer.
    A. URL
    B. CPU
    C. ISP
    D. RAM

19. When computers are interconnected to exchange information, it is referred to as a(n) _____.
    A. network
    B. scanner
    C. Internet
    D. wizard

20. A group of computers and other devices that are connected within the same building is called a(n) _____.
    A. WAN
    B. LAN
    C. WAR
    D. LAW

Sentence Completion

Complete each sentence or statement.

1. _____ memory is the read and write memory that a computer can use for storage, when the computer is working.

2. _____ is a group of computers and other devices that are connected between buildings, cities, and even countries.

3. A(n) _____ uses a light source similar to a photocopier to copy a picture or document placed on its bed and send it through the modem or cable to the computer.

4. A(n) _____ is a company that provides a host access to the Internet.

5. In a word processing software program, font and _____ are the size and style of the typeface; number of characters per inch.

Short Answers

1. Describe the eight basic hardware parts of a computer.

   _____

   _____

   _____

   _____

   _____

   _____

   _____

   _____

2. Explain why menus were developed.

_____

_____

_____

_____

_____

3. List three safeguards for protecting patient privacy.

_____

_____

_____

_____

_____

4. List the four most common tasks of medical practice software.

_____

_____

_____

_____

_____

_____

INTERNET RESEARCH AND CRITICAL THINKING

Keyword: Computers

Search the internet using the above keyword, locating several computer Websites. Compare a minimum of two computers for the most cost-effective yet best computer for a medical office. Compare the size of hard drives, memory capacity, price, and functionality. Create a proposal to present to the physician (instructor) supporting the computer you select. Write one paragraph describing the computer you selected and why you chose it. Cite your source. Be prepared to give a 2-minute oral presentation should your instructor assign you to do so.

WHAT WOULD YOU DO?

If you have accomplished the objectives in this chapter, you will be able to make better choices as a medical assistant. Take a look at this situation and decide what you would do.

Dr. Santos has just hired Terrell, a medical assistant, to transfer demographic and insurance data from the current paper records to the computerized patient accounting system. Terrell's assignment is to ensure that all the information on current patients is up to date in the computer and that the latest updates and additions to the computer program are installed. As each new patient arrives at the office, Terrell has the duty of obtaining information for the data entry. He then must be sure that the appointment has been scheduled into the computer so that medical notes and insurance information will be available as needed. Kate, an established patient, comes to the office and sees the new computer system in operation. Terrell explains that the office is becoming more technologically advanced and that the computer will be used to schedule appointments, store transcription, and manage patient accounts in the future.

Would you be prepared to use the computer to perform data entry, scheduling, and other medical office tasks?

1. **What functions would you expect to be accomplished by the computer?**

2. **What administrative tasks can be done on a computer?**

3. **What clinical tasks can be done on the computer?**

4. How can a computer assist the health care professional who wants more information on uncommon diseases?

_____

_____

_____

_____

_____

5. How is word processing used in a physician's office?

_____

_____

_____

_____

_____

_____

6. What is meant by "backing up" a computer? Why is backing up at the end of the day so important?

_____

_____

_____

_____

_____

7. What are the three types of networks? Which would you expect to find in a small private practice? Which would you probably find in a medical practice that has multiple sites over a large area?

_____

_____

_____

_____

_____

_____

8. **What is the importance of HIPAA in regard to computer use?**

_____

_____

_____

_____

_____

APPLICATION OF SKILLS

Download the AltaPoint Demo software program from the CD-ROM located in the back of the textbook. Access and complete the exercises located on the EVOLVE Website

CHAPTER QUIZ

Multiple Choice

Identify the letter of the choice that best completes the statement or answers the question.

1. To safeguard data files of the medical practice, it is a good practice to back-up data _____.
   A. once a week
   B. monthly
   C. bimonthly
   D. daily

2. Hardware is the mechanical devices and physical components of a computer.
   A. True
   B. False

3. The _____ is the brain of the computer.
   A. CPU
   B. ROM
   C. RAM
   D. OCR

4. The _____ is a pointing device that can either be connected to the computer or be independent.
   A. mouse
   B. trackball
   C. touch pad
   D. all of the above

5. The _____ is the main device a computer uses to store and retrieve information.
   A. RAM
   B. hard drive
   C. CPU
   D. ROM

6. Floppy disks are currently about _____ inches square.
   A. 2½
   B. 3½
   C. 4½
   D. 5¼

7. _____ have high external storage capacity.
   A. Floppies
   B. CDs
   C. Zip drives
   D. ROMs

8. A printed copy is referred to as a _____.
   A. hard copy
   B. soft copy
   C. warm copy
   D. cold copy

9. Messages are transmitted over the Internet when a URL is entered into a browser.
   A. True
   B. False

10. _____ were developed to allow novice computer users to access various options without having to remember specific commands
    A. Prompts
    B. Tutorials
    C. OCR computer systems
    D. Scanners

11. A wizard is a sequence of screens that directs the user through a multiuse software task.
    A. True
    B. False

12. A(n) _____ allow(s) computer users to enter a topic, word, or group of words into a textbox in order locate information.
    A. ISP
    B. URL
    C. search engine
    D. comain name

13. _____ is a system of entering and editing text that requires interaction between a person and a computer.
    A. Spreadsheet
    B. Word processing
    C. Data
    D. None of the above

14. Practice management software can generate in-house reports of patient's entire clinical history.
    A. True
    B. False

15. _____ protocol is the way computers exchange information over the Internet.
    A. ROM
    B. http//:
    C. www.
    D. ISP address

16. Which one of the following is NOT a common Internet domain?
    A. .edu
    B. .com
    C. .mcg
    D. .net

17. Which one of the following is NOT a major consideration when purchasing practice management software?
    A. Physician's preference
    B. Office budget
    C. In-house training availability
    D. Whether it comes with built-in software games to relieve stress

18. Some practice management software programs can be purchased with fully loaded CPT codes.
    A. True
    B. False

19. Currently in medical practices, a _____ is used to back-up practice information.
    A. 3.5-inch floppy disk
    B. VHS tape
    C. CD-ROM
    D. hard drive

20. The purpose of a _____ is to store large amounts of related information, which allows multiple users to manipulate data for various purposes.
    A. word processing document
    B. spreadsheet
    C. database
    D. all of the above

CHAPTER **TWENTY-EIGHT**

Infection Control and Asepsis

VOCABULARY REVIEW:

Matching

Match each term with the correct definition.

A. anaerobes

B. autoclave

C. bacilli

D. Centers for Disease Control and Prevention

E. cocci

F. disinfection

G. exposure incident

H. indirect contact

I. material safety data sheet

J. method of transmission

K. normal flora

L. parasite

M. protozoa

N. rickettsiae

O. Right to Know law

P. route of entry

Q. spirilla

R. sterile

_____ 1. Way in which a microorganism enters the body

_____ 2. Microorganisms that do not require oxygen to grow

_____ 3. Bacteria that appear in chains

_____ 4. Work practices that minimize the possibility of infectious exposure to employees

_____ 5. Federal agency responsible for establishing guidelines to prevent the spread of disease-producing microorganisms

_____ 6. Infectious organism that needs a host to live or survive

_____ 7. Microorganisms that easily transfer to a host because of its location

_____ 8. Fact sheet about chemicals that includes handling precautions and first-aid procedures after a person has been exposed to a chemical

_____ 9. Free from all microorganisms, including spores

_____ 10. Destruction or inhibition of the activity of pathogens, but not of spores

_____ 11. Smallest of all microorganisms, visible only under electron microscopy

S. sterilization strip

T. streptococci

U. surgical asepsis

V. susceptible host

W. transient flora

X. viruses

Y. work practice controls

Z. surgical handwash

_____ 12. Way that microorganisms are passed on to other hosts or objects

_____ 13. Cleaning the hands with an antiseptic solution using a prescribed time and action to remove most microorganisms possible

_____ 14. Equipment that sterilizes objects through the use of steam under pressure or gas

_____ 15. Removal of all microorganisms from an object, including spores

_____ 16. Microorganisms that naturally occur within certain body systems

_____ 17. Contact with blood or other bio-hazardous and infectious materials that occur at work

_____ 18. Microorganisms that live in a particular species of insect and are transmitted through its bite

_____ 19. Rod-shaped bacteria

_____ 20. Person, insect, or animal that can be infected easily by a particular micro-organism

_____ 21. Round or spherical bacteria

_____ 22. Chemical indicator embedded within the center of a wrapped, dense pack that shows conditions for sterilization with in the pack

_____ 23. Method by which microorganisms are transmitted other than by person-to-person contact

_____ 24. Single-celled animals

_____ 25. Hazard communication standard that allows each employee to know of potential exposure problems

_____ 26. Spiral or corkscrew-shaped bacteria

THEORY RECALL

True/False

Indicate whether the sentence or statement is true or false.

_____ 1. Pathogens are not harmful and are not disease-producing microorganisms.

_____ 2. Sanitization destroys pathogens.

_____ 3. Standard Precautions must be observed at all times and for all patients regardless of age, gender, and diagnosis.

_____ 4. To be considered sterile, an item must be free from all microorganisms, including spores.

_____ 5. Steam sterilization is the primary method used to sterilize instruments in the medical office.

Multiple Choice

Identify the letter of the choice that best completes the statement or answers the question.

1. _____ are found in the air we breathe, on our skin, on everything we touch, and even in our food.
   A. Bacteria
   B. Microorganisms
   C. Protozoa
   D. Pathogens

2. _____ are single-celled animals found in contaminated water and decaying material.
   A. Bacteria
   B. Microorganisms
   C. Protozoa
   D. Fungi

3. _____ is the process of making an area clean and free of infection-causing microorganisms.
   A. Medical asepsis
   B. Surgical asepsis
   C. Autoclaving
   D. Disinfection

4. The use of a(n) _____ provides the only true indication that an item is sterile.
   A. autoclave tape
   B. biological indicator
   C. chemical indicator
   D. sterilization strip

5. _____ include yeast and molds.
   A. Bacteria
   B. Fungi
   C. Rickettesiae
   D. Viruses

6. OSHA mandates that employers must provide _____.
   A. an exposure control plan
   B. implementation of engineering controls
   C. PPEs
   D. all of the above

7. The CDC recommends the use of _____-based handrubs by all health care providers during patient care.
   A. alcohol
   B. soap
   C. gel
   D. lotion

8. Antiseptic handrubs, handwashing, antiseptic hand wash, and surgical handwashing are examples of _____.
   A. good hygiene
   B. hand hygiene
   C. Standard Precautions
   D. none of the above

9. _____ reduces the number of microorganisms on an item.
   A. Disinfection
   B. Sanitization
   C. Sterilization
   D. All of the above

10. _____ gloves are used when performing clean procedures.
    A. Nondisposable
    B. Nonsterile disposable
    C. Sterile nondisposable
    D. Sterile disposable

11. When storing autoclaved instruments, the packages with the _____ date are placed up front.
    A. earliest
    B. most recent
    C. oldest
    D. date does not affect how autoclaved instruments are stored

12. _____ are equipment and facilities that minimize the possibility of exposure to microorganisms.
    A. Autoclaves
    B. Engineering controls
    C. Work practice controls
    D. None of the above

13. _____ are microorganisms that need oxygen to live.
    A. Aerobes
    B. Anaerobes
    C. Pathogens
    D. Protozoa

14. _____ are bacteria with a hard wall capsule that is resistant to heat.
    A. Bacilli
    B. Cocci
    C. Staphylococci
    D. Diplococci

15. _____ are bacteria that appear to be corkscrew shaped.
    A. Bacilli
    B. Streptococci
    C. Staphylococci
    D. Spirilla

16. A _____ is an infected person who has disease-causing germs but may not have symptoms of the disease.
    A. carrier
    B. reservoir host
    C. Both A and B
    D. Neither A nor B

17. Non–disease-producing microorganisms are also called _____.
    A. microorganisms
    B. diplococci
    C. fungi
    D. nonpathogens

18. A device that is impregnated with a special dye that changes color when exposed to the sterilization process is a(n) _____.
    A. biological indicator
    B. chemical indicator
    C. alcohol-based hand wash
    D. all of the above

19. A method by which microorganisms are transmitted other than via person-to-person contact is _____.
    A. direct contact
    B. indirect contact
    C. infection control
    D. sanitization

20. ____ is the process of making an area clean and free of infectious materials and spaces.
    A. Medical asepsis
    B. Surgical asepsis
    C. Sanitization
    D. Sterilization

Sentence Completion

Complete each sentence or statement.

1. _____ refers to microorganisms that grow on the surface of the skin that are usually

   nonpathogenic.

2. _____ are parasites that need a host to survive and cannot live outside the body.

3. _____ occurs naturally on the skin and in the body, and they fight off infection when they remain in their normal location.

4. _____ reduces hand contamination by 75%.

5. _____ are nonharmful and are not disease-producing microorganisms.

6. _____ can reproduce only if they are within a living cell.

7. _____ mandates and enforces the use of Standard Precautions.

8. _____ occurs by using heat, steam under pressure, gas, ultraviolet light, or chemicals.

Short Answers

1. List the three primary conditions that must be met for steam sterilization to occur.

_____

_____

2. List and describe the five classifications of bacteria.

_____

_____

_____

_____

3. Describe the chain of infection.

_____

_____

_____

_____

4. Explain the four clinical situations when you would use alcohol-based hand rubs.

_____

_____

_____

_____

5. List four ways to determine whether items were exposed to conditions necessary for sterilization.

_____

_____

_____

_____

CRITICAL THINKING

When you check today's schedule, you notice that Dr. Sondheim has four minor surgical procedures scheduled. The clinic has only two full minor surgery packs, one of which was used yesterday for a laceration repair. You sanitized the instruments before you went home, but you did not autoclave them. It is a good thing that the second surgery is 2 hours from now. You can use the sterilized pack for the first surgery and have the second pack ready before the doctor needs it. In the lab/prep area, you start accumulating all of the supplies you are going to need for the day. You check on the autoclaved pack to make sure the dates are good. The pack is 3 days past the 30-day expiration date.

1. Can you use the 3-day outdated instrument pack? Explain your answer.

_____

_____

_____

2. Explain the steps involved in sterilizing an instrument pack.

_____

_____

_____

_____

INTERNET RESEARCH

Keywords: Medical Asepsis, Personal Protective Equipment, Standard Medical Precautions.

Choose one of the following topics to research: new techniques in medical asepsis, OSHA's specific requirements for use of PPEs, the difference between universal precautions and standard precautions. Cite your source. Be prepared to give a 2-minute oral presentation should your instructor assign you to do so.

WHAT WOULD YOU DO?

If you have accomplished the objectives in this chapter, you will be able to make better choices as a medical assistant. Take another look at this situation and decide what you would do.

Janine is a new medical assistant in the office of Dr. McGee, a specialist in infectious diseases. Janine did her practical experience in a pediatric practice, often caring for children with viral and bacterial infections. As she begins her new employment, Janine asks to see the MSDSs and the current Exposure Control Plan. She also wants to know where the PPEs for her use are stored.

   During patient care, medical workers often come in direct contact with many microorganisms, as Janine will in an office that specializes in infectious diseases. Janine's supervisor wants to be sure she is prepared to protect patients, other staff, and herself from infection. The supervisor reviews with Janine the importance of proper handwashing in infection control. Another important task for Janine will be performing both medical asepsis and surgical asepsis on a regular basis, so the supervisor assesses Janine's ability to perform these skills. The supervisor asks Janine what is done at the end of the day before leaving the office to break the cycle of infection. Janine responds that all medical workers should remove any garments that have been in direct contact with pathogens and nonpathogens and each person should carefully sanitize his or her hands.

Would you be prepared to take the necessary precautions to stop the spread of infection in the medical office?

   1. **What are "MSDSs"? What are "PPEs"? Why are both important to the health care worker?**

   _____

   _____

   _____

   _____

   2. **What is "OSHA," and what are the requirements that a medical office must have to meet the OSHA standards?**

   _____

   _____

   _____

   _____

3. What is included in the "Exposure Control Plan"?

_____

_____

_____

_____

4. What is the "chain of infection," and why is hand sanitization important in breaking this chain?

_____

_____

_____

_____

_____

5. What is the difference between handwashing and hand sanitization in maintaining hand hygiene? Give two indications for the appropriate use of each.

_____

_____

_____

_____

_____

6. What is the difference between medical asepsis and surgical asepsis?

_____

_____

_____

_____

7. What is the difference between sanitization and disinfection?

_____

_____

_____

_____

8. **Is there a degree of sterilization in surgical asepsis? Defend your answer.**

_____

_____

_____

_____

_____

9. **What is a non-pathogen? A pathogen?**

_____

_____

_____

_____

10. **How should Janine handle infectious waste from patients with a bacterial infection who are seen by Dr. McGee?**

_____

_____

_____

_____

APPLICATION OF SKILLS

Procedure Check-off Sheets (*) and Assignments from MACC CD (see Procedure Check-off Sheets for which procedure from the MACC CD to perform).

1. Perform Procedure 28-1: Practice Standard Precautions.*
    A. Develop an exposure and postexposure control plan and identify exposure control mechanisms in a simulated exposure event. Include the following areas:
    • Barrier protection
    • Environmental protection
    • Housekeeping controls
    • Safety training programs
    • Follow-up
    • Documentation
    • Material safety data sheets (MSDSs)
    B. Demonstrate knowledge, by verbal or written communication as required by instructor, an explanation of the basic guidelines approved by OSHA and recommended by the CDC for a postexposure action plan as outlined in procedure sheet 28-1 in textbook.

2. Perform Procedure 28-2: Properly Dispose of Biohazardous Materials.*

3. Perform Procedure 28-3: Perform Proper Handwashing for Medical Asepsis.*

4. Perform Procedure 28-4: Perform Alcohol-Based Hand Sanitization.*

5. Perform Procedure 28-5: Apply and Remove Clean, Disposable (Nonsterile) Gloves.*

6. Perform Procedure 28-6: Sanitize Instruments.*

7. Perform Procedure 28-7: Perform Chemical Sterilization.*

8. Perform Procedure 28-8: Wrap Instruments for the Autoclave.*

9. Perform Procedure 28-9: Sterilize Articles in the Autoclave.*

Student Name _____ Date _____

PROCEDURE 28-1: PRACTICE STANDARD PRECAUTIONS

TASK: Identify and demonstrate the application of standard precautions, as assigned by the instructor. Develop an exposure and postexposure control plan.

CONDITIONS: Given the proper equipment and supplies, the student will be required to role-play the proper method for practicing standard precautions.

NOTE: The student should practice the procedure using the MACC CD in the back of the textbook and then practice and perform the task in the classroom: MACC CD MACC/Clinical skills/Infection control/Practicing Standard Precautions.

EQUIPMENT AND SUPPLIES
- MACC CD/computer
- Personal protective equipment (PPE): eyewear, gown, boots (shoe covers), mask, gloves
- Current Standard Precautions
- Biohazardous waste container
- Puncture-resistant sharps container
- Pen or pencil

STANDARDS: Complete the procedure within _____ minutes and achieve a minimum score of _____ %.

Time began _____   Time ended _____

Steps	Possible Points	First Attempt	Second Attempt
1. Assemble all supplies and equipment.	5		
2. Select the appropriate PPE for the assigned procedure.	10		
3. Identify the body substance isolation (BSI) procedures	10		
4. Apply transmission-based precautions as they apply to the assigned procedure.	10		
5. Explain Standard Precautions as they apply to all body fluids, secretions and excretions, blood, nonintact skin, and mucous membranes.	10		
6. Explain the importance of continuing education as it relates to practices using Standard Precautions.	20		
7. Demonstrate the proper use of the following exposure control devices: • Sharps container • Eyewash stations • Fire extinguishers • Biohazardous waste containers	20		
8. Demonstrate proper documentation of Standard Precautions training including the time requirement for the training or retraining record.	15		

Total Points Possible: 100

Comments: Total Points Earned _____ Divided by _____ Total Possible Points = _____ % Score

Instructor's Signature _____

Student Name _____ Date _____

PROCEDURE 28-2: PROPERLY DISPOSE OF BIOHAZARDOUS MATERIALS

TASK: Identify waste classified as biohazardous and select appropriate containers for proper disposal. Assemble all equipment and demonstrate disposal of actual or simulated waste, following exposure control guidelines.

CONDITIONS: Given the proper equipment and supplies, the student will be required to role-play the proper method for properly disposing of biohazardous materials. The instructor will provide specific instruction on what to dispose of.

NOTE: The student should practice the procedure using the MACC CD in the back of the textbook and then practice and perform the task in the classroom: MACC CD MACC/Clinical skills/Infection control/Practicing Standard Precautions.

EQUIPMENT AND SUPPLIES
- Personal protective equipment (PPE): eyewear, gown, boots (shoe covers), mask, gloves
- Current Standard Precautions
- Biohazardous waste container
- Puncture-resistant sharps container

STANDARDS: Complete the procedure within _____ minutes and achieve a minimum score of _____ %.

Time began _____   Time ended _____

Steps	Possible Points	First Attempt	Second Attempt
1. Assemble all supplies and equipment.	5		
2. Select the appropriate PPE.	5		
3. Verbally communicate a list identifying waste classified as biohazardous.	10		
4. Identify the universal biohazardous symbol and describe the proper use of the biohazardous spill cleanup kits.	10		
5. Explain housekeeping safety controls.	20		
6. Identify and review material safety data sheets (MSDSs). List the various pieces of information included on an MSDS.	20		
7. Document the decontamination of equipment procedures. Keep a decontamination action log.	20		
8. Describe the importance of ongoing safety training.	10		

Total Points Possible: 100

Comments: Total Points Earned _____ Divided by _____ Total Possible Points = _____ % Score

Instructor's Signature _____

Student Name _____ Date _____

PROCEDURE 28-3: PERFORM PROPER HANDWASHING FOR MEDICAL ASEPSIS

TASK: Prevent the spread of pathogens by aseptically washing hands, following Standard Precautions.
CONDITIONS: Given the proper equipment and supplies, the student will be required to demonstrate the
  proper method of performing handwashing for medical asepsis.
*NOTE: The student should practice the procedure using the MACC CD in the back of the textbook and then
  practice and perform the task in the classroom: MACC CD MACC/Clinical skills/Infection
  control/Sanitizing hands.*

EQUIPMENT AND SUPPLIES
- MACC CD/Computer
- Liquid antibacterial soap
- Nailbrush or orange stick
- Paper towels
- Warm running water
- Regular waste container

STANDARDS: Complete the procedure within _____ minutes and achieve a minimum score of _____ %.

Time began _____   Time ended _____

Steps	Possible Points	First Attempt	Second Attempt
1. Assemble all supplies and equipment.	5		
2. Remove rings and watch or push the watch up on the forearm.	5		
3. Stand close to the sink, without allowing clothing to touch the sink.	5		
4. Turn on the faucets, using a paper towel.	5		
5. Adjust the water temperature to warm – not hot or cold. Explain why proper water temperature is important.	10		
6. Discard the paper towel in the proper waste container.	5		
7. Wet hands and wrists under running water, and apply liquid antibacterial soap. Hands must be held lower than the elbows at all times. Must not touch the inside of the sink.	10		
8. Work soap into a lather by rubbing the palms together using a circular motion.	10		
9. Clean the finger nails with a nail brush or an orange stick.	5		
10. Rinse hands thoroughly under running water, holding them in a downward position and allowing soap and water to run off the fingertips.	10		
11. Repeat the procedure if hands are grossly contaminated.	10		
12. Dry the hands gently and thoroughly using a clean paper towel. Discard the paper towel in proper waste container.	10		

Steps	Possible Points	First Attempt	Second Attempt
13. Using a dry paper towel, turn the faucets off, clean the area around the sink, and discard the towel in regular waste container.	10		

Total Points Possible: 100

Comments: Total Points Earned _____ Divided by _____ Total Possible Points = _____ % Score

Instructor's Signature _____

Student Name _____ Date _____

PROCEDURE 28-4: PERFORM ALCOHOL-BASED HAND SANITIZATON

TASK: Apply an alcohol-based hand rub to prevent the spread of pathogens.

CONDITIONS: Given the proper equipment and supplies, the student will be required to demonstrate the proper method of performing alcohol-based hand sanitization for medical asepsis.

NOTE: The student should practice the procedure using the MACC CD in the back of the textbook and then practice and perform the task in the classroom: MACC CD MACC/Clinical skills/Infection control/Sanitizing hands.

EQUIPMENT AND SUPPLIES
- MACC CD/computer
- Alcohol-based hand rub containing 60% to 95% ethanol or isopropanol (gel, foam, lotion)

STANDARDS: Complete the procedure within _____ minutes and achieve a minimum score of _____ %.

Time began _____   Time ended _____

Steps	Possible Points	First Attempt	Second Attempt
1. Assemble all supplies and equipment.	5		
2. Visibly inspect hands for obvious contaminants or debris.	5		
3. Remove rings.	5		
4. Open container and apply product to the palm of one hand, following manufacturer's recommendations regarding the amount of product to use.	10		
5. Close container and replace in specified location.	5		
6. Spread gel evenly, covering all surfaces of hands and fingers, 1 to 1½ inches above the wrist.	10		
7. Rub hands together until hands are dry, approximately 15 to 30 seconds.	10		

Total Points Possible: 50

Comments: Total Points Earned _____ Divided by _____ Total Possible Points = _____ % Score

Instructor's Signature _____

Student Name _____ Date _____

PROCEDURE 28-5: APPLY AND REMOVE CLEAN, DISPOSABLE (NONSTERILE) GLOVES

TASK: Apply and remove disposable (nonsterile) gloves properly.

CONDITIONS: Given the proper equipment and supplies, the student will be required to apply and remove nonsterile disposable gloves.

NOTE: The student should practice the procedure using the MACC CD in the back of the textbook and then practice and perform the task in the classroom: MACC CD MACC/Clinical skills/Infection control/Practicing Standard Precautions.

EQUIPMENT AND SUPPLIES
- MACC CD/computer
- Alcohol-based hand rub
- Nonsterile disposable gloves
- Biohazardous waste container

STANDARDS: Complete the procedure within _____ minutes and achieve a minimum score of _____ %.

Time began _____   **Time ended** _____

Steps	Possible Points	First Attempt	Second Attempt
Applying Gloves			
1. Assemble all supplies and equipment.	5		
2. Select the correct size and style of gloves according to office policy.	5		
3. Sanitize hands as described in Procedure 28-3 or 28-4.	10		
4. Apply gloves and adjust them to ensure a proper fit.	5		
5. Inspect the gloves carefully for tears, holes, or punctures before and after application.	5		
Removing Gloves			
1. Grasp the outside of one glove with the first three fingers of the other hand approximately 1 to 2 inches below the cuff.	10		
2. Stretch the soiled glove by pulling it away from the hand, and slowly pull the glove downward off the hand. Usually the dominant hand is ungloved first.	10		
3. After the glove is pulled free from the hand, ball it in the palm of the gloved hand.	10		
4. Remove the other glove by placing the index and middle fingers of the ungloved hand inside the glove of the gloved hand; turn the cuff downward. Be careful not to touch the outside of the soiled glove.	10		
5. Stretch the glove away from the hand and pull the cuff downward over the hand and over the balled-up glove, turning it inside out with the balled glove inside.	10		

Steps	Possible Points	First Attempt	Second Attempt
6. Carefully dispose of the gloves in a marked biohazardous waste container.	10		
7. Sanitize hands.	10		

Total Points Possible: 100

Comments: Total Points Earned _____ Divided by _____ Total Possible Points = _____ % Score

Instructor's Signature _____

Student Name _____ Date _____

PROCEDURE 28-6: SANITIZE INSTRUMENTS

TASK: Properly sanitize contaminated instruments by cleansing with detergent and water to reduce the number of microorganisms or by using an ultrasound cleaner.

CONDITIONS: Given the proper equipment and supplies, the student will be required to demonstrate the proper method of sanitizing instruments in preparation for autoclaving. The instructor may select the method of sanitization—manual or ultrasonic cleaner or both.

NOTE: The student should practice the procedure using the MACC CD in the back of the textbook and then practice and perform the task in the classroom: MACC CD MACC/Clinical skills/Infection control/Sanitizing and wrapping instruments for the autoclave.

EQUIPMENT AND SUPPLIES
- MACC CD/computer
- Disposable gloves
- Rubber (utility) gloves
- Fluid-resistant laboratory apron
- Lab safety goggles
- Stiff nylon brush
- Container to hold instruments
- Instrument cleaning solution, stain remover, and lubricant
- Ultrasonic cleaner, if applicable
- Material safety data sheet (MSDS) for cleaning solutions
- Towel

STANDARDS: Complete the procedure within _____ minutes and achieve a minimum score of _____ %.

Time began _____   Time ended _____

Steps	Possible Points	First Attempt	Second Attempt
Manual Method			
1. Assemble all supplies and equipment.	5		
2. Review the MSDS for the chemical agent being used.	5		
3. Apply appropriate personal protective equipment (PPE).	5		
4. Apply utility gloves over the disposable gloves.	10		
5. Mix cleaning solution for the instruments, following manufacturer's directions on the label. Alternately, prepare the ultrasound cleaning device, following manufacturer's directions.	10		
6. Remove contaminated instruments from area of use, and place them in a covered container, separating the instruments as appropriate.	10		
7. Rinse all instruments under cool running water to remove organic material.	10		
8. Using a scrub brush and cleaning solution, loosen any debris on the instruments.	10		
9. Check instruments for stain and/or rust and treat appropriately.	10		

Steps	Possible Points	First Attempt	Second Attempt
10. Rinse all instruments.	10		
11. Dry each instrument with a paper towel.	10		
12. Dispose of cleaning solution, drying material, or remaining contaminated material as appropriate.	10		
13. Lubricate hinged instruments as appropriate.	10		
14. Remove and dispose of PPEs as appropriate.	5		
15. Sanitize hands.	5		
Ultrasonic Method			
1. Assemble all supplies and equipment.	5		
2. Review the MSDS for the chemical agent being used.	5		
3. Apply appropriate PPEs.	5		
4. Prepare ultrasonic cleaning solution according to manufacturer's recommendations.	10		
5. Separate sanitized instruments into different types of metals and by delicate and sharp instruments.	10		
6. Open hinged instruments and place in the ultrasonic cleaner, completely submerging them.	10		
7. Turn on the ultrasonic machine and set the timer for the recommended period of time for type of instrument(s).	10		
8. Remove the instruments at the end of the cycle and dry.	10		
9. Change the ultrasonic cleaner according to manufacturer's instructions as appropriate.	5		
10. Cover container between uses.	5		

Total Points Possible: 200

Comments: Total Points Earned _____ Divided by _____ Total Possible Points = _____ % Score

Instructor's Signature _____

Student Name _____ **Date** _____

PROCEDURE 28-7: PERFORM CHEMICAL STERILIZATION

TASK: Properly sterilize items using a chemical agent.
CONDITIONS: Given the proper equipment and supplies, the student will be required to demonstrate the proper method of performing chemical sterilization of instruments.

EQUIPMENT AND SUPPLIES
- Chemical agent, disinfectant
- Material safety data sheet (MSDS)
- Disposable gloves
- Stainless steel or glass container with cover
- Towels
- Articles to be sterilized

STANDARDS: Complete the procedure within _____ minutes and achieve a minimum score of _____ %.

Time began _____   **Time ended** _____

Steps	Possible Points	First Attempt	Second Attempt
1. Assemble all supplies and equipment.	5		
2. Review the MSDS for the chemical agent being used.	5		
3. Apply appropriate personal protective equipment (PPE).	5		
4. Place the sanitized items in the chemical solution for sterilization. Instruments must be completely covered in the chemical agent.	10		
5. Place the airtight lid on the container.	5		
6. Treat the items for the required time.	10		
7. Before using the instruments, remove the items from the chemical and rinse completely. Lift out the stainless steel tray and rinse in a sterile distilled-water bath.	10		
8. Using sterile transfer forceps, remove the items from the tray for use.	10		
9. Dry items before use with a sterile towel.	10		
10. Remove gloves and sanitize hands.	5		

Total Points Possible: 75

Comments: Total Points Earned _____ Divided by _____ Total Possible Points = _____ % Score

Instructor's Signature _____

Student Name _____ Date _____

PROCEDURE 28-8: WRAP INSTRUMENTS FOR THE AUTOCLAVE

TASK: Wrap sanitized instruments for autoclaving.

CONDITIONS: Given the proper equipment and supplies, the student will be required to demonstrate the proper method of wrapping instruments in preparation for autoclaving.

The student should practice the procedure using the MACC CD in the back of the textbook and then practice and perform the task in the classroom: MACC CD MACC/Clinical skills/Infection control/Sanitizing & wrapping instruments for the autoclave.

EQUIPMENT AND SUPPLIES
- MACC CD/computer
- Autoclave wrapping material
- Autoclave tape
- Sterilization indicator strip
- Sterilization pouch
- Waterproof pen
- Ten 4 ¥ 4-inch gauze squares
- One forceps
- One Kelly hemostat
- One S/S operating scissors
- Or other items as designated
- One instrument to be wrapped separately

STANDARDS: Complete the procedure within _____ minutes and achieve a minimum score of _____ %.

Time began _____   Time ended _____

Steps	Possible Points	First Attempt	Second Attempt
1. Assemble all supplies and equipment.	5		
2. Sanitize hands.	5		
3. Place instruments on appropriate size wrapper.	10		
4. Place a sterilization strip in the center of the pack.	10		
5. Wrap instruments in proper manner.	10		
6. Repeat the wrapping process for the outside wrap if applicable.	10		
7. Secure the package with autoclave tape.	10		
8. Label the autoclave tape with a waterproof pen.	10		
9. Set the package aside until it is time to autoclave.	5		
Individual Instrument			
10. Label the pouch.	5		
11. Place the instrument carefully into the sterilization pack in the correct position for appropriate removal.	10		

Steps	Possible Points	First Attempt	Second Attempt
12. Seal the pouch.	5		
13. Set aside the package until it is time to autoclave.	5		

Total Points Possible: 100

Comments: Total Points Earned _____ Divided by _____ Total Possible Points = _____ % Score

Instructor's Signature _____

Student Name _____ **Date** _____

PROCEDURE 28-9: STERILIZE ARTICLES IN THE AUTOCLAVE

TASK: Properly sterilize supplies and medical equipment using an autoclave.

CONDITIONS: Given the proper equipment and supplies, the student will be required to demonstrate sterilization of articles in the autoclave.

The student should practice the procedure using the MACC CD in the back of the textbook and then practice and perform the task in the classroom: MACC CD MACC/Clinical skills/Infection control/Sterilizing articles in the autoclave.

EQUIPMENT AND SUPPLIES
- MACC CD/computer
- Distilled water
- Heat-resistant gloves
- Wrapped packs
- Other autoclavable items as required
- Autoclave with instruction manual
- Autoclave log
- Pen

STANDARDS: Complete the procedure within _____ minutes and achieve a minimum score of _____ %.

Time began _____   **Time ended** _____

Steps	Possible Points	First Attempt	Second Attempt
1. Assemble previously wrapped autoclave packs, other items to sterilize, and all other supplies and equipment.	5		
2. Fill the autoclave reservoir with distilled water.	5		
3. Properly load the autoclave chamber with previously prepared items.	10		
4. Fill chamber with distilled water to fill line.	5		
5. Close the door tightly.	5		
6. Turn the control knob to the "on" or "autoclave" setting to start the autoclave.	10		
7. Check the pressure gauge for appropriate pounds of pressure and proper temperature.	10		
8. Set the timer for the required time.	10		
9. After sterilization is complete, turn the control knob to "vent."	5		
10. Open the door 1/2 to 1 inch when appropriate.	5		
11. Allow items to dry.	5		
12. Use heat-resistant gloves to remove items from the chamber.	5		
13. Turn the autoclave control knob to the "off" position.	5		
14. Inspect each pack for any breaks in sterilization technique.	5		
15. Appropriately store the autoclaved articles.	5		

Steps	Possible Points	First Attempt	Second Attempt
16. Maintain the autoclave log with all required information.	5		

Total Points Possible: 100

Comments: Total Points Earned _____ Divided by _____ Total Possible Points = _____ % Score

Instructor's Signature _____

CHAPTER QUIZ

Multiple Choice

Identify the letter of the choice that best completes the statement or answers the question.

1. Spiral or corkscrew-shaped bacteria are known as _____.
   A. diplococcic
   B. staphylococci
   C. spirilla
   D. spores

2. Microorganisms that naturally occur within certain body systems are known as _____.
   A. nonpathogens
   B. normal flora
   C. pathogens
   D. parasites

3. _____ is the primary method used to sterilize instruments in the medical office.
   A. Autoclaving
   B. Disinfection
   C. Sanitization
   D. Sterilization

4. _____ destroys pathogens.
   A. Autoclaving
   B. Disinfection
   C. Sanitization
   D. Sterilization

5. _____ is the removal of all microorganisms, both pathogenic and nonpathogenic, from an object.
   A. Medical asepsis
   B. Sanitization
   C. Sterilization
   D. Surgical asepsis

6. When drawing blood, sterile gloves are used.
   A. True
   B. False

7. _____ is a primary condition that must be met for steam sterilization to occur.
   A. Appropriate time period depending on size of surgical pack or instrument
   B. Pressure of 15 pounds
   C. Temperature of 250° to 270° F
   D. All of the above

8. _____ provides the only true indication that an item is sterile.
   A. Autoclave tape
   B. Biological indicators
   C. Chemical indicators
   D. Sterilization strips

9. Sanitization occurs by using heat, steam under pressure, gas, UV light, or chemicals.
   A. True
   B. False

10. _____ is hazard communication standard that allows each employee to know of potential exposure problems.
    A. OSHA
    B. Right to Know law
    C. Material safety data sheet
    D. Exposure control plan

11. The way microorganisms are transmitted (passed on, spread) to other hosts is known as _____.
    A. indirect contact
    B. method of transmission
    C. route of entry
    D. none of the above

12. Maintaining the hands in a clean state by using soap and water, antiseptic solution, or alcohol-based hand rubs is known as _____.
    A. antiseptic hand wash
    B. handwashing
    C. hand hygiene
    D. medical asepsis

13. Established policies and procedures that must be followed to minimize the risk of spreading disease-producing microorganisms are known as _____.
    A. infection control
    B. PPE
    C. Right to Know law
    D. workplace controls

14. The federal agency known as the Centers for Disease Control and Prevention enforces the use of safety measures in place under Standard Precautions.
    A. True
    B. False

15. Microorganisms that feed on organic material are known as _____.
    A. fungi
    B. parasites
    C. spirilla
    D. viruses

16. Microorganisms that do not require oxygen to grow are as _____.
    A. aerobic
    B. anaerobic
    C. nonpathogenic
    D. sterile

17. Microorganisms are microscopic animals capable of reproducing.
    A. True
    B. False

18. Paper- or muslin-wrapped autoclaved items can be stored for _____.
    A. 15 days
    B. 30 days
    C. 6 months
    D. 1 year

19. Gloves reduce hand contamination by an average of _____ %.
    A. 50
    B. 65
    C. 70
    D. 75

20. Normal flora refers to organisms that grow on the surface of the skin and are picked up easily by the hands.
    A. True
    B. False

CHAPTER **TWENTY-NINE**

Preparing the Examination Room

VOCABULARY REVIEW

Matching

Match each term with the correct definition.

A. audiometer

B. tuning fork

C. otoscope

D. specimen

E. percussion hammer

F. tape measure

G. ophthalmoscope

H. tongue depressor

I. lubricant

J. penlight

_____ 1. Instrument used to hold the tongue down or move it from side to side when examining the mouth

_____ 2. Agent used to reduce friction by making a surface moist; used to facilitate anal and vaginal examinations

_____ 3. Instrument used to test hearing acuity by air or bone conduction

_____ 4. Instrument used to measure tendon reflexes

_____ 5. Instrument used to examine internal structure of the eye

_____ 6. Electronic instrument used to test hearing

_____ 7. Sample of a larger part, such as body tissue or cells

_____ 8. Instrument used to examine the ear canal and eardrum

_____ 9. Device used to measure body parts and wound length

_____ 10. Instrument used to enhance examination in a cavity and to check for papillary response to light

THEORY RECALL

True/False

Indicate whether the sentence or statement is true or false.

_____ 1. Confidentiality is a key issue for patients.

_____ 2. It is acceptable to leave prescription pads on the counter in examination rooms, because even if a patient took the pad he or she could not use it.

_____ 3. A medical assistant should be present while a patient changes into a gown.

_____ 4. Otoscope may have a short and wide speculum attached and can be used by the physician to examine the nasal area.

_____ 5. Examination tables must be covered with nonpermeable latex as directed by OSHA.

Multiple Choice

Identify the letter of the choice that best completes the statement or answers the question.

1. An instrument used to measure tendon reflexes is a(n) _____.
   A. audiometer
   B. percussion hammer
   C. tape measure
   D. tuning fork

2. The _____ test is used when a patient states hearing is better in one ear than in the other.
   A. audiometer
   B. Rinne
   C. verbal
   D. Weber

3. Appropriate accommodations need to be made in examination rooms to ensure that the room is accessible to all patients, including those in wheelchairs, as directed by _____.
   A. CDC
   B. OSHA
   C. ADA
   D. none of the above

4. Which one of the following is the correct spelling for the medical term for a blood pressure cuff?
   A. Syphgmomanometer
   B. Sphygmomanometer
   C. Syfigmomanometer
   D. None of the above

5. A _____ holds used needles and other sharps for disposal.
   A. biohazardous waste container
   B. puncture-resistant container
   C. sealable stainless steel canister
   D. none of the above

6. _____ requires that all contaminated work surfaces be decontaminated using appropriate disinfectant as soon as possible after a procedure or immediately if potential infectious contamination has occurred.
   A. CDC
   B. Office procedure manual
   C. OSHA
   D. Exposure control plan

7. _____ is(are) used to collect specimens and remove debris.
   A. Cotton-tipped applicator
   B. Lubricant
   C. Sterile saline
   D. Sharp/sharp operating scissors

8. _____ is an instrument used to test hearing acuity through vibration.
   A. Audiometer
   B. Otoscope
   C. Percussion hammer
   D. Tuning fork

9. _____ is an instrument used for viewing a cavity.
   A. Penlight
   B. Tongue depressor
   C. Speculum
   D. None of the above

10. The _____ test compares air conduction with bone conduction.
    A. audiometer
    B. percussion hammer
    C. Rinne
    D. Weber

11. _____ disinfects skin and equipment surfaces.
    A. Sterile saline
    B. Isopropyl alcohol 70%
    C. Johnson & Johnson "Wet Wipes"
    D. None of the above

12. Lubricants used in a medical office should be _____.
    A. water soluble
    B. oil based
    C. consistent with the ingredients of household detergent
    D. none of the above

13. Examination tables and counter surfaces must be cleaned in between patients with _____.
    A. sterile saline
    B. 70% isopropyl alcohol wipe
    C. 10% bleach solution
    D. all of the above

14. All instruments used during an exam must be removed, cleaned, and _____.
    A. sanitized
    B. disinfected
    C. sterilized
    D. all of the above

15. Which one of the following is a specialty item that would be added to an examination tray for a Pap smear?
    A. Sigmoidoscope
    B. Ophthalmoscope
    C. Tuning fork
    D. Vaginal speculum

Sentence Completion

Complete each sentence or statement.

1. _____ measures should be taken to ensure patients do not injure themselves in the office.

2. _____ mandates the privacy and confidentiality of patients.

3. Gloves are always worn when coming in contact with _____.

4. _____ is used for taping the tendon in the elbow, wrist, ankle, and knee to test for

   reflex action.

5. _____ is used to examine the internal structures of the eye.

Short Answers

1. Describe what safety measures need to be taken in the medical office so that patients do not injure themselves.

   _____

   _____

   _____

   _____

2. List equipment for a physical examination typically found in an examination room.

_____

_____

_____

_____

3. List the four major areas of treatment plan preparation that the medical assistant can address.

_____

_____

_____

_____

4. List four general considerations taken when preparing an examination room for a patient.

_____

_____

_____

_____

CRITICAL THINKING

Today is your first day of externship, and the medical assistant that you will be training with has asked you to set up Room 3 for a routine physical exam. List the items you will need to have available for the physician, and describe the preparation of the exam room.

INTERNET RESEARCH

Keywords: Health Insurance Portability and Accountability Act (HIPAA) regulations on patient privacy— Americans With Disabilities Act (ADA) accessibility requirements for medical offices and clinics.

Choose one of the following topics to research: Health Insurance Portability and Accountability Act (HIPAA) regulations on patient privacy— Americans With Disabilities Act (ADA) accessibility requirements for medical offices and clinics. Prepare a one-page report, and cite your source. Be prepared to give a 2-minute oral presentation should your instructor assign you to do so.

WHAT WOULD YOU DO?

If you have accomplished the objectives in this chapter, you will be able to make better choices as a medical assistant. Take another look at this situation and decide what you would do.

Julie, a medical assistant who was not educated in a medical assisting program, has been hired by a local family physician to assist with physical examinations. Today is her second day on the job. Her mentor has called in sick, so Julie is responsible for the clinical area by herself. Another physician, Dr. Johnson, will be performing the invasive procedures, and Julie is expected to have the room and patient ready for Dr. Johnson's examinations. Julie finds the room too warm for her comfort, and she knows that it will be too warm for the physician in a lab coat, so she lowers the thermostat to 67° F. As Mrs. Sito is undressing, Julie barges into the room and leaves the door open. A male patient walks by and sees Mrs. Sito undressed. During the examination Dr. Johnson asks for the ophthalmoscope and otoscope. When he tries to use these, the necessary light will not work, so he asks for a penlight. Julie leaves the room to find the penlight and a tape measure. Dr. Johnson reaches for a cotton-tipped applicator and tongue depressors. Noticing that the supply is low, he asks Julie, "Would you please fill these containers?" Julie immediately departs to fill the jars, leaving Dr. Johnson alone with the patient, who needs a pelvic examination. After Mrs. Sito leaves the room, Julie decides that the table paper does not look used. Thinking she will save the physician some money in supplies, she does not change the paper covering and brings in 5-year-old Joey Novelle, placing him on the table Mrs. Sito has just left. The sink still contains the dirty instruments used for the other patients. Joey's mother tells Dr. Johnson that she has never seen someone placed on dirty table paper, and she does not want her child to see dirty instruments in the sink. At the end of Joey's physical examination, Dr. Johnson takes Julie to his office and explains that if she cannot properly prepare and clean the examination room in the future, he will have to find someone to replace her.

If you worked with Julie, what are some suggestions you would make to help her perform her duties more effectively?

1. **What part did the lack of education in the medical assisting field play in Julie making mistakes?**

   _____

   _____

   _____

2. **What temperature is appropriate for the patient examination room?**

   _____

3. **Why should Julie have been very careful to keep the door closed to the examination room where a patient was placed?**

   _____

   _____

   _____

4. **What is the use of the ophthalmoscope and otoscope?**

   _____

   _____

_____

_____

5. **Should Julie have left the room to fill the containers of cotton-tipped applicators and tongue depressors? Explain your answer.**

_____

_____

_____

_____

6. **Why is changing the examination table's paper covering such an important task?**

_____

_____

_____

_____

7. **Do you think that Joey's mother and Dr. Johnson had a right to be upset?**

_____

_____

_____

8. **What effect did the room's lack of preparation have on the appointments for that day?**

_____

_____

_____

_____

APPLICATION OF SKILLS

1. With a partner, gather the equipment and supplies required to perform a routine physical exam. Explain to your partner what each item is used for.

2. The student should practice the procedure using the MACC CD in the back of the textbook and then practice and perform the task in the classroom: MACC CD MACC/Clinical skills/Patient care/The physical exam/Assisting with a physical exam and maintaining/preparing exam room.

CHAPTER QUIZ

Multiple Choice

Identify the letter of the choice that best completes the statement or answers the question.

1. _____ is used when a patient states that the hearing is better on one side than the other.
   A. Audiometer test
   B. Tuning fork
   C. Rinne test
   D. Weber test

2. _____ is always worn when coming in contact with patient body secretions.
   A. Latex gloves
   B. Powdered gloves
   C. Disposable gloves
   D. Sterile gloves

3. A _____ should be available in the exam room for a patient to access an exam table.
   A. Stepstool
   B. Footrest
   C. Pullout platform
   D. any of the above

4. Prescription pads should not be left on the counter in exam rooms.
   A. True
   B. False

5. The medical assistant should prepare the exam room _____ the patient arrives.
   A. after
   B. before
   C. when
   D. none of the above

6. The Americans With Disabilities Act requires that appropriate accommodations be made in exam rooms so that all patients, including those in wheelchairs, have access.
   A. True
   B. False

7. _____ is a piece of equipment typically kept in exam rooms for physical examination.
   A. Cotton-tipped applicators
   B. Disposable gloves
   C. Tongue depressors
   D. Otoscope

8. Confidentiality is not an issue for most patients.
   A. True
   B. False

9. _____ regulates that all contaminated work surfaces must be decontaminated using an appropriate disinfectant as soon as the patient leaves.
   A. Office policy manual
   B. CDC
   C. Exposure control plan
   D. State law

10. _____ protects the patient's right to privacy.
    A. CDC
    B. OSHA
    C. HIPAA
    D. Office policy

11. Exam table paper needs to be changed _____.
    A. every morning
    B. twice a day
    C. end of the day
    D. after each patient

12. When the medical assistant is preparing the patient for carrying out the treatment plan, the medical assistant should _____.
    A. make sure the patient understands the instructions
    B. make sure the patient's living environment will allow for compliance
    C. make sure the patient is not hearing impaired
    D. all of the above

13. _____ is an instrument for viewing a cavity.
    A. Penlight
    B. Otoscope
    C. Speculum
    D. Tongue depressor

14. _____ is an instrument to view the internal structure of the eye.
    A. Audiometer
    B. Otoscope
    C. Ophthalmoscope
    D. Penlight

15. The medical assistant should stay in the exam room while a patient changes into a gown.
    A. True
    B. False

CHAPTER THIRTY

Body Measurements and Vital Signs

VOCABULARY REVIEW

Matching

Match each term with the correct definition.

A. afebrile

B. apical pulse

C. baseline

D. brachial artery

E. carotid artery

F. diastolic pressure

G. dorsalis pedis artery

H. femoral artery

I. hypotension

J. inspiration

K. popliteal artery

L. pulse rate

M. radial pulse

N. rales

O. respiratory rate

P. rhonchi

Q. sphygmomanometer

R. stridor

_____ 1. Numerical measurement of heartbeats or respirations per minute; characteristic of measuring the pulse or respiration

_____ 2. High-pitched sounds heard when bronchial tubes are narrowed by disease

_____ 3. Without fever

_____ 4. Artery located behind the knee

_____ 5. Area of the eardrum

_____ 6. Pulse rate of less than 60 beats per minute

_____ 7. Instrument used to measure blood pressure

_____ 8. Underarm area

_____ 9. First measurable sound of blood pressure when the heart contracts

_____ 10. Measurement of blood pressure that is below the expected range for the patient's age group

_____ 11. Heartbeat that is taken with a stethoscope over the apex of the heart

_____ 12. Systematic measurement of a patient's temperature, pulse rate, respiration, and blood pressure

428

S. systolic pressure

T. tachycardia

U. tympanic

V. vital signs

W. wheezes

X. axillary

Y. rate

Z. bradycardia

_____ 13. Minimum ("resting") pressure of blood against arteries occurring late in ventricular resting of the heart

_____ 14. Cycle of breathing to include inspiration and expiration in a minute

_____ 15. Measurement of a vital sign that serves as a basis to which all subsequent measurements of that vital sign are compared

_____ 16. Pulse rate above 100 beats per minute

_____ 17. Act of taking a breath or breathing in; inhaling

_____ 18. Artery located in the upper arm

_____ 19. Shrill sound heard on inspiration

_____ 20. Artery located in the thigh

_____ 21. Number of heartbeats per minute

_____ 22. Artery located on both sides of the neck

_____ 23. Low-pitched sounds created as air goes through narrowed bronchi

_____ 24. Artery located in the foot

_____ 25. Breathing sounds of "tissue paper being crumpled" caused by fluid or secretions in the bronchus

_____ 26. Pulse felt at the wrist over the radius

THEORY RECALL

True/False

Indicate whether the sentence or statement is true or false.

_____ 1. Body temperature is the measurement of the amount of heat within a person's body.

_____ 2. It is okay to place a blood pressure cuff over clothing if the patient's sleeve is too tight to pull up.

_____ 3. Children should have their height recorded at each visit.

_____ 4. When recording blood pressures, the systolic number is recorded on the bottom.

_____ 5. It is better to use a smaller blood pressure cuff when in doubt.

Multiple Choice

Identify the letter of the choice that best completes the statement or answers the question.

1. Bradycardia is a pulse rate lower than _____ beats per minute.
   A. 40
   B. 50
   C. 60
   D. 65

2. _____ is a low–pitched sound created as air goes through mucus or narrowed bronchi.
   A. Stridor
   B. Rales
   C. Rhonchi
   D. Wheezes

3. _____ is the most common place to measure pulse rate.
   A. Apical
   B. Brachial pulse
   C. Radial pulse
   D. Popliteal pulse

4. _____ is a measurement of the number of times the heart beats in a minute.
   A. Pulse rate
   B. Pulse
   C. Heart rate
   D. Heartbeat

5. _____ thermometers usually have digital read-outs and are hand held.
   A. Disposable
   B. Electronic
   C. Mercury-free glass
   D. Tympanic

6. The weight of an infant should _____ by 6 months compared with birth weight.
   A. double
   B. triple
   C. quadruple
   D. none of the above

7. Mercury-free glass thermometers have a _____ color-coded end.
   A. red
   B. green
   C. yellow
   D. blue

8. A _____ usually takes 1 to 2 seconds to register.
   A. disposable oral thermometer
   B. temperature-sensitive tape
   C. tympanic thermometer
   D. mercury-free thermometer

9. When taking a patient's pulse, it is best if you take it for _____.
   A. 10 seconds and multiply by 6
   B. 15 seconds and multiply by 4
   C. 30 seconds and multiply by 2
   D. 60 seconds

10. _____ pulse rate is taken over the apex of the heart.
    A. Apical
    B. Brachial
    C. Carotid
    D. Temporal

11. An adult respiratory rate is _____ breaths per minute.
    A. 10 to 15
    B. 16 to 20
    C. 20 to 40
    D. 25 to 40

12. When taking blood pressure, the normal range for adult systolic pressure is _____.
    A. 60 to 90 mm Hg
    B. 90 to 118 mm Hg
    C. 100 to 120 mm Hg
    D. 100 to 140 mm Hg

13. An older adult's height should be measured _____.
    A. every 3 years
    B. every 2 years
    C. every year
    D. every visit

14. "Bradycardia" is _____.
    A. slow breathing
    B. slow heart rate
    C. fast breathing
    D. fast heart rate

15. To take a(n) _____ pulse, a stethoscope must be used.
    A. apical
    B. femoral
    C. radial
    D. temporal

16. _____ is concerned with breathing patterns.
    A. Respiratory rate
    B. Respiratory rhythm
    C. Respiratory depth
    D. None of the above

17. _____ is(are) high-pitched sounds that occur when bronchial tubes are narrowed by disease.
    A. Stridor
    B. Rales
    C. Rhonchi
    D. Wheezing

18. _____ measure(s) body temperature by measuring the body temperature inside the ear canal or the membrane of the ear.
    A. Digital thermometers
    B. Temperature-sensitive tape
    C. Tympanic thermometers
    D. None of the above

19. The head circumference of a child is approximately _____ % of an adult's circumference by 1 year of age.
    A. 70
    B. 75
    C. 80
    D. 85

20. _____ can raise or lower a pulse rate.
    A. Alcohol
    B. Nicotine
    C. Medications
    D. All of the above

Sentence Completion

Complete each sentence or statement.

1. A(n) _____ is an instrument used to listen to body sounds.

2. The heart makes a(n) _____ sound.

3. A(n) _____ temperature is taken under the arm.

4. _____ is the strength or force of each heartbeat.

5. _____ is the temperature scale that uses 0° as the freezing point and 100° as the boiling

point of water.

6. _____ provides documentation of a child's progress of height and weight from infancy.

7. When taking a temperature with _____, apply it to the forehead or on the abdomen.

8. _____ is the time interval between each heartbeat.

9. _____ refers to the strength or force of each heartbeat.

10. _____ is another word for "breathing in."

Short Answers

1. List the four components of vital signs.

_____

_____

2. Describe three examples of volume.

_____

_____

3. List six factors that might influence someone's blood pressure.

_____

_____

_____

_____

4. List five general guidelines for using a stethoscope.

_____

_____

_____

_____

5. List the three characteristics of the pulse that medical assistants should note in documentation.

_____

_____

_____

CRITICAL THINKING

Whitney Carleton is 18 years old and the single parent of a 4-month-old baby girl. She has brought her baby in for a check-up because she feels hot and is crying all the time. Dr. Donaldson has asked you to measure the infant's vital signs. Whitney is a very nervous new mother, and she wants you to explain everything you are going to do to her baby. You ask Whitney if she has taken the baby's temperature. She tells you she has not, she does not have a thermometer nor does she know how to check her temperature. Explain to Whitney how to conduct a rectal exam to determine if her baby's temperature is increased.

INTERNET RESEARCH

Keywords: Hypertension, Growth Charts

Choose one of the following topics to research: Hypertension or Children's Growth Charts. Write a one-page report. Cite your source. Be prepared to give a 2-minute oral presentation should your instructor assign you to do so.

WHAT WOULD YOU DO?

If you have accomplished the objectives in this chapter, you will be able to make better choices as a medical assistant. Take another look at this situation and decide what you would do.

Stephanie works for a general practitioner who sees pediatric as well as adult and geriatric patients. Dr. Karas wants height and weight measurements for patients at each visit, regardless of the patient's age. Dr. Karas also wants head and chest circumference measurements taken for pediatric patients up to age 3 years. Travis, a new patient, is a young teenager who does not want to have his weight and height measured because he is obese. He balks at having his temperature taken, stating that he knows he is not ill and "absolutely does not need to have that done." Stephanie tries explaining to Travis the differences in temperature, pulse, respiration, and blood pressure in different age groups. Finally, Travis agrees to have his temperature taken with a tympanic thermometer. When Stephanie starts to take Travis's blood pressure, he resists and tells her that he is scared and just knows that taking his blood pressure will hurt. Stephanie finally convinces Travis that she needs to take all his vital signs to prepare him for Dr. Karas's examination.

Would you be prepared to explain to a new patient the importance of taking body measurements and vital signs?

1. **Why would Dr. Karas want height and weight measurements on each visit for patients in all age groups?**

_____

_____

2. Why are growth charts important in treating pediatric patients?

_____

_____

_____

3. Why are head and chest circumference measurements important in pediatric patients?

_____

_____

_____

4. How can Stephanie convince Travis that it is important for his height and weight to be taken with each visit? How can she make the weight mensuration less upsetting to Travis?

_____

_____

_____

5. What are the differences in temperature, pulse, respirations, and blood pressure in age groups?

_____

_____

_____

_____

6. How would a tympanic temperature reading differ from an oral temperature?

_____

_____

_____

7. What does Stephanie need to explain to Travis about taking blood pressure?

_____

_____

_____

_____

8. Since Travis is upset, should Stephanie take his blood pressure immediately? Explain your answer.

_____

_____

_____

_____

9. What measurements are included in taking a patient's vital signs?

_____

_____

APPLICATION OF SKILLS

Procedure Check-off Sheets (*) and Assignments from MACC CD (see Procedure Check-off Sheets for which procedure from the MACC CD to perform).

1. Perform Procedure 30-1: Measure Weight and Height of an Adult.*

2. Perform Procedure 30-2: Measure Weight and Length of an Infant.*

3. Perform Procedure 30-3: Measure Head and Chest Circumference of an Infant.*

4. Perform Procedure 30-4: Measure Oral Body Temperature Using a Mercury-Free Glass Thermometer.*

5. Perform Procedure 30-5: Measure Oral Body Temperature Using a Rechargeable Electronic or Digital Thermometer.*

6. Perform Procedure 30-6: Measure Rectal Body Temperature Using a Rechargeable Electronic or Digital Thermometer.*

7. Perform Procedure 30-7: Measure Axillary Body Temperature Using a Rechargeable Electronic or Digital Thermometer.*

8. Perform Procedure 30-8: Measure Body Temperature Using a Tympanic Thermometer.*

9. Perform Procedure 30-9: Measure Body Temperature Using a Disposable Oral Thermometer.*

10. Perform Procedure 30-10: Measure Radial Pulse.*

11. Perform Procedure 30-11: Measure Apical Pulse.*

12. Perform Procedure 30-12: Measure Respiratory Rate.*

13. Perform Procedure 30-13: Measure Blood Pressure.*

Student Name _____ **Date** _____

PROCEDURE 30-1: MEASURE WEIGHT AND HEIGHT OF AN ADULT

TASK: Correctly obtain accurate height and weight measurements on an adult patient.

CONDITIONS: Given the proper equipment and supplies, the student will be required to role-play with another student or an instructor the proper method for measuring the height and weight of an adult patient.

NOTE: The student should practice the procedure using the MACC CD in the back of the textbook and then practice and perform the task in the classroom: MACC CD MACC/Clinical skills/Patient care/Patient preparation/Obtaining height and weight.

EQUIPMENT AND SUPPLIES
- MACC CD/computer
- Paper towel
- Balance scale with bar measure for height
- Patient's medical record
- Pen

STANDARDS: Complete the procedure within _____ minutes and achieve a minimum score of _____ %.

Time began _____   **Time ended** _____

Steps	Possible Points	First Attempt	Second Attempt
Weight			
1. Assemble all supplies and equipment.	5		
2. Sanitize hands.	5		
3. Check the scale to ensure it is properly balanced.	10		
4. Greet and identify the patient.	5		
5. Explain the procedure to the patient.	5		
6. Instruct the patient to remove shoes and empty items from pockets.	10		
7. Assist the patient onto the scale facing forward as necessary.	10		
8. Instruct the patient to stand still and to not hold onto objects for support.	10		
9. Balance the scale by moving the large weight (50-lb increment) first and then the small (1-lb increment) weight until scale is balanced.	5		
10. Read the results.	5		
11. Return the balance weights to the resting position of "0."	5		
12. Record the weight in the patient's medical record.	5		
Height			
1. Instruct the patient to stand erect and look straight ahead, with his or her back to the scale. (The patient must turn around on scale from being weighed.)	10		

Steps	Possible Points	First Attempt	Second Attempt
2. Raise the height bar above the person's head.	5		
3. Open the bar, taking care not to hit the patient's head.	5		
4. Move the bar down gently until it rests level on top of the patient's head.	10		
5. Assist the patient in stepping off the scale as appropriate.	5		
6. Read and record the measurement in the patient's medical record; convert from inches to feet and inches as per office policy.	20		
7. Assist the patient as needed in putting their shoes back on as appropriate.	5		
8. Return the bar to the resting position.	5		
9. Sanitize hands.	5		

Total Points Possible   150

Comments: Total Points Earned _____ Divided by _____ Total Possible Points = _____ % Score

Instructor's Signature _____

Student Name _____ **Date** _____

PROCEDURE 30-2: MEASURE WEIGHT AND LENGTH OF AN INFANT

TASK: Correctly measure the weight and length of an infant to monitor development.

CONDITIONS: Given the proper equipment and supplies, the student will be required to role-play using a mannequin the proper method for measuring the weight and length of an infant.

NOTE: The student should practice the procedure using the MACC CD in the back of the textbook and then practice and perform the task in the classroom: MACC CD MACC/Clinical skills/Patient care/The physical exam/Taking pediatric measurements and plotting on a growth chart.

EQUIPMENT AND SUPPLIES
- MACC CD/computer
- Infant scale with disposable plastic-lined drape or pad cover
- Flexible tape measure
- Infant growth charts, male or female, as appropriate
- Patient's medical record
- Pen
- Ruler

STANDARDS: Complete the procedure within _____ minutes and achieve a minimum score of _____ %.

Time began _____   **Time ended** _____

Steps	Possible Points	First Attempt	Second Attempt
Weight			
1. Assemble all supplies and equipment.	5		
2. Sanitize hands.	5		
3. Unlock the pediatric scale and balance as necessary.	10		
4. Greet the parent or guardian and identify the patient.	10		
5. Explain the procedure to the parent or guardian.	10		
6. Place the plastic-lined disposable drape or pad cover on the scale.	10		
7. Undress the infant, including the diaper.	10		
8. Gently place the infant on his or her back on the scale.	10		
9. Weigh the infant by first moving the pound weight and then the ounce weight until the scale balances.	10		
10. Read the results.	10		
11. Record the infant's weight in the medical record.	10		
12. Return the balance weights to the resting position.	10		
13. Remove the infant from the scale. (If you are measuring the length of the infant on a scale that has length measurement included, do not perform steps 13 and 14 at this time.)	10		
14. Discard the scale drape or pad.	10		

Copyright © 2005 by Elsevier Inc.

Steps	Possible Points	First Attempt	Second Attempt
Length (measured on the infant scale)			
1. Position the infant in the scale by placing the vertex of the infant head against the headboard at the zero mark, asking the parent or guardian to hold the infant in place.	10		
2. Read the length in inches to the nearest fraction of an inch.	10		
3. Record the results.	10		
4. Remove the infant from the scale.	10		
5. Discard the scale drape or pad.	10		
6. Read and record the measurement in the patient's medical record.	10		
Length (measured using the examination table)			
7. Position the infant on his or her back in the center of the examination table.	10		
8. Ask the parent or guardian to hold the infant in place.	5		
9. With a pen, mark a line on the table paper level with the patient's head.	10		
10. Holding the infant, stretch the leg and foot down and place a mark at the heel.	10		
11. Gently remove the infant from the table.	10		
12. Measure the length between the two pen marks using the tape measure.	10		
13. Inform the parent or guardian of the measurements and have the parent or guardian replace the diaper.	10		
14. Discard the protective paper on the examination table in the appropriate container.	10		
15. Sanitize hands.	5		
17. Plot the infant's weight and length on the growth charts and in the patient's medical record.	20		
Total Points Possible	290		

Comments: Total Points Earned _____ Divided by _____ Total Possible Points = _____ % Score

Instructor's Signature _____

Student Name _____ **Date** _____

PROCEDURE 30-3: MEASURE HEAD AND CHEST CIRCUMFERENCE OF AN INFANT

TASK: Accurately measure the head circumference and chest circumference of an infant.

CONDITIONS: Given the proper equipment and supplies, the student will be required to role-play using a mannequin the proper method for measuring the weight and length of an infant.

NOTE: The student should practice the procedure using the MACC CD in the back of the textbook and then practice and perform the task in the classroom: MACC CD MACC/Clinical skills/Patient care/The physical exam/Taking pediatric measurements & plotting on a growth chart.

EQUIPMENT AND SUPPLIES
- MACC CD/computer
- Flexible tape measure
- Infant growth charts, male or female, as appropriate
- Patient's medical record
- Pen
- Ruler

STANDARDS: Complete the procedure within _____ minutes and achieve a minimum score of _____ %.

Time began _____   **Time ended** _____

Steps	Possible Points	First Attempt	Second Attempt
Head Circumference			
1. Assemble all supplies and equipment.	5		
2. Sanitize hands.	5		
3. Greet the parent or guardian and identify the patient.	5		
4. Explain the procedure to the parent or guardian.	5		
5. Position the infant.	5		
6. Position the tape measure around the infant's head above the ears and just over the eyebrows.	10		
7. Read the tape measure to the nearest 1/4 inch.	10		
8. Write the results on the examination paper.	5		
Chest Circumference			
1. Place the tape around the infant's chest at the nipple line.	5		
2. Read the tape measure to the nearest 1/4 inch.	5		
3. Write the results on the examination paper.	5		
4. Hand the infant back to the parent or guardian.	5		
5. Inform the parent or guardian of the measurements and record the results in the patient's medical record.	10		
6. Discard the protective paper on the examination table in the appropriate container if the examination will not be done on the same table.	5		

Steps	Possible Points	First Attempt	Second Attempt
7. Sanitize hands.	5		
8. Plot points on the growth chart and connect the dots using the ruler.	10		

Total Points Possible   100

Comments: Total Points Earned _____ Divided by _____ Total Possible Points = _____ % Score

Instructor's Signature _____

Student Name _____ Date _____

PROCEDURE 30-4: MEASURE ORAL BODY TEMPERATURE USING A MERCURY-FREE GLASS THERMOMETER

TASK: Accurately measure and record a patient's oral temperature.
CONDITIONS: Given the proper equipment and supplies, the student will be required to role-play with another student or an instructor the proper method for measuring an oral body temperature using a mercury-free glass thermometer.

EQUIPMENT AND SUPPLIES
- Mercury-free glass oral thermometer
- Thermometer sheath
- Disposable gloves
- Biohazardous waste container
- Pen
- Patient's medical record

STANDARDS: Complete the procedure within _____ minutes and achieve a minimum score of _____ %.

Time began _____   Time ended _____

Steps	Possible Points	First Attempt	Second Attempt
1. Assemble all supplies and equipment.	5		
2. Sanitize hands.	5		
3. Greet and identify the patient.	5		
4. Explain the procedure to the patient.	5		
5. Determine if the patient has recently had a hot or cold beverage to drink or has smoked.	5		
6. Put on gloves and remove the thermometer from its holder, without touching the bulb end with your fingers.	5		
7. Inspect the thermometer for chips or cracks.	5		
8. Read the thermometer to ensure that the temperature is well below 96.0° F. Shake down thermometer as necessary.	5		
9. Cover the thermometer with a protective thermometer sheath.	5		
10. Ask the patient to open his or her mouth and place the probe tip under the tongue.	5		
11. Ask the patient to hold, not clasp, the thermometer between the teeth and to close the lips snugly around it to form an airtight seal.	5		
12. Leave the thermometer in place for a minimum of 3 minutes.	5		
13. Remove the thermometer and read the results.	10		
14. Holding the thermometer by the stem, remove the protective sheath and discard in a biohazardous waste container.	5		
15. Sanitize the thermometer following the manufacturer's recommendations.	5		

Copyright © 2005 by Elsevier Inc.

Steps	Possible Points	First Attempt	Second Attempt
16. Remove gloves and discard in biohazardous waste container.	5		
17. Return the thermometer to its storage container.	5		
18. Sanitize hands.	5		
19. Document the results in the patient's medical record.	5		

Total Points Possible   100

Comments: Total Points Earned _____ Divided by _____ Total Possible Points = _____ % Score

Instructor's Signature _____

Student Name _____   Date _____

PROCEDURE 30-5: MEASURE ORAL BODY TEMPERATURE USING A RECHARGEABLE ELECTRONIC OR DIGITAL THERMOMETER

TASK: Accurately measure and record a patient's oral temperature.

CONDITIONS: Given the proper equipment and supplies, the student will be required to role-play with another student or an instructor the proper method for measuring an oral body temperature using a rechargeable electronic or digital thermometer.

NOTE: The student should practice the procedure using the MACC CD in the back of the textbook and then practice and perform the task in the classroom: MACC CD MACC/Clinical skills/Patient care/The physical exam/Obtaining digital oral, digital rectal & tympanic body temperatures

EQUIPMENT AND SUPPLIES
- MACC CD/computer
- Rechargeable electronic or digital thermometer
- Probe cover
- Waste container
- Pen
- Patient's medical record

STANDARDS: Complete the procedure within _____ minutes and achieve a minimum score of _____ %.

Time began _____   **Time ended** _____

Steps	Possible Points	First Attempt	Second Attempt
1. Assemble all supplies and equipment.	5		
2. Sanitize hands.	5		
3. Greet and identify the patient.	5		
4. Explain the procedure to the patient.	5		
5. Remove the thermometer unit from its rechargeable base, and attach the blue collar probe for measuring oral temperature.	10		
6. Remove the thermometer probe cover from the probe holder and attach to thermometer probe.	5		
7. Ask the patient to open his or her mouth. Place the probe tip under the tongue.	10		
8. Ask the patient to close his or her mouth.	5		
9. When the alert signal is seen or heard, remove the probe from the patient's mouth.	10		
10. Read the result in the LED window of the unit.	10		
11. Dispose of the thermometer tip.	5		
12. Return the probe to the stored position on the thermometer.	5		
13. Place the thermometer unit back on the rechargeable base.	5		

Steps	Possible Points	First Attempt	Second Attempt
14. Sanitize hands.	5		
15. Document results in the patient's medical record.	10		

Total Points Possible 100

Comments: Total Points Earned _____ Divided by _____ Total Possible Points = _____ % Score

Instructor's Signature _____

Student Name _____ **Date** _____

PROCEDURE 30-6: MEASURE RECTAL BODY TEMPERATURE USING A RECHARGEABLE ELECTRONIC OR DIGITAL THERMOMETER

TASK: Accurately measure and record a patient's rectal temperature.

CONDITIONS: Given the proper equipment and supplies, the student will be required to role-play with a mannequin the proper method for measuring the rectal temperature using a rechargeable electronic or digital thermometer.

NOTE: The student should practice the procedure using the MACC CD in the back of the textbook and then practice and perform the task in the classroom: MACC CD MACC/Clinical skills/Patient care/Patient preparation/Obtaining digital oral, digital rectal, & tympanic body temperature.

EQUIPMENT AND SUPPLIES
- MACC CD/computer
- Rechargeable electronic or digital thermometer
- Probe cover
- Disposable gloves
- Lubricant
- Biohazardous waste container
- Pen
- Patient's medical record
- Soft tissue
- Gauze squares

STANDARDS: Complete the procedure within _____ minutes and achieve a minimum score of _____ %.

Time began _____   **Time ended** _____

Steps	Possible Points	First Attempt	Second Attempt
1. Assemble all supplies and equipment.	5		
2. Sanitize hands.	5		
3. Greet and identify the patient.	5		
4. Explain the procedure to the patient.	5		
5. Remove the thermometer unit from its rechargeable base, and attach the red collar probe for measuring rectal temperature.	5		
6. Remove the thermometer probe cover from the probe holder and attach to thermometer probe.	5		
7. Place a plastic-lined disposable drape or pad cover on the table.	5		
8. Put on disposable gloves.	5		
9. Undress the child, including the diaper. (Position an adult patient in the Sim's position and properly drape. Expose the rectal area of an adult patient.)	5		
10. Squeeze approximately 1 inch of lubricant onto a gauze square; lubricate the first 2 inches of the probe cover for an adult and 1 inch for a child.	5		

Steps	Possible Points	First Attempt	Second Attempt
11. If patient is a child, have the parent or guardian (classmate) hold the child firmly but comfortably so that the child lies still, to avoid injury to the rectal wall.	5		
12. Insert the tip about 1 to 2 inches for an adult or 1/2 inch for a child.	5		
13. When the alert signal is seen or heard, read the results in the LED window of the unit.	5		
14. Remove the probe cover.	5		
15. Return the probe to the stored position on the thermometer.	5		
16. Place the thermometer unit back on the rechargeable base.	5		
17. Wipe the patient's anal area with tissue.	5		
18. Remove soiled gloves and discard in a biohazardous waste container.	5		
19. Sanitize hands.	5		
20. Document results in the patient's medical record using ® to indicate rectal temperature was obtained.	5		

Total Points Possible   100

Comments: Total Points Earned _____ Divided by _____ Total Possible Points = _____ % Score

Instructor's Signature _____

Student Name _____ Date _____

PROCEDURE 30-7: MEASURE AXILLARY BODY TEMPERATURE USING A RECHARGEABLE ELECTRONIC OR DIGITAL THERMOMETER

TASK: Accurately measure and record a patient's axillary temperature.

CONDITIONS: Given the proper equipment and supplies, the student will be required to role-play with another student or an instructor the proper method for measuring the axillary temperature using a rechargeable electronic or digital thermometer.

EQUIPMENT AND SUPPLIES
- Rechargeable electronic or digital thermometer
- Probe cover
- Waste container
- Pen
- Patient's medical record

STANDARDS: Complete the procedure within _____ minutes and achieve a minimum score of _____ %.

Time began _____   Time ended _____

Steps	Possible Points	First Attempt	Second Attempt
1. Assemble all supplies and equipment.	5		
2. Sanitize hands.	5		
3. Greet and identify the patient.	5		
4. Explain the procedure to the patient.	5		
5. Remove the thermometer unit from its rechargeable base, and attach the probe with the blue collar for measuring axillary temperature.	10		
6. Remove the thermometer probe from the probe holder and attach thermometer cover.	5		
7. Remove the patient's clothing as needed to access the axillary region.	5		
8. Pat the axilla and axillary area dry as needed.	5		
9. Place the probe into the center of the patient's armpit.	5		
10. Instruct the patient to hold the arm snugly across the chest until the thermometer sends the alert signal that the temperature has been taken.	5		
11. When the alert signal is seen or heard, remove the probe from the patient's armpit.	5		
12. Read the results in the LED window of the unit.	10		
13. Dispose of the probe cover.	5		
14. Return the probe to the stored position on the thermometer.	5		
15. Place the thermometer unit back on the rechargeable base.	5		

Steps	Possible Points	First Attempt	Second Attempt
16. Sanitize hands.	5		
17. Document results in the patient's medical record.	10		
Total Points Possible	100		

Comments: Total Points Earned _____ Divided by _____ Total Possible Points = _____ % Score

Instructor's Signature _____

Student Name _____ Date _____

PROCEDURE 30-8: MEASURE BODY TEMPERATURE
USING A TYMPANIC THERMOMETER

TASK: Accurately measure and record a patient's temperature using a tympanic thermometer.

CONDITIONS: Given the proper equipment and supplies, the student will be required to role-play with another student the proper method for measuring the tympanic temperature using a tympanic thermometer.

NOTE: The student should practice the procedure using the MACC CD in the back of the textbook and then practice and perform the task in the classroom: MACC CD MACC/Clinical skills/Patient care/Patient preparation/Obtaining digital oral, digital rectal, and tympanic body temperature.

EQUIPMENT AND SUPPLIES
- MACC CD/computer
- Tympanic thermometer
- Disposable probe cover
- Pen
- Patient's medical record
- Biohazardous waste container

STANDARDS: Complete the procedure within _____ minutes and achieve a minimum score of _____ %.

Time began _____   Time ended _____

Steps	Possible Points	First Attempt	Second Attempt
1. Assemble all supplies and equipment.	5		
2. Sanitize hands.	5		
3. Greet and identify the patient.	5		
4. Explain the procedure to the patient.	5		
5. Remove the thermometer from the charger.	5		
6. Check to be sure the mode for interpretation of temperature is set to "oral" mode.	10		
7. Check the lens probe to be sure it is clean and not scratched.	5		
8. Turn on the thermometer.	5		
9. Insert the probe firmly into a disposable plastic probe cover.	5		
10. Wait for a digital "READY" display.	5		
11. With the hand that is not holding the probe, pull adult patient's ear up and back to straighten the ear canal. For a small child, pull the patient's ear down and back to straighten the ear canal.	10		
12. Insert the probe into the patient's ear and tightly seal the ear canal opening.	10		
13. Position the probe.	5		
14. Depress the activation button.	5		
15. Release the activation button and wait 2 seconds.	5		
16. Remove the probe from the ear and read the temperature.	5		

Copyright © 2005 by Elsevier Inc.

Steps	Possible Points	First Attempt	Second Attempt
17. Note the reading, making sure that the screen displays "oral" as the mode of interpretation.	5		
18. Discard the probe cover in a biohazardous waste container.	5		
19. Replace the thermometer on the charger base.	5		
20. Sanitize hands.	5		
21. Document results in the patient's medical record using ⓣ to indicate a tympanic temperature was obtained.	10		

Total Points Possible   125

Comments: Total Points Earned _____ Divided by _____ Total Possible Points = _____ % Score

Instructor's Signature _____

Student Name _____ Date _____

PROCEDURE 30-9: MEASURE BODY TEMPERATURE USING A DISPOSABLE ORAL THERMOMETER

TASK: Accurately measure and record a patient's oral temperature using a disposable thermometer.
CONDITIONS: Given the proper equipment and supplies, the student will be required to perform the proper method for measuring an oral temperature using a disposable oral thermometer.

EQUIPMENT AND SUPPLIES
- Disposable thermometer
- Disposable gloves
- Biohazardous waste container
- Pen
- Patient's medical record

STANDARDS: Complete the procedure within _____ minutes and achieve a minimum score of _____ %.

Time began _____   Time ended _____

Steps	Possible Points	First Attempt	Second Attempt
1. Assemble all supplies and equipment.	5		
2. Sanitize hands.	5		
3. Greet and identify the patient.	5		
4. Explain the procedure to the patient.	5		
5. Put on disposable gloves.	5		
6. Open the thermometer packaging.	5		
7. Place the thermometer under the patient's tongue and wait 60 seconds.	5		
8. Remove the thermometer and read the results by looking at the colored dots.	5		
9. Discard the thermometer and gloves in a biohazardous waste container.	5		
10. Sanitize hands.	5		
11. Document results in the patient's medical record.	10		

Total Points Possible   60

Comments: Total Points Earned _____ Divided by _____ Total Possible Points = _____ % Score

Instructor's Signature _____

Student Name _____ **Date** _____

PROCEDURE 30-10: MEASURE RADIAL PULSE

TASK: Accurately measure and record the rate, rhythm, and quality of a patient's pulse.

CONDITIONS: Given the proper equipment and supplies, the student will be required to role-play with another student or an instructor the proper method for measuring a patient's radial pulse.

NOTE: The student should practice the procedure using the MACC CD in the back of the textbook and then practice and perform the task in the classroom: MACC CD MACC/Clinical skills/Patient care/Patient preparation/Obtaining pulse & respiration.

EQUIPMENT AND SUPPLIES
- MACC CD/computer
- Watch with a second hand
- Patient's medical record
- Pen

STANDARDS: Complete the procedure within _____ minutes and achieve a minimum score of _____ %.

Time began _____   **Time ended** _____

Steps	Possible Points	First Attempt	Second Attempt
1. Assemble all supplies and equipment.	5		
2. Sanitize hands.	5		
3. Greet and identify the patient.	5		
4. Explain the procedure to the patient.	5		
5. Observe the patient for any signs that may indicate an increase or a decrease in the pulse rate due to external conditions.	5		
6. Position the patient.	5		
7. Place the index and middle fingertips over the radial artery while resting the thumb on the back of the patient's wrist.	10		
8. Apply moderate, gentle pressure directly over the site until the pulse can be felt.	10		
9. Count the pulse for 60 seconds.	10		
10. Sanitize hands.	5		
11. Document the results in the patient's chart; include the pulse rate, rhythm, and volume.	10		

Total Points Possible   75

Comments: Total Points Earned _____ Divided by _____ Total Possible Points = _____ % Score

Instructor's Signature _____

Student Name _____ **Date** _____

PROCEDURE 30-11: MEASURE APICAL PULSE

TASK: Accurately measure and record the rate, rhythm, and quality of a patient's pulse.

CONDITIONS: Given the proper equipment and supplies, the student will be required to role-play with another student or an instructor the proper method for measuring a patient's apical pulse.

EQUIPMENT AND SUPPLIES
- Watch with a second hand
- Stethoscope
- Alcohol wipe
- Patient's medical record
- Pen

STANDARDS: Complete the procedure within _____ minutes and achieve a minimum score of _____ %.

Time began _____   **Time ended** _____

Steps	Possible Points	First Attempt	Second Attempt
1. Assemble all supplies and equipment.	5		
2. Sanitize hands.	5		
3. Greet and identify the patient.	5		
4. Explain the procedure to the patient.	5		
5. Clean the earpieces of the stethoscope with an alcohol wipe.	5		
6. Position the patient in a supine or sitting position.	10		
7. Position the stethoscope over apex of heart.	10		
8. Count the number of beats for 1 full minute.	10		
9. Clean the stethoscope earpieces and diaphragm with an alcohol wipe.	5		
10. Sanitize hands.	5		
11. Document the results in the patient's chart; include the pulse rate, rhythm, and volume.	10		

Total Points Possible   75

Comments: Total Points Earned _____ Divided by _____ Total Possible Points = _____ % Score

Instructor's Signature _____

Student Name _____ Date _____

PROCEDURE 30-12: MEASURE RESPIRATORY RATE

TASK: Accurately measure and record a patient's respiratory rate.

CONDITIONS: Given the proper equipment and supplies, the student will be required to role-play with another student the proper method for measuring a patient's respiratory rate.

NOTE: The student should practice the procedure using the MACC CD in the back of the textbook and then practice and perform the task in the classroom: MACC CD MACC/Clinical skills/Patient care/Patient preparation/Obtaining pulse and respiration.

EQUIPMENT AND SUPPLIES
- MACC CD/computer
- Watch with a second hand
- Patient's medical record
- Pen

STANDARDS: Complete the procedure within _____ minutes and achieve a minimum score of _____ %.

Time began _____   **Time ended** _____

Steps	Possible Points	First Attempt	Second Attempt
1. Assemble all supplies and equipment.	5		
2. Sanitize hands.	5		
3. Greet and identify the patient.	5		
4. Explain the procedure to the patient.	5		
5. Count each respiration for 30 seconds and multiply by 2. (If breathing pattern is inaccurate, count for 1 full minute.)	15		
6. Sanitize hands.	5		
7. Document the results in the patient's chart; include the respiratory rate, rhythm, and depth. Document any irregularities found.	10		
Total Points Possible	50		

Comments: Total Points Earned _____ Divided by _____ Total Possible Points = _____ % Score

Instructor's Signature _____

Student Name _____ **Date** _____

PROCEDURE 30-13: MEASURE BLOOD PRESSURE

TASK: Accurately measure and record a patient's blood pressure by palpation and auscultation.

CONDITIONS: Given the proper equipment and supplies, the student will be required to role-play with another student the proper method for measuring a patient's blood pressure.

NOTE: The student should practice the procedure using the MACC CD in the back of the textbook and then practice and perform the task in the classroom: MACC CD MACC/Clinical skills/Patient care/Patient preparation/Obtaining blood pressure.

EQUIPMENT AND SUPPLIES
- MACC CD/computer
- Stethoscope
- Aneroid sphygmomanometer in proper size for patient
- Alcohol wipe
- Patient's medical record
- Pen

STANDARDS: Complete the procedure within _____ minutes and achieve a minimum score of _____ %.

Time began _____   **Time ended** _____

Steps	Possible Points	First Attempt	Second Attempt
1. Assemble all supplies and equipment.	5		
2. Sanitize hands.	5		
3. Greet and identify the patient.	5		
4. Explain the procedure to the patient.	5		
5. Position the patient comfortably in a sitting or supine position.	5		
6. Palpate the brachial artery.	10		
7. Position the blood pressure cuff; wrap the cuff snugly and evenly around the patient's arm and secure the end.	10		
8. Position the aneroid gauge for direct viewing at a distance of no more than 3 feet.	10		
9. Measure the systolic pressure by palpation.	15		
10. Deflate the cuff completely and wait at least 60 seconds before reinflating.	10		
11. Clean the stethoscope.	5		
12. Place the earpieces of the stethoscope in your ears, with the earpieces directed slightly forward.	5		
13. Position the head of the stethoscope over the brachial artery of the arm.	5		
14. Close the valve to the manometer.	5		
15. Pump the cuff at a smooth rate to approximately 20 to 30 mm Hg above the palpated systolic pressure	10		
16. Loosen the thumbscrew slightly to open the valve and release the pressure on the cuff, slowly and steadily.	10		

Steps	Possible Points	First Attempt	Second Attempt
17. Obtain the systolic reading.	10		
18. Continue to release the air from the cuff at a moderately slow rate.	5		
19. Listen for the disappearance of the Korotkoff sounds; obtain diastolic pressure.	10		
20. Release the air remaining in the cuff quickly by loosening the thumbscrew to open the valve completely.	5		
21. Remove the earpieces of the stethoscope from your ears, and remove the cuff from the patient's arm.	5		
22. Sanitize hands.	5		
23. Document the results in the patient's chart.	10		
24. Clean the earpieces and diaphragm with an alcohol wipe, and properly store the equipment.	5		

Total Points Possible   75

Comments: Total Points Earned _____ Divided by _____ Total Possible Points = _____ % Score

Instructor's Signature _____

CHAPTER QUIZ:

Multiple Choice

Identify the letter of the choice that best completes the statement or answers the question.

1. The birth weight of an infant should _____ in the first 6 months.
   A. double
   B. triple
   C. quadruple
   D. stay the same

2. Children should have their height recorded _____.
   A. each month
   B. every 6 months
   C. every visit
   D. every year

3. Growth charts provide information on the height and weight pattern of a child from infancy.
   A. True
   B. False

4. When the ventricles contract, the first measurable pressure is the _____ pressure.
   A. blood
   B. diastolic
   C. systolic
   D. none of the above

5. The mercury-free thermometer tip color, _____, signifies that it is to be used orally.
   A. blue
   B. green
   C. red
   D. yellow

6. It is better to use a larger cuff when in doubt of which size to use.
   A. True
   B. False

7. _____ is(are) a low-pitched sound created as air goes through mucus.
   A. Stridor
   B. Rales
   C. Rhonchi
   D. Wheezes

8. An infant's head circumference is approximately _____ % of an adult's head circumference by age 1.
   A. 50
   B. 60
   C. 70
   D. 80

9. Hypotension is a blood pressure that exceeds the acceptable range for the patient's age group.
   A. True
   B. False

10. _____ is the number of times the heart beats in a minute.
    A. Pulse
    B. Pulse rate
    C. Heart rate
    D. None of the above

11. When using a(n) _____, the temperature typically registers within 60 seconds.
    A. disposable oral thermometer
    B. temperature-sensitive tape
    C. tympanic thermometer
    D. electronic thermometer

12. Adults have a respiration rate of _____.
    A. 10 to 15
    B. 16 to 20
    C. 20 to 25
    D. 22 to 28

13. Normal adult systolic range is _____ mm Hg.
    A. 80 to 100
    B. 90 to 110
    C. 100 to 120
    D. 110 to 125

14. Respiratory rate can be described as being normal, slow, or rapid.
    A. True
    B. False

15. A heart rate greater than _____ is considered to be tachycardia.
    A. 80
    B. 90
    C. 95
    D. 100

16. It is recommended the medical assistant takes a patient's pulse for _____.
    A. 15 seconds and multiply by 4
    B. 20 seconds and multiply by 3
    C. 30 seconds and multiply by 2
    D. 60 seconds

17. The _____ artery is the most common place for a pulse to be measured in an adult.
    A. apical
    B. brachial
    C. femoral
    D. radial

18. When listening to the heart with a stethoscope, the sound you hear is _____.
    A. lupp-dupp
    B. lubb-dubb
    C. lubb-dupp
    D. none of the above

19. A blood pressure can be measured over clothes.
    A. True
    B. False

20. The _____ pulse must be taken with a stethoscope.
    A. apical
    B. brachial
    C. popliteal
    D. radial

CHAPTER THIRTY-ONE

Medical History Taking

VOCABULARY REVIEW:

Matching

Match each term with the correct definition.

A. charting

B. demographics

C. familial

D. Health Insurance Portability and Accountability Act (HIPAA)

E. hereditary

F. objective information

G. past history

H. release of information

I. review of systems

J. social history

K. subjective information

L. symptoms

M. chief complaint

N. open-ended questions

O. signs

_____ 1. Step-by-step review of each body system

_____ 2. Biographical data; personal information

_____ 3. Subjective data reported by the patient

_____ 4. Able to be seen or measured

_____ 5. Summary of a patient's prior health

_____ 6. Found in family member

_____ 7. Overview of a patient's lifestyle

_____ 8. Documenting what is observed or what is told by the patient

_____ 9. Not able to be seen or measured

_____ 10. Government act mandating that appropriate measures be taken to protect a patient's personal information

_____ 11. Legal form signed by a patient that indicates who can see the patient's health records

_____ 12. Acquired through genetic makeup

_____ 13. Reason why the patient wants to see the physician

_____ 14. Questions that require more than a "yes" or "no" answer

_____ 15. Observable evidence that can be seen or measured

THEORY RECALL

True/False

Indicate whether the sentence or statement is true or false.

_____ 1. The first step in interviewing any patient is to ensure the interview is private and free of interruptions.

_____ 2. Information that can be measured or observed is called objective information.

_____ 3. Effective communication slows down the medical assistant in her or his search for necessary information.

_____ 4. It is important to be reactive to shocking details the patient tells the medical assistant.

_____ 5. The medical assistant must report what is seen, heard, felt, and smelled.

Multiple Choice

Identify the letter of the choice that best completes the statement or answers the question.

1. Charting must be _____.
   A. clear
   B. correct
   C. nonjudgmental
   D. all of the above

2. Personal data section of a medical history is completed by the _____.
   A. physician
   B. medical assistant
   C. patient
   D. insurance company
   E. either B or C

3. Symptoms that cannot be seen are referred to as _____ information.
   A. assessment
   B. objective
   C. subjective
   D. present illness

4. The medical assistant should start the charting with _____.
   A. a clean progress note sheet
   B. the date and time
   C. a pen, blue ink only
   D. a bottle of white-out in hand to make necessary corrections

5. When interviewing the patient, the medical assistant should _____.
   A. be quick, efficient, and to the point
   B. relay personal stories to make the patient feel more at ease
   C. show genuine concern for the patient
   D. make assumptions as to the patient's answers

6. The _____ section contains more description about the current illness.
   A. social history
   B. present illness
   C. past history
   D. family history

7. The review of systems starts _____.
   A. as the patient walks in the door
   B. at the patient's feet and moves upward
   C. at the patient's head and moves downward
   D. none of the above

8. The medical assistant should ask _____.
   A. only the 13 standard questions of a physical exam
   B. yes or no questions
   C. open-ended questions
   D. direct questions

9. _____ is a brief statement of only one or two signs or symptoms.
   A. CC
   B. PH
   C. SH
   D. PI

10. _____ statements that pertain to the patient are key to providing a good database for the patient's physical examination.
    A. Encoding
    B. Charting
    C. Expanding on
    D. None of the above

11. The physician's treatment plan is based on _____.
    A. latest trends in technology
    B. laboratory findings only
    C. information gathered during history taking and physical exam
    D. physical exam only

12. Patients have _____ to expect that their confidential information is being protected.
    A. the right
    B. the privilege
    C. guarantees
    D. laws

Sentence Completion

Complete each sentence or statement.

1. _____ is an inventory of a patient's immediate family.

2. _____ information includes the patient's name, address, date of birth, and telephone number.

3. _____ is an expansion of the patient's chief complaint.

4. _____ must be completed before a patient's chart can be shared with another physician.

5. _____ presents an overview of the patient's lifestyle.

Short Answers

1. List six pieces of information that need to be included when gathering the patient's past history.

   _____

   _____

   _____

2. List the four areas on which observations are based.

   _____

   _____

   _____

   _____

3. List the seven sections of the medical history form.

   _____

   _____

   _____

4. List five items the medical assistant should remember about charting.

   _____

   _____

   _____

   _____

   _____

CRITICAL THINKING

Melinda was your eighth patient after lunch. The last thing you felt like doing was taking Melinda back to the exam room. Melinda always had a zillion questions and a story for everything. Trying to get to the reason Melinda was in to see the physician was always a challenge.

"Hey, Claire, will you take Melinda back?"

"No way. It's your turn," replied Claire. "I did it last week; it is your turn."

"Oh, all right." "Good afternoon, Melinda. How are you today?" Cindy asked as she went to retrieve Melinda from the waiting area.

"I'm fine, and you?" Melinda wasn't even smiling. She was shuffling her feet and staring at the ground all the way back to the exam room.

"What's wrong, Melinda? You don't seem to be yourself today."

"No, dear, I'm just fine; don't you worry."

But Cindy was worried that what Melinda was saying did not coincide with how she was acting.

1. Describe what verbal and nonverbal communication is occurring between Cindy and Melinda.

2. If you had to guess, what do you think is going on with Melinda, based just on the brief exchange given here.

INTERNET RESEARCH

Keyword: Verbal and Nonverbal Communication

Choose one of the following topics to research: Effective communication, What nonverbal communication tells the health care provider. Cite your source. Be prepared to give a 2-minute oral presentation should your instructor assign you to do so.

WHAT WOULD YOU DO?

If you have accomplished the objectives in this chapter, you will be able to make better choices as a medical assistant. Take another look at this situation and decide what you would do.

Dr. Walker, an obstetrician/gynecologist and internal medicine physician, has hired Jenny to assist with taking medical histories for his patients. Dr. Walker sees many patients who have high-risk pregnancies because of an infectious disease. Sarah, a new patient who is 4 months' pregnant, has been referred to Dr. Walker because she is at risk for several infectious diseases. Jenny goes to the waiting room and starts to ask Sarah questions about her pregnancy and her past medical history. Sarah tells Jenny that she does not want to discuss this with a medical assistant and would rather give the information to Dr. Walker. Jenny adamantly tells Sarah that if she does not want to cooperate, Dr. Walker will not see her as a patient. Sarah begins to cry but starts telling her history to Jenny. Trying to impress Sarah during the interview, Jenny uses medical terminology to ask questions, and she never looks at Sarah or makes any observations about Sarah's remarks. After the history taking, Sarah is escorted to the examination room, where her vital signs are taken. After discussing her previous illnesses and family history, Dr. Walker examines Sarah and orders several laboratory tests, including tests for HIV and for syphilis. His tentative diagnosis is "possible HIV infection," and he confirms her pregnancy of 4 months. On leaving the office, Sarah makes an appointment for 2 weeks to discuss her test results and final diagnosis with Dr. Walker.

What should Jenny have done differently as a medical assistant initially taking Sarah's history?

1. **Did Jenny handle the taking of the medical history correctly? Where should the history have been taken?**

2. **What actions would cause Sarah to think that Jenny is incompetent in taking a medical history?**

3. **Why is effective communication between the patient and the medical assistant so important when taking a medical history?**

4. **What is the "chief complaint," and how should it be documented?**

5. **What are signs? What are symptoms?**

6. What is the correct name for the "tentative diagnosis"? What is the difference between this diagnosis and the "final diagnosis"?

_____

_____

_____

_____

_____

7. Why would it be incorrect for the insurance coder to use the tentative diagnosis on the insurance claim form? What could be the repercussions if the laboratory tests are negative?

_____

_____

_____

_____

_____

8. Why would it have been important for Jenny to observe Sarah during the taking of the medical history?

_____

_____

_____

_____

APPLICATION OF SKILLS

Procedure Check-off Sheets (*) and Assignments from MACC CD (see Procedure Check-off Sheets for which procedure from the MACC CD to perform).

Perform Procedure 31-1: Complete a Medical History Form.*

Perform Procedure 32-2: Recognize and Respond to Verbal and Nonverbal Communication.*

Student Name _____ **Date** _____

PROCEDURE 31-1: COMPLETE A MEDICAL HISTORY FORM

TASK: Obtain and record a patient's medical history using verbal and nonverbal communication skills and applying the principles of accurate documentation in the patient's medical record.

CONDITIONS: Given the proper equipment and supplies, the student will be required to role-play with another student or an instructor the proper method for obtaining and recording a patient's medical history.

NOTE: The student should practice the procedure using the MACC CD in the back of the textbook and then practice and perform the task in the classroom. MACC CD MACC/Clinical skills/Patient care/Patient preparation/Obtaining & recording a medical history.

EQUIPMENT AND SUPPLIES
- MACC CD/computer
- Medical history form
- Patient's medical record
- Pen (red and black ink)
- Clipboard
- Quiet private area

STANDARDS: Complete the procedure within _____ minutes and achieve a minimum score of _____ %.

Time began _____   **Time ended** _____

Steps	Possible Points	First Attempt	Second Attempt
1. Assemble all supplies and equipment.	5		
2. Greet and identify the patient.	5		
3. Escort the patient to a quiet, comfortable room that is well lit and affords privacy.	5		
4. Explain why information is needed and reassure the patient that the information will be kept confidential.	10		
5. Seat the patient, and then sit near the patient at eye level.	5		
6. Review the completed portion of the medical history form, looking for omissions or incomplete answers. Verify information as needed.	15		
7. Speak clearly and distinctly; maintain eye contact as appropriate with the patient.	10		
8. Remember to record all information legibly in black ink.	5		
9. Ask the patient to state the reason for today's visit.	10		
10. Record the information briefly and concisely, using the patient's own words as much as possible.	20		
11. Ask the patient about prescription, over-the-counter, and herbal medications or treatments; record all medications the patient is taking.	10		

Steps	Possible Points	First Attempt	Second Attempt
12. Inquire about allergies to medications, food, and other substances; record any allergies in red ink on every page of the history form. Record no allergies as appropriate.	10		
13. Review and record information in all sections of the family history form.	10		
14. Thank the patient for providing the information.	10		
15. Review the record for errors prior to giving to the physician.	10		
16. Use the information to complete the patient's record as directed.	10		

Total Points Possible   150

Comments: Total Points Earned _____ Divided by _____ Total Possible Points = _____ % Score

Instructor's Signature _____

Student Name _____ Date _____

PROCEDURE 31-2: RECOGNIZE AND RESPOND TO VERBAL AND NONVERBAL COMMUNICATION

TASK: Recognize and respond to basic verbal and nonverbal communication.

CONDITIONS: Given the proper equipment and supplies, the student will be required to role-play with another student the proper method for recognizing and responding to basic verbal and nonverbal communication.

NOTE: The student should practice the procedure using the MACC CD in the back of the textbook and then practice and perform the task in the classroom. MACC CD MACC/ Professionalism/ Communication/ Recognizing & responding to verbal/nonverbal communication.

EQUIPMENT AND SUPPLIES
• No equipment or supplies required

STANDARDS: Complete the procedure within _____ minutes and achieve a minimum score of _____ %.

Time began _____   Time ended _____

Steps	Possible Points	First Attempt	Second Attempt
1. Greet the patient, smile to welcome the patient, and introduce yourself.	5		
2. Verify the patient's name and use it with a courtesy title, unless instructed otherwise by the patient.	5		
3. Establish a comfortable physical environment while respecting individual ethnic and cultural differences.	5		
4. Verify the patient feels comfortable.	5		
5. Establish the topic of discussion as directed.	5		
6. Observe the patient for nonverbal communication cues.	10		
7. Ask open-ended questions. Verify that the patient understands the questions.	10		
8. Practice active listening; provide feedback.	10		
9. Near the end of the discussion, provide the patient the opportunity to ask questions or provide further clarifications.	10		
10. Thank the patient for his or her comments and signal the end of the discussion.	10		

Total Points Possible   75

Comments: Total Points Earned _____ Divided by _____ Total Possible Points = _____ % Score

Instructor's Signature _____

CHAPTER QUIZ

Multiple Choice

Identify the letter of the choice that best completes the statement or answers the question.

1. The medical assistant must ensure _____ in order to obtain a good interview with a patient.
   A. confidentiality
   B. privacy
   C. an interruption-free environment
   D. all of the above

2. Symptoms that cannot be measured are known as (the) _____.
   A. chief complaint
   B. objective information
   C. present illness
   D. subjective information

3. A release of information form must be on file in order for a patient's information to be released to another physician.
   A. True
   B. False

4. _____ gives an overview of the patient's eating, drinking, smoking, and exercise habits.
   A. Family history
   B. Past history
   C. Review of systems
   D. Social history

5. _____ provide(s) observable information that can be measured.
   A. Chief complaint
   B. Signs
   C. Symptoms
   D. Past history

6. When charting, the medical assistant must be _____.
   A. clear and concise
   B. judgmental and critical
   C. selective and indecisive
   D. quick and decisive

7. _____ information includes a patient's name, address, date of birth, and gender.
   A. Familial
   B. Social
   C. Demographic
   D. Past history

8. The ROS starts with the _____.
   A. feet
   B. head
   C. when the patient walks in the door
   D. none of the above

9. The medical assistant only has to report what he or she hears to the physician.
   A. True
   B. False

10. Identification of a disease or condition based on review of signs and symptoms, laboratory reports, history, and procedures is known as the _____.
   A. chief complaint
   B. diagnosis
   C. objective information
   D. past history

11. _____ should be held in the strictest confidence.
   A. Family history
   B. Social history
   C. Past history
   D. All of the above

12. A medical assistant is allowed to chart his or her opinions about the patient's present history.
   A. True
   B. False

13. Information that can be measured or observed is _____.
   A. objective
   B. subjective
   C. assessment
   D. social history

14. _____ are observable evidence that can be seen or measured.
   A. Signs
   B. Symptoms

15. _____ is acquired through genetic makeup.
   A. Heredity
   B. Social history
   C. Environmental history
   D. None of the above

CHAPTER THIRTY-TWO
Assisting With the Physical Examination

VOCABULARY REVIEW

Matching

Match each term with the correct definition.

A. accommodation

B. auscultation

C. BSE

D. crepitus

E. diaphoresis

F. distention

G. erythema

H. gingivitis

I. goniometer

J. herpes simplex

K. jaundice

L. lithotomy position

M. macrotia

N. murmur

O. pallor

P. patent

Q. percussion

R. perforation

_____ 1. Patient's back is on the table; horizontal recumbent position

_____ 2. Crackling sound heard in the lungs or joints

_____ 3. Paleness

_____ 4. Humming or low-pitched fluttering sound of the heart heard on auscultation

_____ 5. Viral infection of the lip-skin junction; cold sore

_____ 6. Rattling sounds heard in the lungs, usually at the base

_____ 7. Ability of the eye to see objects in the distance and then adjust to a close object

_____ 8. Ability to see at different distances

_____ 9. Patient assumes the dorsal recumbent position first; then the buttocks are moved to the end of the table and the feet are placed in stirrups

_____ 10. Decrease in hearing ability resulting from aging

_____ 11. Swollen

S.   PERRLA

T.   presbycusis

U.   prone position

V.   rhonchi

W.   Sims' position

X.   supine position

Y.   thrill

Z.   tinnitus

AA.   turgor

BB.   vertigo

CC.   visual acuity

DD.   sitting position

_____ 12. Tapping to check for reflexes or sounds of body cavities

_____ 13. Ringing in the ears

_____ 14. Listening for signs using a stethoscope

_____ 15. Open; not obstructed

_____ 16. Patient is first in the supine position, then turns onto left side with the right leg sharply bent upward

_____ 17. Skin resiliency

_____ 18. Ears larger than 10 cm

_____ 19. Yellowish appearance to the skin and eyes

_____ 20. Pupils equal, round, and reactive to light and accommodation

_____ 21. Excessive perspiration

_____ 22. Palpable vibration

_____ 23. Device used to measure joint movements and angles

_____ 24. Breast-self examination

_____ 25. Dizziness

_____ 26. Inflammation of the gums

_____ 27. Tear or hole in an organ or body part

_____ 28. Reddish discoloration of the skin

_____ 29. Patient lies on the abdomen with the head turned slightly to the side

_____ 30. Patient's body is at a 90-degree angle

THEORY RECALL

True/False

Indicate whether the sentence or statement is true or false.

_____ 1. When the medical assistant is positioning and draping the patient, he or she should always consider the patient's comfort and minimize the area of exposure.

_____ 2. When a patient is in semi-Fowler's position, the table must be at a 90-degree angle.

_____ 3. The medical assistant must assist the elderly patient with disrobing.

_____ 4. The receptionist is responsible for having the patient ready in a room for the medical assistant.

_____ 5. A patient can withdraw consent for an examination after the form has been put into the chart.

Multiple Choice

Identify the letter of the choice that best completes the statement or answers the question.

1. The _____ position helps the patient breathe easier.
   A. dorsal recumbent
   B. knee-chest
   C. Fowler's
   D. Sims'

2. _____ is the medical term for "ringing of the ears."
   A. Crepitus
   B. Tinnitus
   C. Presbycusis
   D. Vertigo

3. (A) _____ must be provided if the examination is beyond a wellness physical.
   A. chaperone
   B. gown
   C. patient's informed consent
   D. none of the above

4. Failure to secure consent for a procedure such as a colonoscopy is considered _____.
   A. assault and battery
   B. an OSHA violation
   C. dangerous
   D. consent is not required for a colonoscopy

5. The _____ position is most often used to begin a physical exam because the upper extremities are clearly accessible.
   A. horizontal recumbent
   B. sitting
   C. Sims'
   D. standing

6. When a patient is in full-Fowler's position, the table will be at a _____-degree angle.
   A. 30
   B. 45
   C. 60
   D. 90

7. The _____ position can be used for rectal examination and enema administration.
   A. knee-chest
   B. prone
   C. Sims'
   D. supine

8. The physician uses a(n) _____ to examine the interior of the eye.
   A. otoscope
   B. ophthalmoscope
   C. speculum
   D. none of the above

9. The _____ chart is used to test a person's ability to read at a prescribed near distance.
   A. Jaeger
   B. Ishihara
   C. Snellen
   D. rotating E chart

10. When using the Snellen eye chart, the patient should be _____ feet from the chart.
    A. 10
    B. 15
    C. 20
    D. 25

11. The patient's type of gown will be decided by _____.
    A. patient's preference
    B. procedure to be performed
    C. the AMA
    D. all of the above

12. Patients have the right to refuse treatment.
    A. True
    B. False

13. _____ is a yellowish discoloration of the skin and eyes.
    A. Bruit
    B. Cyanosis
    C. Jaundice
    D. Erythema

14. _____ is a low-pitched fluttering sound made by the heart.
    A. Rales
    B. Thrill
    C. Turgor
    D. Murmur

15. _____ is the touching or feeling of body organs, lymph nodes, and tissue.
    A. Auscultation
    B. Palpation
    C. Percussion
    D. Turgor

16. Patient _____ must be the prime consideration for the medical assistant during positioning of the patient.
    A. safety
    B. ethnicity
    C. body size
    D. modesty

17. The _____ eye chart has rows of letters.
    A. Jaeger
    B. Ishihara
    C. Snellen
    D. none of the above

18. The _____ position is most often used for nonflexible sigmoidoscopy.
    A. Sims'
    B. Fowler's
    C. knee-chest
    D. dorsal recumbent

19. When a physician needs to determine the patient's coordination and balance through observation, the patient would be in the _____ position.
    A. dorsal recumbent
    B. sitting
    C. prone
    D. standing

20. _____ is a visual viewing of all body parts and surface areas for symmetry.
    A. Palpation
    B. Auscultation
    C. Inspection
    D. Percussion

21. _____ is when a patient has trouble focusing and vision is blurred. The shape of the cornea or lens prevents light from projecting onto the retina.
    A. Hypermetropia
    B. Myopia
    C. Presbyopia
    D. Astigmatism

22. Which method of vision testing works best for preschoolers?
    A. Jaeger
    B. Ishihara
    C. Snellen
    D. None of the above

23. Of the following, which item would NOT be used for a distance visual acuity test?
    A. Eye occluder
    B. Snellen eye chart
    C. Ophthalmoscope
    D. All would be used

24. The medical assistant's major role in preparing a patient for a _____ is to have the patient gowned, appropriately positioned, and draped for the physician.
    A. CPX
    B. BMI
    C. CXR
    D. PXR

25. Which one of the following items is NOT required for a routine physical examination?
    A. Tape measure
    B. Vaginal speculum
    C. Percussion hammer
    D. Tuning fork

Sentence Completion

Complete each sentence or statement.

1. _____ involves the use of a stethoscope to detect sounds of the heart, respiratory system, and intestines.

2. The _____ position is the best position for the Pap smear and pelvic examination.

3. _____ involves the use by the physician of his or her hands to locate and touch major organs and lymph nodes to detect tenderness in an area.

4. The _____ eye chart tests for distant visual acuity.

5. The _____ aids physicians in checking the appearance of the eardrum and ear canal.

Short Answers

1. List the nine examination positions with which a medical assistant should be familiar.

   _____

   _____

   _____

   _____

2. Describe the three types of the Snellen charts, and give one example of why each would be used.

   _____

   _____

   _____

   _____

   _____

   _____

3. Explain the difference between implied and informed consent.

_____

_____

_____

_____

CRITICAL THINKING

Magdalena Jimenez has recently moved to the United States; her mother is enrolling her in school and has made an appointment for a school physical. Magdalena does not speak English and her mother speaks very little. You do not speak Spanish. Describe how you would proceed with Magdalena's physical exam. Which Snellen chart would you use to assess Magdalena's visual acuity?

INTERNET RESEARCH

Keywords: Visual Acuity Testing, Physical Exams.

Based on your Internet research, write a one-page paper on your topic of choice. Cite your source. Be prepared to give a 2-minute oral presentation should your instructor assign you to do so.

WHAT WOULD YOU DO?

If you have accomplished the objectives in this chapter, you will be able to make better choices as a medical assistant. Take a look at this situation and decide what you would do.

Beth is a medical assistant in the office of Dr. Havidiz, a family practitioner. Dr. Havidiz treats many low-income families, and many women in the community see him for gynecological visits. Holly, a new patient, comes to see Dr. Havidiz for a possible vaginal infection. Her demeanor shows her fear of the doctor's office, especially since this is the first time she has seen Dr. Havidiz. Dr. Havidiz was called to the hospital to see a critically ill patient earlier in the day, so appointments are delayed.

There is an available examination room when Holly arrives, so Beth takes her to the room and tells her to undress completely. Beth does not tell Holly how to put on the gown, but she stands in the room and watches Holly undress. While Holly is undressing, Beth asks the questions necessary to obtain the medical history. Beth then places Holly on the examination table in the lithotomy position and immediately leaves the room, giving the impression that she is in a great hurry. After 15 minutes, Holly has discomfort in her back but dares not move from the position because she does not want to delay the examination. After 30 minutes, Holly wonders just how much longer it will take for Dr. Havidiz to come and check her. Finally, Dr. Havidiz arrives and the examination begins.

During the examination, Beth leaves the room to answer a personal phone call, leaving Dr. Havidiz and Holly alone. As Holly leaves the office, she is in tears from back pain and appears to be very upset. Beth shows no sympathy or empathy for Holly. Two days later, Holly asks that her records be transferred to another physician and tells Dr. Havidiz that she has never been treated as rudely as she was in his office.

How might this situation have been avoided?

1. **How did Beth invade Holly's privacy?**

   _____

   _____

   _____

2. **Under what conditions should Beth have taken Holly's history?**

   _____

   _____

3. **Why was it important to tell Holly how to put on the gown for the examination? How should the drape have been applied?**

   _____

   _____

   _____

   _____

4. **What examination methods would you expect the medical assistant to use while preparing Holly for an examination?**

   _____

   _____

   _____

   _____

5. **What methods of examination would you expect the physician to use during the examination?**

   _____

   _____

   _____

   _____

6. **What positions should have been used for Holly while she was waiting for the pelvic exam? What positions are inappropriate for a long wait? What explanation should Beth have given when placing Holly in the position?**

_____

_____

_____

_____

_____

_____

7. **How should Beth have handled the delay?**

_____

_____

_____

8. **Why is it unethical for Beth to leave the room during the physical examination?**

_____

_____

_____

9. **Do you think that Holly had a legitimate complaint to Dr. Havidiz about her treatment? Explain your answer.**

_____

_____

_____

_____

APPLICATION OF SKILLS

Procedure Check-off Sheets (*) and Assignments from MACC CD (see Procedure Check-off Sheets for which procedure from the MACC CD to perform).

Perform Procedure 32-1: Assist with the Physical Examination.*

Perform Procedure 32-2: Sitting Position.*

Perform Procedure 32-3: Recumbent Position.*

Perform Procedure 32-4: Lithotomy Position.*

Perform Procedure 32-5: Sims' Position.*

Perform Procedure 32-6: Prone Position.*

Perform Procedure 32-7: Knee-Chest Position.*

Perform Procedure 32-8: Fowler's Position.*

Perform Procedure 32-9: Assess Distance Visual Acuity Using a Snellen Chart.*

Perform Procedure 32-10: Assess Color Vision Using the Ishihara Test.*

Perform Procedure 32-11: Assess Near Vision Using a Jaeger Card.*

Student Name _____ Date _____

PROCEDURE 32-1: ASSIST WITH THE PHYSICAL EXAMINATION

TASK: Prepare a patient and assist the physician or health care practitioner with a general physical examination.

CONDITIONS: Given the proper equipment and supplies, the student will be required to role-play with another student or an instructor the proper method for assisting with a general physical examination.

NOTE: The student should practice the procedure using the MACC CD in the back of the textbook and then practice and perform the task in the classroom: MACC CD MACC/Clinical skills/Patient care/The physical exam/Assisting with a physical exam & maintaining and preparing exam room.

EQUIPMENT AND SUPPLIES
- MACC CD/computer
- Examination table
- Table paper
- Patient gown
- Drape
- Urine specimen container
- Snellen chart
- Patient's medical record
- Balance scale
- Tongue depressor
- Plastic-backed paper towel
- Stethoscope
- Sphygmomanometer
- Otoscope
- Ophthalmoscope
- Pen (red and black ink)

STANDARDS: Complete the procedure within _____ minutes and achieve a minimum score of _____ %.

Time began _____   **Time ended** _____

Steps	Possible Points	First Attempt	Second Attempt
1. Sanitize hands.	5		
2. Assemble equipment and supplies.	5		
3. Obtain the patient's medical record.	5		
4. Greet and identify the patient.	5		
5. Explain the procedure to the patient.	5		
6. Measure weight and height, and document the results.	10		
7. Measure visual acuity and document the results.	10		
8. Have the patient obtain a urine sample (if office policy).	5		
9. Escort the patient to the examination room.	5		
10. Measure the patient's vital signs, and document the results.	10		

Steps	Possible Points	First Attempt	Second Attempt
11. Provide a gown and drape to the patient and allow the patient to change into the gown. Inform the physician when the patient is ready, and make the patient's medical record available to the physician.	10		
12. Assist physician with eye exam.	10		
13. Assist physician with ear exam.	10		
14. Assist physician with nasal exam.	10		
15. Assist physician with throat exam.	10		
16. Assist physician with heart and lung exam.	10		
17. Assist physician with testing and examination of the upper extremity reflexes.	10		
18. Position the patient as required.	10		
19. Assist the patient from the examination table as appropriate.	10		
20. Allow the patient time to change from gown to street clothes.	10		
21. Allow time for further discussion between the physician and patient regarding prescriptions, medications, and a return visit. Ask the patient if he or she has any questions.	10		
22. Document any instructions given to the patient in the medical record.	10		
23. Clean the examination room according to Standard Precautions and take used equipment to appropriate place for sanitization.	10		
24. Sanitize hands.	5		

Total Points Possible   200

Comments: Total Points Earned _____ Divided by _____ Total Possible Points = _____ % Score

Instructor's Signature _____

Student Name _____ Date _____

PROCEDURE 32-2: SITTING POSITION

TASK: Properly position and drape the patient for examination of the head, neck, chest, and upper extremities and measurement of vital signs.

CONDITIONS: Given the proper equipment and supplies, the student will be required to role-play with another student or an instructor the proper method for positioning the patient in the sitting position.

NOTE: The student should practice the procedure using the MACC CD in the back of the textbook and then practice and perform the task in the classroom: Medical Assisting Competency Challenge CD MACC/Clinical skills/Patient care/The physical exam/Assisting with a physical exam & maintaining and preparing exam room.

EQUIPMENT AND SUPPLIES
- MACC CD/computer
- Examination table
- Table paper
- Patient gown
- Drape

STANDARDS: Complete the procedure within _____ minutes and achieve a minimum score of _____ %.

Time began _____   Time ended _____

Steps	Possible Points	First Attempt	Second Attempt
1. Sanitize hands.	5		
2. Assemble equipment and supplies.	5		
3. Greet and identify the patient.	5		
4. Explain the procedure to the patient.	5		
5. Provide a gown for the patient and instruct the patient to change into the gown with opening in the back.	5		
6. Pull out the footrest of the table, and assist the patient to a sitting position.	5		
7. Drape the patient for modesty.	5		
8. When the examination is complete, assist the patient from the table.	5		
9. Clean the examination room according to Standard Precautions.	5		
10. Sanitize hands.	5		

Total Points Possible   50

Comments: Total Points Earned _____ Divided by _____ Total Possible Points = _____ % Score

Instructor's Signature _____

Student Name _____   **Date** _____

PROCEDURE 32-3: RECUMBENT POSITION

TASK: Properly position and drape the patient for catheter insertion, examinations of the abdomen, and general examination procedures.

CONDITIONS: Given the proper equipment and supplies, the student will be required to role-play with another student or an instructor the proper method for positioning the patient in the recumbent position.

NOTE: The student should practice the procedure using the MACC CD in the back of the textbook and then practice and perform the task in the classroom: MACC CD MACC/Clinical skills/Patient care/The physical exam/Assisting with a physical exam & maintaining and preparing exam room.

EQUIPMENT AND SUPPLIES
- Examination table
- Table paper
- Patient gown
- Drape

STANDARDS: Complete the procedure within _____ minutes and achieve a minimum score of _____ %.

Time began _____   **Time ended** _____

Steps	Possible Points	First Attempt	Second Attempt
1. Sanitize hands.	5		
2. Assemble equipment and supplies.	5		
3. Greet and identify the patient.	5		
4. Explain the procedure to the patient.	5		
5. Provide a gown for the patient and instruct the patient to change into the gown with opening in the back.	5		
6. Pull out the footrest of the table, and assist the patient to a sitting position.	10		
7. Place the patient in the recumbent position.	10		
8. Drape the patient as appropriate.	10		
9. When the examination is complete, assist the patient from the recumbent position and into a sitting position. Assist the patient from the table.	5		
10. Clean the examination room according to Standard Precautions.	10		
11. Sanitize hands.	5		

Total Points Possible   75

Comments: Total Points Earned _____ Divided by _____ Total Possible Points = _____ % Score

Instructor's Signature _____

Student Name _____ Date _____

PROCEDURE 32-4: LITHOTOMY POSITION

TASK: Properly position and drape the patient in the lithotomy position for a vaginal, pelvic, or rectal examination

CONDITIONS: Given the proper equipment and supplies, the student will be required to role-play with another student or an instructor the proper method for positioning the patient in the lithotomy position.

NOTE: The student should practice the procedure using the MACC CD in the back of the textbook and then practice and perform the task in the classroom: MACC CD MACC/Clinical skills/Patient care/The physical exam/Assisting with a physical exam & maintaining and preparing exam room.

EQUIPMENT AND SUPPLIES
- Examination table
- Table paper
- Patient gown
- Drape

STANDARDS: Complete the procedure within _____ minutes and achieve a minimum score of _____ %.

Time began _____   **Time ended** _____

Steps	Possible Points	First Attempt	Second Attempt
1. Sanitize hands.	5		
2. Assemble equipment and supplies.	5		
3. Greet and identify the patient.	5		
4. Explain the procedure to the patient.	5		
5. Provide a gown for the patient and instruct the patient to change into the gown with opening in the back.	5		
6. Pull out the footrest of the table, and assist the patient to a sitting position.	10		
7. Place the patient in the supine position.	10		
8. Drape the patient as appropriate.	10		
9. Pull out the stirrups and place the patient in the lithotomy position. Place both legs in the stirrups at the same time.	10		
10. Have the patient slide the buttocks to the edge of the table.	10		
11. When the examination is complete, assist the patient from the lithotomy position into the supine position and into a sitting position. Support both legs and remove from stirrups at the same time. Assist the patient from the table.	10		

Steps	Possible Points	First Attempt	Second Attempt
12. Clean the examination room according to Standard Precautions.	10		
13. Sanitize hands.	5		

Total Points Possible   100

Comments: Total Points Earned _____ Divided by _____ Total Possible Points = _____ % Score

Instructor's Signature _____

Student Name _____ **Date** _____

PROCEDURE 32-5: SIMS' POSITION

TASK: Properly position and drape the patient for a vaginal or rectal examination.

CONDITIONS: Given the proper equipment and supplies, the student will be required to role-play with another student or an instructor the proper method for positioning the patient in the Sims' position.

NOTE: The student should practice the procedure using the MACC CD in the back of the textbook and then practice and perform the task in the classroom: MACC CD MACC/Clinical skills/Patient care/The physical exam/Assisting with a physical exam & maintaining and preparing exam room.

EQUIPMENT AND SUPPLIES
- MACC CD/computer
- Examination table
- Table paper
- Patient gown
- Drape

STANDARDS: Complete the procedure within _____ minutes and achieve a minimum score of _____ %.

Time began _____   **Time ended** _____

Steps	Possible Points	First Attempt	Second Attempt
1. Sanitize hands.	5		
2. Assemble equipment and supplies.	5		
3. Greet and identify the patient.	5		
4. Explain the procedure to the patient.	5		
5. Provide a gown for the patient and instruct the patient to change into the gown with opening in the back.	5		
6. Pull out the footrest of the table, and assist the patient to a sitting position.	10		
7. Place the patient in the supine position.	10		
8. Drape the patient as appropriate so rectal area can be viewed while providing patient modesty.	10		
9. Place the patient in Sims' position.	10		
10. Adjust the drape as the physician examines the anal area.	10		
11. When the examination is complete, assist the patient from the Sims' position into the supine position and into a sitting position. Assist the patient from the examination table.	10		

Steps	Possible Points	First Attempt	Second Attempt
12. Clean the examination room according to Standard Precautions.	10		
13. Sanitize hands.	5		

Total Points Possible	100		

Comments: Total Points Earned _____ Divided by _____ Total Possible Points = _____ % Score

Instructor's Signature _____

Student Name _____ Date _____

PROCEDURE 32-6: PRONE POSITION

TASK: Properly position and drape the patient for examination of the back.

CONDITIONS: Given the proper equipment and supplies, the student will be required to role-play with another student or an instructor the proper method for positioning the patient.

NOTE: The student should practice the procedure using the MACC CD in the back of the textbook and then practice and perform the task in the classroom: MACC CD MACC/Clinical skills/Patient care/The physical exam/Assisting with a physical exam & maintaining and preparing exam room.

EQUIPMENT AND SUPPLIES
• MACC CD/computer
• Examination table
• Table paper
• Patient gown
• Drape

STANDARDS: Complete the procedure within _____ minutes and achieve a minimum score of _____ %.

Time began _____   **Time ended** _____

Steps	Possible Points	First Attempt	Second Attempt
1. Sanitize hands.	5		
2. Assemble equipment and supplies.	5		
3. Greet and identify the patient.	5		
4. Explain the procedure to the patient.	5		
5. Provide a gown for the patient and instruct the patient to change into the gown with opening in the back.	5		
6. Pull out the footrest of the table, and assist the patient to a sitting position.	10		
7. Place the patient in the supine position.	10		
8. Drape the patient as appropriate for patient modesty.	10		
9. Place the patient in the prone position.	10		
10. Adjust the drape as necessary.	10		
11. When the examination is complete, assist the patient from the prone position into the supine position and into a sitting position. Assist the patient from the examination table.	10		

Steps	Possible Points	First Attempt	Second Attempt
12. Clean the examination room according to Standard Precautions.	10		
13. Sanitize hands.	5		
Total Points Possible	100		

Comments: Total Points Earned _____ Divided by _____ Total Possible Points = _____ % Score

Instructor's Signature _____

Student Name _____ Date _____

PROCEDURE 32-7: KNEE-CHEST POSITION

TASK: Properly position and drape the patient for a proctological examination.

CONDITIONS: Given the proper equipment and supplies, the student will be required to role-play with another student or an instructor the proper method for positioning the patient in the knee-chest position.

NOTE: The student should practice the procedure using the MACC CD in the back of the textbook and then practice and perform the task in the classroom: MACC CD MACC/Clinical skills/Patient care/The physical exam/Assisting with a physical exam & maintaining and preparing exam room.

EQUIPMENT AND SUPPLIES
- Examination table
- Table paper
- Patient gown
- Drape
- Tissue

STANDARDS: Complete the procedure within _____ minutes and achieve a minimum score of _____ %.

Time began _____   **Time ended** _____

Steps	Possible Points	First Attempt	Second Attempt
1. Sanitize hands.	5		
2. Assemble equipment and supplies.	5		
3. Greet and identify the patient.	5		
4. Explain the procedure to the patient.	5		
5. Provide a gown for the patient and instruct the patient to change into the gown with opening in the back.	5		
6. Pull out the footrest of the table, and assist the patient to a sitting position.	10		
7. Place the patient in the supine position.	10		
8. Drape the patient as appropriate for patient modesty.	10		
9. Place the patient in the prone position.	10		
10. Have the patient bend the arms at the elbows and rest them alongside the head.	10		
11. Place the patient in the knee-chest position.	10		
12. Adjust the drape as the physician exams the rectal area.	10		
13. Wipe the rectal area with tissue as appropriate following the exam to remove excess lubricant.	10		
14. When the examination is complete, assist the patient from the knee-chest position into the prone position, into a supine position, and into a sitting position. Assist the patient from the examination table.	10		

Steps	Possible Points	First Attempt	Second Attempt
15. Clean the examination room according to Standard Precautions.	10		
16. Sanitize hands.	5		

Total Points Possible   130

Comments: Total Points Earned _____ Divided by _____ Total Possible Points = _____ % Score

Instructor's Signature _____

Student Name _____ Date _____

PROCEDURE 32-8: FOWLER'S POSITION

TASK: Properly position and drape the patient for examination of the head, chest, abdomen, and extremities.

CONDITIONS: Given the proper equipment and supplies, the student will be required to role-play with another student or an instructor the proper method for positioning the patient in Fowler's position.

NOTE: The student should practice the procedure using the MACC CD in the back of the textbook and then practice and perform the task in the classroom: MACC CD MACC/Clinical skills/Patient care/The physical exam/Assisting with a physical exam & maintaining and preparing exam room.

EQUIPMENT AND SUPPLIES
- Examination table
- Table paper
- Patient gown
- Drape

STANDARDS: Complete the procedure within _____ minutes and achieve a minimum score of _____ %.

Time began _____   **Time ended** _____

Steps	Possible Points	First Attempt	Second Attempt
1. Sanitize hands.	5		
2. Assemble equipment and supplies.	5		
3. Greet and identify the patient.	5		
4. Explain the procedure to the patient.	5		
5. Provide a gown for the patient and instruct the patient to change into the gown with opening in the back.	5		
6. Pull out the footrest of the table, and assist the patient to a sitting position.	10		
7. Place the patient in Fowler's position or semi-Fowler's position, supporting head with pillow as appropriate.	10		
8. Drape the patient as appropriate for patient modesty and exam being performed.	10		
9. When the examination is complete, assist the patient from the examination table. Raise head of table as appropriate.	10		
10. Clean the examination room according to Standard Precautions.	10		
11. Sanitize hands.	5		

Total Points Possible   80

Comments: Total Points Earned _____ Divided by _____ Total Possible Points = _____ % Score

Instructor's Signature _____

Student Name _____ Date _____

PROCEDURE 32-9: ASSESS DISTANCE VISUAL ACUITY USING A SNELLEN CHART

TASK: Accurately measure visual acuity using a Snellen eye chart, and document the procedure in the patient's medical record.

CONDITIONS: Given the proper equipment and supplies, the student will be required to measure visual acuity using a Snellen chart.

NOTE: The student should practice the procedure using the MACC CD in the back of the textbook and then practice and perform the task in the classroom: Medical Assisting Competency Challenge CD MACC/Clinical skills/ Patient care/The physical exam/Measuring visual acuity.

EQUIPMENT AND SUPPLIES
- MACC CD/computer
- Snellen eye chart
- Eye occlluder
- Well-lit examination room
- Floor mark (20 feet from chart)
- Patient's medical record
- Pen

STANDARDS: Complete the procedure within _____ minutes and achieve a minimum score of _____ %.

Time began _____   Time ended _____

Steps	Possible Points	First Attempt	Second Attempt
1. Sanitize hands.	5		
2. Assemble equipment and supplies.	5		
3. Greet and identify the patient.	5		
4. Explain the procedure to the patient.	5		
5. Ask the patient if he or she is wearing contact lenses, and observe for eyeglasses.	10		
6. Place the patient in a comfortable position 20 feet from the chart.	10		
7. Select the appropriate Snellen chart for the patient and position the center of the chart at the patient's eye level. Stand next to the chart during the test to indicate to the patient the line to be identified.	10		
8. Ask the patient to cover the left eye with the eye occluder, keeping the eye open.	10		
9. Measure the visual acuity of the right eye by asking the patient to identify verbally each letter (or picture or rotating "E" direction) in the row on the Snellen chart, starting with the 20/70 line.	10		
10. Proceed up or down the chart as necessary.	10		
11. Observe the patient for any unusual symptoms while he or she is reading the letters, such as squinting, tilting the head, or watering eyes.	10		

Steps	Possible Points	First Attempt	Second Attempt
12. Repeat the procedure to test the left eye by covering the right eye.	10		
13. Record the results appropriately, indicating the errors for each eye.	10		
14. Repeat the procedure without covering either eye.	10		
15. If appropriate, repeat the procedure without corrective lenses.	10		
16. Chart the procedure.	10		
17. Sanitize or discard the occluder as appropriate.	5		
18. Sanitize hands.	5		

Total Points Possible   150

Comments: Total Points Earned _____ Divided by _____ Total Possible Points = _____ % Score

Instructor's Signature _____

Student Name _____ Date _____

PROCEDURE 32-10: ASSESS COLOR VISION USING THE ISHIHARA TEST

TASK: Measure color visual acuity accurately using the Ishihara color-blindness test.

CONDITIONS: Given the proper equipment and supplies, the student will be required to role-play with another student or an instructor the proper method for measuring color visual acuity using the Ishihara color-blindness test.

EQUIPMENT AND SUPPLIES
- Ishihara color plate book
- Cotton swab
- Well-lit examination room (natural light preferred)
- Watch with second hand
- Patient's medical record
- Pen or pencil

STANDARDS: Complete the procedure within _____ minutes and achieve a minimum score of _____ %.

Time began _____   Time ended _____

Steps	Possible Points	First Attempt	Second Attempt
1. Sanitize hands.	5		
2. Assemble equipment and supplies.	5		
3. Greet and identify the patient.	5		
4. Explain the procedure to the patient.	5		
5. In a well-lit room, use the first plate in the book as an example, and instruct the patient on how the examination will be conducted using the plate.	10		
6. Hold the color plates 30 inches from the patient.	10		
7. Ask the patient to identify the number on the plate or, using a cotton-tipped swab, to trace the winding path.	10		
8. Record the results for each plate, and continue until the patient has viewed and responded to all 11 plates.	10		
9. Appropriately record the results in the patient's medical record.	10		
10. Return the Ishihara book to its proper place.	10		
11. Discard cotton-tipped swab as appropriate.	5		
12. Sanitize hands.	5		

Total Points Possible   90

Comments: Total Points Earned _____ Divided by _____ Total Possible Points = _____ % Score

Instructor's Signature _____

Student Name _____ **Date** _____

PROCEDURE 32-11: ASSESS NEAR VISION USING THE JAEGER CARD

TASK: Measure near visual acuity accurately using the Jaeger near-vision acuity card, and document the procedure in the patient's medical record.

CONDITIONS: Given the proper equipment and supplies, the student will be required to role-play with another student or an instructor the proper method for assessing near vision using the Jaeger card.

EQUIPMENT AND SUPPLIES
- Jaeger card
- Occluder
- Well-lit examination room
- Patient's medical record
- Pen

STANDARDS: Complete the procedure within _____ minutes and achieve a minimum score of _____ %.

Time began _____ **Time ended** _____

Steps	Possible Points	First Attempt	Second Attempt
1. Sanitize hands.	5		
2. Assemble equipment and supplies.	5		
3. Greet and identify the patient.	5		
4. Explain the procedure to the patient.	5		
5. In a well-lit room, seat the patient in a comfortable position.	10		
6. Provide the patient with the Jaeger card and instruct the patient to hold the card 14 to 16 inches away from the eyes. Measure the distance for accuracy.	15		
7. Ask the patient to read out loud the paragraphs on the card; cover the left eye and then the right eye with the occluder.	15		
8. Document the number at which the patient stopped reading for each eye.	10		
9. Return the Jaeger card to its proper storage place.	10		
10. Sanitize or discard the occluder as appropriate.	10		
11. Sanitize hands.	10		

Total Points Possible　　　　　　　　　100

Comments: Total Points Earned _____ Divided by _____ Total Possible Points = _____ % Score

Instructor's Signature _____

CHAPTER QUIZ

Multiple Choice

Identify the letter of the choice that best completes the statement or answers the question.

1. _____ is the position that helps the patient breathe better when in respiratory distress.
   A. Dorsal recumbent
   B. Lithotomy
   C. Fowler's
   D. Sims'

2. _____ is used by the physician to check the nervous system.
   A. Auscultation
   B. Palpation
   C. Percussion
   D. Inspection

3. The medical assistant must choose the right type and size of gown for the examination being preformed.
   A. True
   B. False

4. _____ is another name for "ringing in the ears."
   A. Crepitus
   B. Turgor
   C. Tinnitus
   D. Vertigo

5. Listening for body sounds, usually with a stethoscope, is called _____.
   A. auscultation
   B. inspection
   C. palpation
   D. thrill

6. Patients cannot withdraw their consent once it has been given and documented in their chart.
   A. True
   B. False

7. Bluish coloration of the skin due to lack of oxygen is called _____.
   A. bruit
   B. cyanosis
   C. jaundice
   D. gingivitis

8. _____ is(are) crackling sounds heard in the lungs, usually at the base.
   A. Bruit
   B. Crepitus
   C. Rales
   D. Rhonchi

9. Taking a patient's pulse is done by palpation.
   A. True
   B. False

10. The _____ position is most often used for a colonoscopy.
    A. dorsal recumbent
    B. knee-chest
    C. Fowler's
    D. prone

11. Color vision is tested with the _____ test.
    A. Ishihara
    B. Jaeger
    C. Snellen
    D. rotating E chart

12. A patient in the supine position whose head is at a 45-degree angle is in the _____ position.
    A. dorsal recumbent
    B. full-Fowler's
    C. semi-Fowler's
    D. supine

13. The physician uses a(n) _____ to visualize the eardrum or tympanic membrane.
    A. ophthalmoscope
    B. otoscope
    C. speculum
    D. none of the above

14. Ears smaller than 4 cm are known as macrotia.
    A. True
    B. False

15. The back and lower extremities can be examined with the patient in the _____ position.
    A. lithotomy
    B. prone
    C. sitting
    D. standing

16. Observation of the reaction of the pupils to the exposure of direct light is documented using which one of the following acronyms?
    A. PUPIL
    B. PERRLA
    C. AAOLX3
    D. None of the above

17. A device used to measure joint movements and angles is called a _____.
    A. flexible cloth tape measure
    B. yardstick
    C. goniometer
    D. pelvimeter

18. Decrease in hearing ability resulting from aging is called _____.
    A. myopia
    B. presbyopia
    C. presbycusis
    D. tinnitus

19. Medical term for "dizziness" is _____.
    A. tinnitus
    B. turgor
    C. macrotia
    D. vertigo

20. The medical term for "excessive sweating" is _____.
    A. diaphoresis
    B. crepitus
    C. gingivitis
    D. turgor

CHAPTER THIRTY-THREE

Electrocardiography

VOCABULARY REVIEW

Matching

Match each term with the correct definition.

A. alternating current interference

B. amplifier

C. arrhythmia

D. artifact

E. atrioventricular node

F. augmented leads

G. baseline

H. bipolar leads

I. bundle branches

J. bundle of His

K. cardiac cycle

L. electrocardiogram

M. galvanometer

N. interval

O. ischemia

P. myocardial infarction

Q. normal sinus rhythm

R. paroxysmal atrial tachycardia

_____ 1. Condition in which the ventricles receive an impulse prematurely and contract early

_____ 2. Knot of specialized cells in the lower portion of the right atrium that produces the heart's electrical impulses

_____ 3. ECG pattern that represents heart-specific electrical activity

_____ 4. ECG pattern that shows the length of a wave with a segment

_____ 5. Graphic picture of the heart's electrical activity

_____ 6. Body tremors caused by voluntary or involuntary muscle movement

_____ 7. Electrical interference that appears as small, uniform spikes on ECG paper

_____ 8. Sudden onset and ending of atrial tachycardia

_____ 9. Normal, small upward curve that occasionally follows a complete ECG cycle after PQRST

_____ 10. Standard limb leads

_____ 11. Rhythm measurement that starts at the SA node, occurs within an established time frame, and follows an expected, established pattern

S. PR interval

T. premature ventricular contraction

U. Purkinje fibers

V. QRS complex

W. repolarization

X. somatic tremor

Y. standardization

Z. stylus

AA. tracing

BB. U wave

CC. ventricular fibrillation

DD. wandering baseline

EE. wave

_____ 12. Cardiac fibers that receive impulses from the bundle branches and take them throughout the heart muscle

_____ 13. Abnormal heart rate, rhythm, and conduction system

_____ 14. Device that detects and converts the amplified electrical signal into a tracing on the ECG machine

_____ 15. Heated device that records the heart's activity on heat-sensitive graph paper

_____ 16. Small band of atypical cardiac muscle fibers that receive electrical impulses from the AV node

_____ 17. Resting phase of the ECG cycle

_____ 18. Line that separates the various cardiac waves; representative of the space between heartbeats while the heart is "resting"; also called isoelectric line

_____ 19. Time interval between atrial contraction and the beginning of ventricular contraction

_____ 20. Life-threatening condition of ventricular twitching that causes inefficient pumping action, stopping blood circulation

_____ 21. Device on the electrocardiograph that magnifies or enlarges the heart's electrical impulses so they can be recorded

_____ 22. Poor blood supply to body tissue causing a lack of oxygen to that tissue

_____ 23. ECG pattern that shows when the impulse moves through the ventricle and reaches the Purkinje fibers, depicting contraction of both ventricles

_____ 24. Shift on the ECG tracing from the baseline or center of the paper

_____ 25. Unwanted changes in an ECG tracing caused by movement, machine malfunction, or other factors

_____ 26. Heart attack, death of the heart tissue, caused by blockage of the heart's blood vessels

_____ 27. One heartbeat, one contraction/relaxation phase of the heart

_____ 28. Recording of the ECG cycle

_____ 29. Leads that measure cardiac activity from one electrode on the body at a time; recordings are augmented so they can be read

_____ 30. Bundle of cardiac fibers that receive electrical impulses from the bundle of His

_____ 31. Process of ensuring that an ECG taken on one machine will compare to a tracing taken on another machine

THEORY RECALL

True/False

Indicate whether the sentence or statement is true or false.

_____ 1. Electrocardiography is a painless, noninvasive procedure often done as a part of a routine examination.

_____ 2. The QRS complex shows the time interval between the ventricular contraction and the beginning of ventricular relaxation.

_____ 3. Artifact occurs when a tracing shifts from the baseline, or center of the paper, and moves over the ECG paper.

_____ 4. The medical assistant must never interpret the ECG.

_____ 5. Repolarization is a discharge of electrical energy that causes contraction.

Multiple Choice

Identify the letter of the choice that best completes the statement or answers the question.

1. Leads I, II, and III are called _____ leads.
   A. augmented
   B. bipolar
   C. chest
   D. precordial

2. In standard limb leads or bipolar leads, the _____ is always negative.
   A. right arm
   B. right leg
   C. left arm
   D. left leg

3. Lead _____ is considered to be the rhythm strip.
   A. I
   B. II
   C. III
   D. IV

4. The resting phase of the heart is also known as _____ .
   A. depolarization
   B. polarization
   C. relaxation
   D. repolarization

5. _____ shows how long it takes for the electrical impulse to go from the SA node to the AV node.
   A. QT interval
   B. QRS complex
   C. PR interval
   D. PR segment

6. _____ measure the activity of one electrode on the body surface.
   A. Bipolar leads
   B. Chest leads
   C. Standard limb leads
   D. Unipolar leads

7. _____ results from excessive electrical impulses from external sources and appears as small, uniform spikes on the ECG tracing.
   A. AC interference
   B. Artifact
   C. Arrhythmia
   D. Wandering baseline

8. Arrhythmia can mean abnormality in _____ .
   A. conduction
   B. heart rate
   C. heart rhythm
   D. all of the above

9. The _____ wave is represented by a downward deflection following the P wave.
   A. Q
   B. R
   C. S
   D. T

10. _____ wave indicates the resting phase of the heart.
    A. P
    B. Q
    C. S
    D. T

11. _____ represents the time interval between the atrial contraction and the beginning of ventricular stimulation.
    A. QT interval
    B. PR segment
    C. ST segment
    D. QRS

12. The first electrical impulse shown on an ECG is the _____ wave.
    A. T
    B. P
    C. S
    D. U

13. _____ is defined by three or more consecutive PVCs.
    A. Ventricular fibrillation
    B. Ventricular tachycardia
    C. Paroxysmal atrial tachycardia
    D. None of the above

14. _____ is the most life threatening of all arrhythmias.
    A. Premature ventricular contraction
    B. Premature atrial contraction
    C. Ventricular tachycardia
    D. Ventricular fibrillation

15. _____ is a condition in which an electrical impulse in the atria starts before the next expected heartbeat.
    A. PAC
    B. PVC
    C. PAT
    D. NRS

16. When performing a Holter monitor ECG, the test should be conducted over a(n) _____ hour period.
    A. 8- to 12-
    B. 12- to 24-
    C. 24- to 48-
    D. 48- to 60-

17. The SA node is located in the _____ .
    A. lower right atrium
    B. upper right atrium
    C. lower left atrium
    D. upper left atrium

18. Sinus bradycardia is a heartbeat of less than _____ .
    A. 50
    B. 60
    C. 80
    D. 100

19. Standardization mark is a mark made on the ECG paper that indicates the ECG can be interpreted against other ECGs.
    A. True
    B. False

20. A stylus records the motion on graph paper located in the machine by burning the impression on the heat-sensitive paper.
    A. True
    B. False

Sentence Completion

Complete each sentence or statement.

1. _____ is a rhythmic cycle of a contraction and a relaxation process of the heart.

2. _____ is the process of making certain that an ECG taken on one machine will compare with a tracing taken on another machine.

3. _____ is an abnormally rapid heartbeat.

4. _____ is an exercise electrocardiography that is performed to determine if the heart is receiving enough blood during a time of stress.

5. The _____ wave is a small upward curve that may occasionally occur following a normal ECG tracing.

6. _____ are small devices made of a conductive material that are used to pick up the electrical activity of the heart generated by the myocardial cells.

7. _____ is a body tremor caused by voluntary or involuntary muscle movement.

8. A(n) _____ is worn and the diary is kept for a prescribed amount of time to evaluate heart activity over a period of time.

9. On an ECG tracing, the _____ indicates time and shows an entire wave with a segment.

10. The _____ magnifies the heart's electrical signal so that it can be recorded.

Short Answers

1. List and explain where precordial leads are placed.

   _____

   _____

   _____

2. List five problems an electrocardiography can detect.

   _____

   _____

   _____

   _____

   _____

3. Explain the procedures for preparing a patient for a Holter monitor.

   _____

   _____

   _____

   _____

   _____

4. Explain the placement of the electrodes on the skin.

   _____

   _____

   _____

   _____

   _____

CRITICAL THINKING

Ruth Darcy is a 78-year-old patient who is in the office today for a refill check on her heart medication. She looks a little diaphoretic and pale, when you go to escort her back to the examination room. "Ruth, how are you feeling today?" You ask. "Not one of my better days, dear. Definitely not one of my better days. Got a little pain in my chest; probably just indigestion from the sandwich I had at lunch. It feels awfully hot in here." You escort Ms. Darcy to the exam room and then go notify the doctor that Ms.

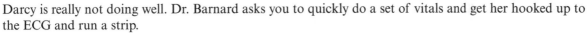

Darcy is really not doing well. Dr. Barnard asks you to quickly do a set of vitals and get her hooked up to the ECG and run a strip.

Ms. Darcy's blood pressure is 220/98, her pulse is 112, and her respirations are 24.

1. Describe your conversation/explanation of the procedure with Ms. Darcy as you are getting her ready for the ECG.

2. Describe the steps of preparing Ms. Darcy for the ECG and the procedure for running the ECG.

INTERNET RESEARCH

Keywords: Einthoven's Triangle, History of Electrocardiogram

Choose one of these topics to research: Einthoven's triangle or History of electrocardiogram. Write a one-page report. Cite your source(s). Be prepared to give a 2-minute oral presentation should your instructor assign you to do so.

WHAT WOULD YOU DO?

If you have accomplished the objectives in this chapter, you will be able to make better choices as a medical assistant. Take a look at this situation and decide what you would do.

Jim, a 55-year-old longtime smoker who is also overweight, has taken his grandchildren to the beach for the day. Mary, Jim's wife, notices that Jim is a little short of breath and seems to rub his chest often, so she asks if he is okay. Jim tells Mary that he thinks that he needs to get to a doctor because he has chest pain that is not subsiding. They drop off the children and immediately go to the medical office.

On arrival, Jim tells Gomez, the medical assistant, about his chest pain, which now seems to be in his left arm and left jaw. Gomez tells Jim that it is "probably just indigestion" and lets Jim sit in the waiting room. Finally, observing that Jim is very short of breath and is clasping his chest, Gomez asks the attending physician, Dr. Startz, if he can obtain an electrocardiogram.

Receiving approval for the ECG, Gomez quickly loads the paper into the electrocardiograph, not taking the necessary care to prevent markings on the ECG paper. Jim has suntan oil on his body, and his chest is relatively hairy, so the electrodes do not attach with sufficient pressure to stay on the skin when the leads are placed on the tabs. Gomez places the electrodes in a haphazard manner, with no consideration of the way the tabs are facing. By this time, Jim is scared and experiencing a great deal of pain, which is causing diaphoresis, trembling, and twisting. Jim starts to sing and talk to relieve his tension, and the ECG has many artifacts. In a hurry to get the ECG to Dr. Startz because of Jim's declining condition, Gomez does not notice that the ECG also contains a wandering baseline. Even the rhythm strip is not readable.

On examination, Dr. Startz realizes the seriousness of Jim's condition and immediately sends him to the hospital, where another ECG and admission to the CICU are ordered. At the end of the day, Dr. Startz is upset and tells Gomez that if he cannot get a presentable ECG in an emergency situation, he might lose his job.

If you were the medical assistant in this situation, what would you have done?

1. **What are Jim's risk factors for coronary artery disease?**

_____

_____

_____

2. What symptoms did Jim have at the beach and later in the medical office?

_____

_____

_____

_____

3. Since Jim came to the office complaining of chest pain, what would have been the appropriate action for Gomez to take?

_____

_____

_____

_____

4. Why does ECG paper need to be handled carefully?

_____

_____

_____

_____

5. How should Gomez have prepared Jim's chest for the ECG, and what effect did no preparation have on the ECG tracing?

_____

_____

_____

_____

_____

_____

6. What is an "artifact"? What actions by Jim caused the artifacts on the ECG?

_____

_____

_____

_____

7. What is a "wandering baseline," and what does this indicate?

_____

_____

_____

_____

8. How should the electrodes be turned when placed on the body?

_____

_____

_____

_____

9. How does a medical assistant obtain a rhythm strip on an ECG? What does the rhythm strip show?

_____

_____

_____

_____

10. What is the role of the medical assistant in obtaining an ECG tracing?

_____

_____

_____

_____

APPLICATION OF SKILLS

Procedure Check-off Sheets (*) and Assignments from MACC CD (see Procedure Check-off Sheets for which procedure from the MACC CD to perform).

1. Perform Procedure 33-1: Obtain a 12-Lead Electrocardiogram (ECG) Using a Single-Channel Electrocardiograph.*

2. Perform Procedure 33-2: Obtain a 12-Lead Electrocardiogram (ECG) Using a Three-Channel Electrocardiograph.*

3. Perform Procedure 33-3: Apply and Remove a Holter Monitor.*

Student Name _____ Date _____

PROCEDURE 33-1: PERFORM A 12-LEAD ELECTROCARDIOGRAM (ECG) USING A SINGLE-CHANNEL ELECTROCARDIOGRAPH

TASK: Obtain an accurate 12-lead ECG tracing by running a single-channel electrocardiograph with manual capacity.

CONDITIONS: Given the proper equipment and supplies, the student will be required to obtain an accurate 12-lead ECG tracing.

NOTE: The student should practice the procedure using the MACC CD in the back of the textbook and then practice and perform the task in the classroom: MACC CD MACC/Clinical skills/Diagnostic testing/Patient testing/Performing an electrocardiogram.

EQUIPMENT AND SUPPLIES
- MACC CD/computer
- Single-channel electrocardiograph with lead wires
- ECG paper
- Disposable electrodes (self-adhesive)
- ECG mounting form and mounting supplies such as an ECG paper cutter, if applicable
- Examination table with foot stool or step
- Alcohol wipes (70% isopropyl)
- 4 × 4-inch gauze squares
- Disposable razor
- Patient gown
- Drape
- Blanket (optional)
- Small pillow

STANDARDS: Complete the procedure within _____ minutes and achieve a minimum score of _____ %.

Time began _____   **Time ended** _____

Steps	Possible Points	First Attempt	Second Attempt
1. Sanitize hands.	5		
2. Assemble equipment and supplies.	5		
3. Greet and identify the patient.	5		
4. Explain the procedure to the patient.	5		
5. Ask the patient to remove all possible sources of electrical interference.	5		
6. Prepare the patient by removing clothes as appropriate; drape and gown the patient.	5		
7. Position the patient in a relaxed position, being sure to prevent stress from the position. Ask patient to remain still and not talk.	10		
8. Prepare the patient's skin for electrode placement; remove hair, oil, etc. as appropriate.	10		
9. Position the ECG machine and turn it "on."	5		
10. Label the beginning of the ECG paper with the patient's name, date, time, and current cardiovascular medications, or input the information directly into the machine.	5		

Steps	Possible Points	First Attempt	Second Attempt
11. Properly apply the limb electrodes.	10		
12. Properly apply the chest electrodes.	10		
13. Connect the lead wires to the electrodes.	5		
14. Standardize the ECG machine.	10		
15. Record ECG as appropriate for machine.	10		
16. Ask the patient to lie as still as possible during the tracing; correct artifacts as necessary. If the ECG reading is not accurate, run the lead again.	10		
17. If an arrhythmia or abnormal tracing occurs during the procedure, notify the nurse or physician immediately.	5		
18. Disconnect the patient from the electrocardiograph by removing all of the lead wires and electrodes when an accurate ECG has been obtained.	5		
19. Discard electrodes and any other waste material in the appropriate waste container.	5		
20. Thank the patient and allow the patient to dress.	5		
21. Sanitize hands.	5		
22. Document any special information on the ECG tracing.	10		
23. Cut and mount the ECG as appropriate.	5		
24. Handle the recording carefully, and place the mounted recording in the appropriate place to be reviewed by the physician.	5		
25. Document the procedure.	10		
26. Clean and return all equipment to its proper place.	5		

Total Points Possible   175

Comments: Total Points Earned _____ Divided by _____ Total Possible Points = _____ % Score

Instructor's Signature _____

Student Name _____ Date _____

PROCEDURE 33-2: OBTAIN A 12-LEAD ELECTROCARDIOGRAM (ECG) USING A THREE-CHANNEL ELECTROCARDIOGRAPH

TASK: Obtain an accurate 12-lead ECG tracing by running a three-channel electrocardiograph.

CONDITIONS: Given the proper equipment and supplies, the student will be required to obtain an accurate 12-lead ECG tracing.

EQUIPMENT AND SUPPLIES
- Three-channel electrocardiograph with lead wires
- ECG paper
- Disposable electrodes (self-adhesive)
- ECG mounting form and mounting supplies such as an ECG paper cutter, if applicable
- Examination table with foot stool or step
- Alcohol wipes (70% isopropyl)
- 4 × 4-inch gauze squares
- Disposable razor
- Patient gown
- Drape
- Blanket (optional)
- Small pillow

STANDARDS: Complete the procedure within _____ minutes and achieve a minimum score of _____ %.

Time began _____   Time ended _____

Steps	Possible Points	First Attempt	Second Attempt
1. Sanitize hands.	5		
2. Assemble equipment and supplies.	5		
3. Greet and identify the patient.	5		
4. Explain the procedure to the patient.	5		
5. Ask the patient to remove all possible sources of electrical interference.	5		
6. Prepare the patient by removing clothes as appropriate; drape and gown the patient.	5		
7. Position the patient in a relaxed position, being sure to prevent stress from the position. Ask patient to remain still and not talk.	5		
8. Prepare the patient's skin for electrode placement; remove hair, oil, etc. as appropriate.	10		
9. Position the ECG machine and turn it "on".	5		
10. Turn on the electrocardiograph, and enter the patient data using the soft-touch keypad. Label the beginning of the ECG paper with the patient's name, date, time, and current cardiovascular medications.	5		
11. Properly apply the limb electrodes.	10		
12. Properly apply chest electrodes.	10		
13. Connect the lead wires to the electrodes.	5		
14. Press the "Start" or "Auto" button on the machine and run the ECG tracing.	10		

Steps	Possible Points	First Attempt	Second Attempt
15. Record ECG as appropriate for machine.	10		
16. Ask the patient to lie as still as possible during the tracing; correct artifacts as necessary. If the ECG reading is not accurate, run the lead again.	10		
17. If an arrhythmia or abnormal tracing occurs during the procedure, notify the nurse or physician immediately.	5		
18. Disconnect the patient from the electrocardiograph by removing all of the lead wires and electrodes when an accurate ECG has been obtained.	5		
19. Discard electrodes and any other waste material in the appropriate waste container.	5		
20. Thank the patient and allow the patient to dress.	5		
21. Sanitize hands.	5		
22. Document any special information on the ECG tracing.	10		
23. Cut and mount the ECG as appropriate.	10		
24. Handle the recording carefully, and place the mounted recording in the appropriate place to be reviewed by the physician.	5		
25. Document the procedure.	10		
26. Clean and return all equipment to its proper place.	5		

Total Points Possible   175

Comments: Total Points Earned _____ Divided by _____ Total Possible Points = _____ % Score

Instructor's Signature _____

Student Name _____ Date _____

PROCEDURE 33-3: APPLY AND REMOVE A HOLTER MONITOR

TASK: Demonstrate the correct procedure for applying and removing a Holter monitor.

CONDITIONS: Given the proper equipment and supplies, the student will be required to role-play with another student or an instructor the proper method for applying and removing a Holter monitor for patient instruction.

EQUIPMENT AND SUPPLIES
- Holter monitor with battery
- Blank magnetic tape
- Patient activity diary
- Carrying case
- Disposable razor
- Belt or shoulder strap
- Disposable electrodes (self-adhesive)
- Nonallergenic tape
- Electrode cable with lead wires
- Gauze squares
- Alcohol wipes (70% isopropyl)

STANDARDS: Complete the procedure within _____ minutes and achieve a minimum score of _____ %.

Time began _____   Time ended _____

Steps	Possible Points	First Attempt	Second Attempt
Applying the Monitor			
1. Sanitize hands.	5		
2. Assemble equipment and supplies.	5		
3. Greet and identify the patient.	5		
4. Explain the procedure to the patient.	5		
5. Prepare the equipment, being sure that all batteries are charged adequately and a blank tape is in the machine.	10		
6. Place the patient in either a sitting position or a supine position on the examination table.	5		
7. Locate and prepare the skin at electrode placement sites.	5		
8. Prepare and apply the electrodes.	5		
9. Repeat Step 8 until all electrodes are firmly applied.	5		
10. Attach lead wires to the electrodes, and place a strip of adhesive nonallergenic tape over the wires just below each electrode.	5		
11. Connect the lead wires to the electrode cable, and tape the cable to the patient's chest.	5		
12. Check the recorder's effectiveness by using the start-up procedure recommended by the manufacturer.	10		
13. Instruct the patient to redress while being careful not to pull on the lead wires.	5		

Steps	Possible Points	First Attempt	Second Attempt
14. Insert the recorder into its carrying case and strap it over the patient's clothing using a waist belt or shoulder strap.	5		
15. Set the Holter monitor and record the start time.	10		
16. Complete the patient identification section to the patient's activity diary.	10		
17. Give the diary to the patient and provide verbal and written instructions on the use of the monitor and proper documentation. Be sure the date and time of application are recorded.	10		
18. Ask the patient if he or she has any questions or would like clarification of any instructions.	5		
19. Instruct the patient on when to return for removal of the monitor.	5		
20. Sanitize hands.	5		
21. Remind the patient not to forget the diary.	5		
22. Document the procedure.	10		
Removing the Monitor			
23. Sanitize hands.	5		
24. Assist the patient with removing clothing from the waist up.	5		
25. Turn off the monitor; remove the monitor strap and detach it from the lead wires.	5		
26. Remove the lead wires and electrodes from the patient.	5		
27. Clean the skin at the electrode sites.	5		
28. Allow the patient to redress and assist the patient as necessary.	5		
29. Obtain the activity diary from the patient.	5		
30. Sanitize hands.	5		
31. Place the cassette in the computerized analyzer for recording.	10		
32. Attach the patient activity diary printout to the patient's medical record, chart the time that the monitor was returned, and give the results of diary to the physician.	10		

Total Points Possible   200

Comments: Total Points Earned _____ Divided by _____ Total Possible Points = _____ % Score

Instructor's Signature _____

CHAPTER QUIZ

Multiple Choice

Identify the letter of the choice that best completes the statement or answers the question.

1. It is perfectly acceptable for the medical assistant to provide the patient a clue as to the results of the ECG.
   A. True
   B. False

2. When attaching electrodes, the _____ is always positive.
   A. left leg
   B. left arm
   C. right leg
   D. right arm

3. An _____ is a wave on an ECG caused by something other than the electrical activity of the heart.
   A. artifact
   B. interference
   C. AC interference
   D. none of the above

4. A _____ occurs when an electrical impulse starts before the next expected beat.
   A. PAC
   B. PAT
   C. PVC
   D. QRS

5. _____ is a sudden onset of tachycardia measuring 150 to 250 beats per minute.
   A. PAC
   B. PAT
   C. PVC
   D. QRS

6. _____ is the most deadly of all arrhythmias.
   A. V tach
   B. V fib
   C. PVC
   D. None of the above

7. _____ is the resting phase of the cardiac cycle.
   A. Contraction
   B. Depolarization
   C. Polarization
   D. Repolarization

8. The _____ wave represents the first electrical impulse.
   A. P
   B. Q
   C. R
   D. S

9. _____ enlarge(s) the heart's electrical signal so it can be recorded.
   A. Leads
   B. Stylus
   C. Galvanometer
   D. Amplifier

10. The rhythm strip is lead _____ .
    A. I
    B. II
    C. III
    D. IV

11. _____ results from electrolyte imbalances, caffeine, stress, cardiac disease, and emotions.
    A. PAC
    B. PVC
    C. PAT
    D. V fib

12. Leads I, II, and III are called _____ leads.
    A. augmented
    B. precordial
    C. standard
    D. chest

13. Holter monitoring is an ECG that is monitored over a(n) _____ hour period of time.
    A. 8- to 10-
    B. 12- to 24-
    C. 24- to 48-
    D. 48- to 60-

14. The _____ represents the time between atrial contraction and the beginning of ventricular stimulation.
    A. P wave
    B. ST interval
    C. PR interval
    D. QRS complex

15. _____ wave represents the resting phase of the cardiac cycle.
    A. S
    B. P
    C. T
    D. U

16. A device that detects and converts the amplified electrical signal into a tracing on the ECG machine is the _____ .
    A. galvanometer
    B. pacemaker
    C. amplifier
    D. electrodes

17. The _____ is a rhythm measurement that starts at the SA node, occurs within an established time frame, and follows an expected, established form.
    A. PVC
    B. PAC
    C. PAT
    D. NSR

18. Unwanted changes in an ECG tracing caused by movement, machine malfunction, or other reasons is called _____ .
    A. polarization
    B. ischemia
    C. artifacts
    D. arrhythmia

19. _____ are leads that measure cardiac activity from one electrode on the body at a time; recordings are augmented so they can be read.
    A. Augmented leads
    B. Ischemic leads
    C. Laser leads
    D. Baseline leads

20. A small band of atypical cardiac muscle fibers that receive electrical impulses from the AV node is _____ .
    A. SA node
    B. Purkinje fibers
    C. bundle of His
    D. myocardium

CHAPTER **THIRTY-FOUR**

Radiography and Diagnostic Imaging

VOCABULARY REVIEW

Matching

Match each term with the correct definition.

A. angiogram

B. caliper

C. claustrophobia

D. computer imaging

E. contrast medium

F. dosimeter

G. fluoroscopic imaging

H. intravenous pyelogram

I. lower gastrointestinal series

J. magnetic resonance imaging

K. mammography

L. nuclear medicine

M. open MRI

N. positron emission tomography

O. radiograph

P. radiopaque

Q. tomography

R. tracer

_____ 1. Use of high-frequency sound waves to produce images

_____ 2. X-ray technique used to detect abnormalities of the breast

_____ 3. Diagnostic radiograph of the blood vessels using a contrast medium

_____ 4. Techniques that use radioactive material for patient diagnosis and treatment

_____ 5. Special photographic film that blackens in response to light

_____ 6. Radiographic imaging in which the view allows the radiologist to view image in motion

_____ 7. Procedure in which a sugar tracer is injected into the body and picked up by cancer cells that send out signals that can be picked up by a camera, forming pictures of various body parts

_____ 8. Radiopaque substance that enhances an image

_____ 9. Able to be seen using an x-ray technique

_____ 10. Procedure in which strong magnetic field and radio waves are used to produce images to view body structures

_____ 11. Fear of closed places

S. transducer

T. ultrasonography

U. upper gastrointestinal series

V. x-ray tube

W. digital radiographic imaging

X. computed tomography

Y. x-ray film

Z. ultrasound

_____ 12. Radiographic examination of the esophagus, stomach, and upper small intestine during and after the introduction of a contrast medium

_____ 13. Device that monitors the quantity of an x-ray exposure to health care workers

_____ 14. Picture or image created on film when exposed to x-rays

_____ 15. Hinged instrument that measures thickness or diameter

_____ 16. Radiographic examination of the lower intestinal tract during and after introduction of a contrast medium

_____ 17. Special radiographic medium that tags body cells, such as cancer cells

_____ 18. Vacuum tube that creates x-radiation

_____ 19. Radiography using computer imaging instead of conventional film or screen imaging

_____ 20. Imaging of soft tissue and internal organs using high-frequency sound waves

_____ 21. Radiographic view of the kidneys using contrast dye injected intravenously

_____ 22. Techniques that display images with the use of contrast media

_____ 23. Imaging table with more space used for MRI versus the enclosed narrow magnet tube

_____ 24. Device that is moved over the skin to record sound waves

_____ 25. Computerized procedure that views the target organ or body area from different angles in a three-dimensional view

_____ 26. Radiography that views the body or organ as a whole in a cross-sectional view

THEORY RECALL

True/False

Indicate whether the sentence or statement is true or false.

_____ 1. There is no advance preparation required for a patient to have a standard x-ray procedure.

_____ 2. It is perfectly acceptable for a patient to move during an x-ray procedure, because the exposure time is of short duration.

_____ 3. Typical contrast media are barium and iodine.

_____ 4. A sugar tracer is used when performing a CT scan.

_____ 5. All states allow medical assistants to perform x-ray procedures.

Multiple Choice

Identify the letter of the choice that best completes the statement or answers the question.

1. _____ is the use of radiography to see the body or an organ as a whole in a cross-sectional or "slice" view.
   A. MRI
   B. PET
   C. Tomography
   D. Ultrasonography

2. When a patient is scheduled for a head and chest CT with contrast, the patient instructions should include _____.
   A. a normal diet
   B. no food or fluids for 8 hours
   C. no food or water 24 hours prior to exam
   D. fast for 6 hours

3. The PET scan can be used to help in the diagnosis of _____.
   A. Alzheimer's
   B. oncological conditions
   C. neurological conditions
   D. all of the above

4. _____ is a radiograph of the gallbladder.
   A. Cholecystogram
   B. Upper GI series
   C. Mammogram
   D. All of the above

5. _____ is a branch of medicine dealing with radiation.
   A. Radiograph
   B. Radiology
   C. Nuclear medicine
   D. Ultrasonography

6. Which one of the following is NOT a typical route for administration of a contrast medium?
   A. enema
   B. injection
   C. swallowed (oral)
   D. inhalation

7. A(n) _____ x-ray provides an image of the lungs, heart, and large blood vessels.
   A. chest
   B. nuclear
   C. MRI
   D. fluoroscopy

8. _____ uses high-frequency sound waves to create an image.
   A. Fluoroscopic imaging
   B. Mammography
   C. Ultrasonography
   D. Tomography

9. A(n) _____ chest x-ray has the patient facing the tube and the film holder at the back of the patient.
   A. AP
   B. PA
   C. lateral
   D. oblique

10. Before performing an MRI, it is important for the medical assistant to ask the patient about _____.
    A. pregnancy
    B. metal medical devices that the patient may have on or in them
    C. whether they can lay still for 30 minutes
    D. all of the above

11. The medical assistant should _____ when performing an x-ray.
    A. stand in the room with the patient for support
    B. stand in front of a lead barrier for better visualization
    C. stand behind a lead barrier for personal safety
    D. any of the above are acceptable depending on office policy

12. When preparing for a PET scan, the patient must fast _____ hours before the procedure.
    A. 6
    B. 12
    C. 24
    D. 48

13. If a report from the radiologist is not received within _____, the medical assistant must make a follow-up call.
    A. 1 day
    B. 3 days
    C. 5 days
    D. 1 week

14. _____ allows the physician to see, in detail, the inside of the body without the use of x-rays.
    A. CT
    B. PET
    C. MRI
    D. Lower GI series

15. In a(n) _____ chest x-ray, the x-ray beam is directed at an angle through the body part.
    A. PA
    B. AP
    C. lateral
    D. oblique

Sentence Completion

Complete each sentence or statement.

1. _____ is a problem for some patients who are not comfortable in enclosed areas.

2. All employees working in the area of x-ray must wear a(n) _____ to monitor the amount of x-ray exposure.

3. When a patient is having a procedure requiring contrast medium, make sure you ask them about _____ allergies.

4. An instrument that is moved over the skin to record sound waves during an ultrasound procedure is called a(n) _____.

5. _____ is used in ultrasonography, magnetic resonance imaging, computer tomography, and nuclear medicine.

6. If the patient is of childbearing age, it is important for the medical assistant to ask _____.

7. _____ is(are) techniques used to produce a picture image that does not involve radiation.

8. _____ tissue does not absorb electromagnetic energy, so it does not appear on an x-ray film.

9. _____ is an imaging method that can evaluate the entire body with a single procedure.

10. _____ is an x-ray of breast tissue.

Short Answers

1. Explain the patient preparation for a mammogram.

_____

_____

_____

_____

_____

2. Explain the two items the medical assistant must inform the patient of before the procedure.

_____

_____

CRITICAL THINKING

Dr. Goldberg has ordered an MRI on Mrs. Frankle. What instructions would you give Mrs. Frankle for preparing for the procedure? Your instructor may require that you verbally answer this question in a role-play format, providing you with the opportunity to practice your patient education skills.

INTERNET RESEARCH

Keywords: History of Radiography, Roentgen, MRI

Choose one of these topics to research: History of radiography; Roentgen; MRI. Write a one-page report. Cite your source. Be prepared to give a 2-minute oral presentation should your instructor assign you to do so.

WHAT WOULD YOU DO?

If you have accomplished the objectives in this chapter, you will be able to make better choices as a medical assistant. Take a look at this situation and decide what you would do.

Suzanne is a medical assistant who works for Dr. Sahara. Dr. Sahara has a medical office with the equipment for basic radiography. She sends her patients to specialized radiographic offices when more extensive testing is necessary. Dr. Sahara informs Suzanne that she has ordered these diagnostic imaging tests: (1) gallbladder ultrasound for middle-aged Mr. Donnolly, (2) baseline mammography for 40-year-old Mrs. Martens, (3) MRI for Mrs. Smith because of a possible brain lesion, and (4) chest radiograph for Mr. Charles, a patient with parkinsonism, because of possible pneumonia. Mr. Charles's chest x-ray film is inconclusive, so Dr. Sahara sends him back for a CT scan. When the CT scan is suspicious, Dr. Sahara orders a PET scan for Mr. Charles 2 days later, and the results come back positive for cancer. Would you be able to prepare patients for these procedures?

Could you answer patient questions concerning the procedures?

1. What protective equipment and safety features should Suzanne use when she is taking x-ray films in Dr. Sahara's office?

_____

_____

_____

_____

2. If Suzanne were asked to perform "AP, PA, oblique, and lat" views of a forearm, in what positions would she place the arm?

_____

_____

_____

3. What preparation would be needed for Mr. Donnolly's ultrasound of the gallbladder? Why would contrast media be used when the original x-ray films of the gallbladder were taken?

_____

_____

_____

_____

4. What does the white area on an x-ray film indicate? The gray area? The black area?

_____

_____

_____

5. What preparation is necessary for Mrs. Martens' mammogram? What would happen if she were not prepared for the test?

_____

_____

_____

_____

_____

6. **Why was MRI used for diagnosing a possible brain lesion?**

_____

_____

_____

7. **What patient preparation is necessary for a chest radiograph?**

_____

_____

_____

8. **Why did Dr. Sahara order a CT scan when the chest x-ray was inconclusive?**

_____

_____

_____

9. **What does the PET scan show that is not in evidence with MRI? What is used as the tracer for cancer cells?**

_____

_____

_____

10. **How would Mr. Charles's parkinsonism affect his x-ray films and MR images?**

_____

_____

_____

_____

11. **What role does the medical assistant play in scheduling patients for imaging tests?**

_____

_____

_____

_____

12. **What should Suzanne do if the x-ray report on the PET scan does not arrive within the week?**

_____

_____

_____

_____

CHAPTER QUIZ

Multiple Choice

Identify the letter of the choice that best completes the statement or answers the question.

1. _____ is a branch of medicine dealing with radioactive substances.
   A. Radiograph
   B. Radiography
   C. Radiology
   D. None of the above

2. Muscle tissue can absorb as much electromagnetic energy as bones.
   A. True
   B. False

3. _____ is an imaging method that can evaluate the entire body through the use of a sugar tracer.
   A. CT
   B. MRI
   C. PET
   D. X-ray

4. A(n) _____ provides an image of the lungs, heart, and large blood vessels.
   A. chest x-ray
   B. mammogram
   C. MRI
   D. CAT scan

5. The medical assistant should stand _____ a lead screen when taking an x-ray.
   A. beside
   B. behind
   C. in front of
   D. between the patient and

6. The Medical Practice Policy and state laws will determine if the medical assistant is allowed to take x-rays.
   A. True
   B. False

7. Before instilling a contrast medium, the medical assistant should _____.
   A. establish the patient is not pregnant.
   B. ask about allergies to shellfish
   C. ask the patient if they have a ride with them
   D. none of the above

8. In patient preparation of a PET scan, the patient should _____.
   A. fast for at least 6 hours
   B. avoid food and fluids for at least 8 hours prior to the procedure
   C. advise and remove all metal medical devices
   D. should avoid caffeine for several days before the procedure

9. _____ is an image created through the use of high-frequency sound waves.
   A. CT
   B. Mammogram
   C. MRI
   D. Ultrasound

10. When a patient is scheduled for a chest x-ray, the preparation should include _____.
    A. fasting minimally for 6 hours
    B. no drink or food for 8 hours
    C. NOT emptying the bladder before the procedure
    D. no advance preparation is required

11. _____ is used to see the body or a whole organ in a cross-sectional view.
    A. PET
    B. MRI
    C. Tomography
    D. X-ray

12. The radiology report should be received no later than _____ from the time the procedure was performed.
    A. 2 hours
    B. 8 hours
    C. 2 days
    D. 1 week

13. A transducer is a device moved over the skin to record sound waves.
    A. True
    B. False

14. When taking a(n) _____ chest view x-ray, the patient is facing the film holder, and the x-ray tube is to the back.
    A. AP
    B. PA
    C. lateral
    D. oblique

15. _____ allows for the introduction of contrast media and may include movement of that contrast media through the body.
    A. Fluoroscopy
    B. MRI
    C. Mammography
    D. X-ray

CHAPTER THIRTY-FIVE

Therapeutic Procedures

VOCABULARY REVIEW

Matching

Match each term with the correct definition.

A. ambulation device

B. bandage turns

C. cast

D. cerumen

E. cold therapy

F. compress

G. coupling agent

H. elastic bandage

I. figure-eight turn

J. gait patterns

K. goniometer

L. heating pad

M. immobilization

N. instillation

O. irrigation

P. orthopedist

Q. patent

R. pressure ulcer

_____ 1. Limb immobilizer made of fiberglass used for simple fractures and sprains

_____ 2. Physician whose specialty is to correct musculoskeletal disorders

_____ 3. Bandage containing elastic that stretches and molds to the body part to which it is applied

_____ 4. Plaster or fiberglass mold applied to immobilize a body part

_____ 5. Process of placing medication into an area as prescribed by a physician

_____ 6. Bandage turn used for a stump or the head that begins with a circular turn and progresses back and forth, overlapping each turn until the area is covered

_____ 7. Procedure that requires a body part to be immersed in water warm enough to increase blood flow to an area or cold enough to slow blood flow to the area

_____ 8. Any device that assists a patient to walk

_____ 9. Patterns of walking used with crutches

_____ 10. Lightweight mobility device providing a stable platform that is used when a patient needs optimal stability and support

S. recurrent turn

T. soak

U. stockinette

V. synthetic cast

W. therapeutic procedures

X. tubular gauze

Y. ultrasound therapy

Z. walker

AA. Kling-type bandage

BB. forearm crutches

_____ 11. Therapy using ice or cold application to reduce or prevent swelling by decreasing circulatory flow to the injured body part

_____ 12. Water-soluble lotion or gel used to transmit energy provided by an ultrasound wand

_____ 13. Gauze bandage made in a tubular shape that can be used to cover rounded body parts

_____ 14. Earwax

_____ 15. Bandage turn that is applied on a slant and progresses upward and then downward to support a dressing or joint

_____ 16. Ulcer created when the skin over a bony area has contact and pressure with an irritating source for long periods

_____ 17. Electrical device that delivers a set temperature of heat for heat therapy

_____ 18. Knitted cotton material used over extremities to cover an area before application of cast material

_____ 19. Method of arranging a bandage on a body part

_____ 20. Prevention of movement; inability to move

_____ 21. Open; not obstructed

_____ 22. Instrument used to measure angles

_____ 23. Therapy that uses high-frequency sound waves to produce heat and vibrations to aid in the healing of inflammation in soft tissue

_____ 24. Folded pad of soft absorbent material used for hot or cold therapy

_____ 25. Washing of or rinsing out an area to remove foreign matter

_____ 26. Procedures done to enhance the body's healing processes and assist in patient mobility

_____ 27. Gauze bandaging material that stretches and molds to irregular-shaped areas

_____ 28. Devices that provide contact with the hand and forearm

THEORY RECALL

True/False

Indicate whether the sentence or statement is true or false.

_____ 1. Of all ambulatory devices, a cane provides the most support for the patient.

_____ 2. Ear treatments are never performed as part of an ear examination.

_____ 3. All irrigation solutions must be sterile.

_____ 4. An air cast is used primarily for immobilization.

_____ 5. It is acceptable for the patient to scratch an itch underneath the cast if the patient is very careful.

Multiple Choice

Identify the letter of the choice that best completes the statement or answers the question.

1. There are _____ basic bandage turns used either for support or to secure a dressing.
   A. two
   B. four
   C. five
   D. eight

2. _____ is an application to the skin used to treat an infectious condition or to treat a traumatized body part and promote circulation.
   A. Cold therapy
   B. Heat therapy
   C. Ultrasound
   D. None of the above

3. [A] _____ is(are) prescribed when the patient needs optimal stability and support and yet still be mobile.
   A. cane
   B. Crutches
   C. walker
   D. all of the above

4. A _____ bandage is used on areas that are uniform in width, such as fingers and wrists.
   A. circular
   B. figure eight
   C. recurrent
   D. spiral turn

5. When performing ultrasound to an affected area, [a(n)] _____ must be used.
   A. ambulatory device
   B. coupling agent
   C. increased wattage
   D. pressure

6. _____ crutch(es) is(are) used by patients with poor arm strength.
   A. Forearm
   B. One
   C. Platform
   D. Would not be able to use crutches

7. _____ finger(s) width should fit between the crutch pads and the axilla.
   A. One
   B. Two
   C. Three
   D. Four

8. The _____-point gait is less stable than the four-point gait but much quicker for the patient.
   A. one
   B. two
   C. three
   D. none of the above

9. Usually a(n) _____ applies a cast.
   A. orthopedist
   B. medical assistant
   C. physician
   D. specially trained nurse

10. The advantage of applying a fiberglass cast versus a plaster cast is that _____.
    A. it is easier to put on
    B. it is lighter in weight
    C. it is more supportive
    D. a plaster cast comes in only one color

11. When fitting a patient with crutches, the elbow flex should be _____ degrees.
    A. 5 to 10
    B. 10 to 15
    C. 15 to 25
    D. 25 to 30

12. When performing eye irrigation, the medical assistant should rinse _____.
    A. toward the center of the eye
    B. toward the inner corner of the eye
    C. toward the outer corner of the eye
    D. with patient's head tilted forward

13. A _____ turn bandage is used when the area to be bandaged is of varying widths, such as the forearm and the lower calf of the leg.
    A. figure eight
    B. recurrent
    C. spiral
    D. spiral reverse turn

14. _____ is(are) a device used when full weight cannot be placed on an injured area.
    A. Cane
    B. Crutches
    C. Walker
    D. None of the above

15. When instilling eardrops, it is important to remember to instill the drops toward the _____ of the canal.
    A. bottom
    B. center
    C. roof
    D. It does not matter which way the drops are instilled.

16. A chemical hot or cold pack has an active life of _____ minutes.
    A. 15
    B. 10 to 15
    C. 30 to 45
    D. 30 to 60

17. Heat compresses promote _____.
    A. increased circulation
    B. faster removal of waste products
    C. new cell growth
    D. all of the above

18. A plaster cast will completely dry in approximately _____ hours.
    A. 12
    B. 24
    C. 48
    D. 72

19. When irrigating an ear of an adult patient, the medical assistant should straighten the ear canal by gently pulling the ear _____.
    A. upward and backward
    B. downward and forward
    C. upward and forward
    D. downward and backward

20. An ear irrigation is performed to _____.
    A. introduce medication into the ear canal
    B. dislodge materials such as insects and earwax
    C. chill the tympanic membrane
    D. all of the above

Sentence Completion

Complete each sentence or statement.

1. _____ is the medical name for "earwax."

2. The application of _____ reduces or prevents swelling.

3. _____ uses high-frequency waves.

4. A(n) _____ is used to open up a cast.

5. _____ bandage is most frequently used for a stump area or for the head.

6. A(n) _____ is a hand-held device that provides minimal support for walking.

7. A(n) _____ bandage application is when each turn overlaps the previous turn.

8. After a bandage or cast has been applied, it is very important that the medical assistant check

   for _____ below the bandaged area.

9. _____ is cotton material applied over the stockinette to protect the skin and to prevent

   pressure sores over bony areas.

10. A(n) _____ turn bandage is most often used to hold a dressing in place or support a

    joint area.

Short Answers

1. Explain and describe the five stages involved in the application of a cast.

   _____

   _____

   _____

2. List three uses for bandages.

   _____

   _____

   _____

3. List and explain the three types of bandages most commonly used in a medical office.

_____

_____

_____

_____

4. List and explain the four different gait patterns

_____

_____

_____

_____

_____

_____

CRITICAL THINKING

Samuel Olsen is a 10-year-old patient who has fallen at the school playground and injured his left arm. His mother brings him in to the clinic and the physician orders AP, Lat of the left forearm both proximal and distal views. You take the x-rays, and the physician diagnoses a fractured ulna and would like for you to set up for a fiberglass cast. List the materials you will need to assemble for the cast, and briefly describe your role as a medical assistant in casting.

INTERNET RESEARCH

Keywords: Heat and/or Cold Therapy; Fractures

Choose one of these topics to research: Heat and/or cold therapy; Fractures. Write a one-page report. Cite your source. Be prepared to give a 2-minute oral presentation should your instructor assign you to do so.

WHAT WOULD YOU DO?

If you have accomplished the objectives in this chapter, you will be able to make better choices as a medical assistant. Take a look at this situation and decide what you would do.

A multispecialty practice has medical assistants who work with each of the specialists. Allene, a medical assistant who has not had the benefit of training, works with Dr. Sumar, an ophthalmologist. Gerald, a graduate of a medical-assisting program, works with Dr. Herzog, an orthopedist. The ophthalmologist and the otolaryngologist share the same examination room, but they use it on different days. Allene is not very busy one day, so she decides to clean the medicine cabinet and rearrange the drugs. She moves the ophthalmic medications to the spot where the otic medications are usually stored, and vice versa.

When Dr. Sumar treats a patient with conjunctivitis the next day, Allene hands him an otic preparation for the eye instillation. Luckily, Dr. Sumar reads the label on the medication before instilling the drops into the patient's eye. Later in the day, Dr. Sumar reprimands Allene for handing him the otic drops. Gerald is the person who communicates to the orthopedic patients the necessity of correct application of the bandaging as well as the care of a cast after its application. For those who need cold or heat therapy, Gerald is responsible for the applications as ordered by Dr. Herzog, and Gerald also performs the ultrasound treatments as indicated. During ultrasound treatments, Gerald is very careful to have sufficient coupling agent and to keep the head of the machine moving at all times.

Would you be able to step into the role of Allene or Gerald and perform their duties successfully?

1. **Why is it important for ophthalmic and otic preparations to remain in the same storage places?**

_____

_____

_____

2. **What is the danger of placing otic medications into the patient's eye?**

_____

_____

_____

3. **Would the ear patient have a problem if the ophthalmic preparation had been used for the ear instillation?**

_____

_____

_____

4. **What reasons do you believe led to Allene's reprimand? What actions during the cleaning process could have caused the medication error?**

_____

_____

_____

_____

_____

5. Why is it important for Gerald to teach patients to apply bandages from distal to proximal?

_____

_____

_____

6. What does Gerald need to teach a patient about caring for a plaster cast?

_____

_____

_____

_____

_____

7. Why is it important for Gerald to keep the head of the ultrasound machine moving at all times?

_____

_____

_____

_____

_____

8. Why should Gerald be concerned if the patient complains of heat during an ultrasound treatment?

_____

_____

_____

_____

_____

APPLICATION OF SKILLS

Perform Procedure 35-1: Perform an Ear Irrigation.

Perform Procedure 35-2: Perform an Ear Instillation.

Perform Procedure 35-3: Perform an Eye Irrigation.

Perform Procedure 35-4: Perform an Eye Instillation.

Perform Procedure 35-5: Apply a Tubular Gauze Bandage.

Perform Procedure 35-6: Apply an Ice Bag.

Perform Procedure 35-7: Apply a Cold Compress.

Perform Procedure 35-8: Apply a Chemical Cold Pack.

Perform Procedure 35-9: Apply a Hot Water Bag.

Perform Procedure 35-10: Apply a Heating Pad.

Perform Procedure 35-11: Apply a Hot Compress.

Perform Procedure 35-12: Apply a Hot Soak.

Perform Procedure 35-13: Administer an Ultrasound Treatment.

Perform Procedure 35-14: Measure for Axillary Crutches.

Perform Procedure 35-15: Instruct the Patient in Crutch Gaits.

Perform Procedure 35-16: Instruct the Patient in the Use of a Walker.

Perform Procedure 35-17: Instruct the Patient in the Use of a Cane.

Perform Procedure 35-18: Assist in Plaster-of-Paris or Fiberglass Cast Application.

Student Name _____ **Date** _____

PROCEDURE 35-1: PERFORM AN EAR IRRIGATION

TASK: Irrigate the external ear canal to remove cerumen.
CONDITIONS: Given the proper equipment and supplies, the student will be required to perform proper irrigation of an external ear to remove cerumen.

EQUIPMENT AND SUPPLIES
- Irrigating solution (may use warm tap water)
- Container to hold irrigating solution (sterile)
- Disposable gloves
- Irrigating syringe or Reiner's ear syringe
- Ear basin for drainage
- Disposable barrier drape
- Cotton balls
- Otoscope with probe cover
- Biohazardous waste container
- Gauze squares
- Towel
- Patient's medical record

STANDARDS: Complete the procedure within _____ minutes and achieve a minimum score of _____ %.

Time began _____   **Time ended** _____

Steps	Possible Points	First Attempt	Second Attempt
1. Sanitize hands.	5		
2. Assemble equipment and supplies.	5		
3. Obtain the patient's medical record.	5		
4. Escort the patient to the examination room, greet and identify the patient, and ask the patient to have a seat on the end of the examination table.	5		
5. After the physician has examined the patient's ear, verify the physician's order and obtain the correct solution as ordered.	5		
6. Explain the procedure to the patient.	10		
7. Warm the irrigating solution to body temperature by running the container under warm tap water.	5		
8. Put on disposable gloves.	5		
9. Examine the ear.	15		
10. Position the patient by tilting the head slightly forward and toward the affected ear.	15		
11. Place a water-resistant disposable barrier on the patient's shoulder on the affected side. Provide an ear basin, and ask the patient to hold the basin snugly against the head underneath the affected ear.	10		
12. Using the solution ordered to perform the irrigation, moisten cotton balls or 2 × 2-inch gauze squares and clean the outer ear.	10		
13. Pour the warmed solution into the sterile basin.	5		

Steps	Possible Points	First Attempt	Second Attempt
14. Fill the ear-irrigating syringe with the ordered solution, being sure to expel air bubbles from the syringe.	10		
15. Straighten the ear canal as appropriate for age.	10		
16. Irrigate the ear by inserting the tip of the irrigating syringe into the ear and injecting the irrigating solution toward the roof of the canal.	15		
17. Irrigate until the solution has been used or until the desired results have been achieved. Save solution for physician to observe if appropriate.	10		
18. Examine the ear canal with the otoscope at the end of the procedure. Gently dry the outside of the ear with a cotton ball or 2×2-inch gauze squares.	10		
19. Explain the patient that the ear may feel sensitive for a few hours. Have the patient lie on the examination table with the affected ear down for approximately 15 minutes.	10		
20. Remove gloves and sanitize the hands.	5		
21. Inform the physician that procedure is complete. Provide otoscope for inspection as appropriate.	5		
22. Provide clarification of questions as appropriate.	5		
23. Escort the patient to the reception area.	5		
24. Document the procedure.	10		
25. Clean the equipment and examination room.	5		

Total Points Possible   200

Comments: Total Points Earned _____ Divided by _____ Total Possible Points = _____ % Score

Instructor's Signature _____

Student Name _____ Date _____

PROCEDURE 35-2: PERFORM AN EAR INSTILLATION

TASK: Properly instill prescribed medication in the affected ear(s).
CONDITIONS: Given the proper equipment and supplies, the student will be required to demonstrate the proper method for instilling prescribed medication into an affected ear.

EQUIPMENT AND SUPPLIES
- Irrigating solution (may use warm tap water)
- Cotton balls
- Disposable gloves
- Patient's medical record

STANDARDS: Complete the procedure within _____ minutes and achieve a minimum score of _____ %.

Time began _____   **Time ended** _____

Steps	Possible Points	First Attempt	Second Attempt
1. Sanitize hands.	5		
2. Assemble equipment and supplies.	5		
3. Obtain the patient's medical record.	5		
4. Verify the physician's order.	5		
5. Escort the patient to the examination room, greet and identify the patient, and ask the patient to have a seat on the end of the examination table.	5		
6. Explain the procedure to the patient.	5		
7. Put on disposable gloves.	5		
8. Warm the medication, if necessary, and draw the medication into a dropper.	10		
9. Position the ear.	5		
10. Instill the medication in the ear as ordered by physician using correct methodology.	10		
11. Instruct the patient to rest on the unaffected side for approximately 5 minutes.	5		
12. If appropriate, place cotton ball in ear canal.	5		
13. Remove gloves and sanitize the hands.	5		
14. Provide the patient with verbal and written follow-up instructions. Allow for questions.	5		
15. Escort the patient to the reception area.	5		
16. Document the procedure.	10		
17. Clean the equipment and examination room.	5		

Total Points Possible   100

Comments: Total Points Earned _____ Divided by _____ Total Possible Points = _____ % Score

Instructor's Signature _____

Student Name _____ Date _____

PROCEDURE 35-3: PERFORM AN EYE IRRIGATION

TASK: Irrigate the patient's eye(s) to remove foreign particles and to soothe irritated tissue.
CONDITIONS: Given the proper equipment and supplies, the student will be required to demonstrate the proper method for irrigating the patient's eye(s).

EQUIPMENT AND SUPPLIES
- Sterile irrigating solution
- Sterile container for solution
- Sterile bottled solution with syringe tip, eye wash cup, or appropriate equipment for eye irrigation
- Disposable gloves (powder free)
- Basin for the returned solution
- Sterile cotton balls or sterile gauze squares
- Disposable moisture-resistant towel
- Biohazardous waste container
- Patient's medical record
- Tissues

STANDARDS: Complete the procedure within _____ minutes and achieve a minimum score of _____ %.

Time began _____   Time ended _____

Steps	Possible Points	First Attempt	Second Attempt
1. Sanitize hands.	5		
2. Assemble equipment and supplies.	5		
3. Obtain the patient's medical record.	5		
4. Obtain correct solution ordered by physician.	5		
5. Escort the patient to the examination room, greet and identify the patient, and ask the patient to have a seat on the end of the examination table.	5		
6. Explain procedure to patient.	5		
7. Warm the irrigating solution to body temperature by running the container under warm running tap water (98.6° to 100°F).	5		
8. Explain the procedure to the patient.	5		
9. Position the patient and apply moisture-resistant barrier to shoulder of affected side.	5		
10. Put on disposable gloves.	5		
11. Remove any debris or discharge from the patient's eyelid using moisturized cotton balls. Wipe from inner to outer canthus.	10		
12. Prepare the irrigating solution.	10		
13. Expose the lower conjunctiva by separating the eyelids with the gloved index finger and thumb, and ask the patient to stare at a fixed spot.	10		
14. Irrigate the affected eye(s) from inner to outer canthus.	10		

Steps	Possible Points	First Attempt	Second Attempt
15. Continue with the irrigation until the correct amount of solution has been used or as ordered by the physician.	10		
16. Dry the eyelids from the inner to the outer canthus using dry cotton balls or dry gauze squares.	10		
17. Wipe the face and neck as needed.	5		
18. Remove gloves and sanitize the hands.	5		
19. Provide any further follow-up instructions. (Inform the patient that the eyes[s] may be red and irritated. If it lasts 2 days or longer, report it to the office.) Allow for questions.	10		
20. Escort the patient to the reception area.	5		
21. Document the procedure.	10		
22. Clean the equipment and examination room.	5		

Total Points Possible   150

Comments: Total Points Earned _____ Divided by _____ Total Possible Points = _____ % Score

Instructor's Signature _____

Student Name _____ Date _____

PROCEDURE 35-4: PERFORM AN EYE INSTILLATION

TASK: Properly instill prescribed medication in the affected eye(s).
CONDITIONS: Given the proper equipment and supplies, the student will be required to perform a proper instillation of eye medication.

EQUIPMENT AND SUPPLIES
- Ophthalmic drops with sterile eyedropper, or ophthalmic ointment as ordered by physician
- Sterile cotton balls, or sterile gauze squares
- Tissues
- Disposable gloves (powder free)
- Patient's medical record

STANDARDS: Complete the procedure within _____ minutes and achieve a minimum score of _____ %.

Time began _____   Time ended _____

Steps	Possible Points	First Attempt	Second Attempt
1. Sanitize hands.	5		
2. Assemble equipment and supplies.	5		
3. Obtain the patient's medical record and verify order.	5		
4. Obtain correct "ophthalmic" medication.	5		
5. Escort the patient to the examination room, greet and identify the patient, and ask the patient to have a seat on the end of the examination table.	10		
6. Explain the procedure to the patient.	10		
7. Place the patient in a sitting or supine position.	5		
8. Put on disposable powder-free gloves and prepare the medication.	5		
9. Prepare the eye for instillation (ask the patient to stare at a fixed spot during the instillation).	10		
10. Expose the lower conjunctival sac of the eye to be treated.	5		
11. Instill the medication according to physician's order. Instill drops in the center of the lower conjunctival sac of the affected eye, or place a thin ribbon of ointment along the length of the lower conjunctival sac from inner to outer canthus, holding the tip of the dropper or ointment tube approximately 1/2 inch above the eye sac, never allowing the applicator to touch the eye.	15		
12. Discard any unused solution from the eye dropper, and replace the dropper into the bottle.	10		
13. Ask the patient to close the eyes gently and rotate the eye. Ask patient to not squeeze the eyelids.	15		

Steps	Possible Points	First Attempt	Second Attempt
14. Blot-dry the eyelids from the inner to the outer canthus with a dry gauze square to remove any excess medication. Use a separate tissue for each eye.	10		
15. Remove gloves and sanitize the hands.	5		
16. Provide verbal and written follow-up instructions.	5		
17. Document the procedure.	15		
18. Clean the equipment and examination room.	10		

Total Points Possible   150

Comments: Total Points Earned _____ Divided by _____ Total Possible Points = _____ % Score

Instructor's Signature _____

Student Name _____ Date _____

PROCEDURE 35-5: APPLY A TUBULAR GAUZE BANDAGE

TASK: Properly apply a gauze bandage to the affected area.

CONDITIONS: Given the proper equipment and supplies, the student will be required to demonstrate the proper method for applying a tubular gauze bandage.

EQUIPMENT AND SUPPLIES
- Tube gauze applicator
- Roll of tubular gauze
- Adhesive tape
- Patient's medical record

STANDARDS: Complete the procedure within _____ minutes and achieve a minimum score of _____ %.

Time began _____   Time ended _____

Steps	Possible Points	First Attempt	Second Attempt
1. Sanitize hands.	5		
2. Assemble equipment and supplies.	5		
3. Obtain the patient's medical record.	5		
4. Escort the patient to the examination room, greet and identify the patient, and seat the patient on the end of the examination table.	5		
5. Explain the procedure to the patient.	5		
6. Prepare the bandage according to manufacturer's directions and the necessary length for the needed bandage.	10		
7. Gently slide the applicator over the proximal end of the appendage.	5		
8. Anchor the bandage at the proximal end of the appendage, pulling the applicator away from the proximal end toward the distal portion.	10		
9. Pull the applicator approximately 1 inch past the distal end of the patient's appendage.	5		
10. Rotate the applicator one full turn to anchor the bandage.	5		
11. Push the applicator toward the proximal end.	5		
12. Repeat steps 8 through 11 until desired layers of gauze have been applied.	20		
13. Remove the applicator, and trim the excess gauze as needed.	5		
14. Secure the bandage with adhesive tape or by securing the length of tube gauze remaining on the applicator around the patient's wrist or ankle.	10		
15. Provide instructions on care of bandage.	10		

Copyright © 2005 by Elsevier Inc.

Steps	Possible Points	First Attempt	Second Attempt
16. Document the procedure.	10		
17. Clean the equipment and examination room.	5		

Total Points Possible 125

Comments: Total Points Earned _____ Divided by _____ Total Possible Points = _____ % Score

Instructor's Signature _____

Student Name _____ Date _____

PROCEDURE 35-6: APPLY AN ICE BAG

TASK: Properly apply an ice bag to a swollen area.
CONDITIONS: Given the proper equipment and supplies, the student will be required to properly perform applying an ice bag.

EQUIPMENT AND SUPPLIES
- Ice bag with protective covering
- Small pieces of ice (ice chips or crushed ice)
- Patient's medical record
- Towel or protective covering

STANDARDS: Complete the procedure within _____ minutes and achieve a minimum score of _____ %.

Time began _____   Time ended _____

Steps	Possible Points	First Attempt	Second Attempt
1. Sanitize hands.	5		
2. Assemble equipment and supplies.	5		
3. Obtain the patient's medical record.	5		
4. Escort the patient to the examination room, and greet and identify the patient.	5		
5. Explain the procedure to the patient.	10		
6. Properly fill the bag one-half to two-thirds full with ice chips or crushed ice.	5		
7. Remove air from bag and replace cap.	5		
8. Dry the outside of the bag and place in protective covering.	5		
9. Apply ice bag to the affected area, asking patient if the temperature is tolerable. Check patient after approximately 5 minutes.	15		
10. Leave bag in place for 20 to 30 minutes or as ordered by physician.	10		
11. Refill the bag with ice and change protective covering as needed.	5		
12. Sanitize hands.	5		
13. Provide written and verbal follow-up instructions to the patient.	5		
14. Document the procedure.	10		
15. Properly sanitize and store ice bag covering.	5		

Total Points Possible   100

Comments: Total Points Earned _____ Divided by _____ Total Possible Points = _____ % Score

_Instructor's Signature_____

Student Name _____ Date _____

PROCEDURE 35-7: APPLY A COLD COMPRESS

TASK: Properly apply a cold compress to an affected area.

CONDITIONS: Given the proper equipment and supplies, the student will be required to apply a cold compress.

EQUIPMENT AND SUPPLIES
- Ice cubes
- Washcloths or gauze squares (compress)
- Basin
- Towel
- Ice bag
- Patient's medical record

STANDARDS: Complete the procedure within _____ minutes and achieve a minimum score of _____ %.

Time began _____   Time ended _____

Steps	Possible Points	First Attempt	Second Attempt
1. Sanitize hands.	5		
2. Assemble equipment and supplies.	5		
3. Obtain the patient's medical record.	5		
4. Escort the patient to the examination room, and explain the procedure to the patient.	5		
5. Prepare the cold water by adding ice for the compress.	5		
6. Prepare and apply the cold compress.	5		
7. Prepare an ice bag and cover the compress in accordance with office policy.	5		
8. Ask the patient if the temperature is tolerable.	5		
9. Prepare compress and repeat application for prescribed duration.	10		
10. Periodically check the patient's skin for signs of blueness or numbness. Check for increased pain at site. Notify physician as necessary. Ask the patient if the site is painful.	15		
11. Add ice as needed to keep water cold.	5		
12. At end of prescribed time, dry the affected area.	5		
13. Sanitize hands.	5		
14. Provide written and verbal follow-up instructions. Allow for questions from patient.	5		
15. Document the procedure.	10		

16. Properly care for the equipment and return to storage. Clean the equipment and examination room.　　　5

Total Points Possible　　　100

Comments: Total Points Earned _____ Divided by _____ Total Possible Points = _____ % Score

*Instructor's Signature*_____

Student Name _____ **Date** _____

PROCEDURE 35-8: APPLY A CHEMICAL COLD PACK

TASK: Properly activate and apply a chemical cold pack.
CONDITIONS: Given the proper equipment and supplies, the student will be required to activate and apply a chemical cold pack.

EQUIPMENT AND SUPPLIES
- Chemical cold pack
- Protective covering
- Patient's medical record

STANDARDS: Complete the procedure within _____ minutes and achieve a minimum score of _____ %.

Time began _____   **Time ended** _____

Steps	Possible Points	First Attempt	Second Attempt
1. Sanitize hands.	5		
2. Assemble equipment and supplies.	5		
3. Obtain the patient's medical record.	5		
4. Greet and identify the patient; escort the patient to the examination room.	5		
5. Explain the procedure to the patient.	10		
6. Follow manufacturer's instructions to activate the cold pack.	10		
7. Apply a cover to the pack and apply to the proper area.	15		
8. Administer cold therapy for the prescribed time.	10		
9. Discard the bag in the appropriate waste receptacle.	10		
10. Sanitize the hands.	5		
11. Provide verbal and written follow-up instructions.	10		
12. Document the procedure.	10		

Total Points Possible   100

Comments: Total Points Earned _____ Divided by _____ Total Possible Points = _____ % Score

Instructor's Signature _____

Student Name _____ Date _____

PROCEDURE 35-9: APPLY A HOT WATER BAG

TASK: Fill and apply a hot water bag to an affected area.
CONDITIONS: Given the proper equipment and supplies, the student will be required to apply a hot water bag.

EQUIPMENT AND SUPPLIES
- Hot water bag with protective covering
- Pitcher to hold water
- Bath thermometer
- Patient's medical record

STANDARDS: Complete the procedure within _____ minutes and achieve a minimum score of _____ %.

Time began _____   **Time ended** _____

Steps	Possible Points	First Attempt	Second Attempt
1. Sanitize hands.	5		
2. Assemble equipment and supplies.	5		
3. Obtain the patient's medical record.	5		
4. Greet and identify the patient. Escort the patient to the examination room.	5		
5. Explain the procedure to the patient.	10		
6. Prepare the water to be used in the hot water bag.	10		
7. Fill the hot water bag one-third to one-half full.	5		
8. Expel excess air.	5		
9. Dry the outside of the bag and test for leakage.	5		
10. Cover with protective covering and place the hot water bag on the affected area. Be sure patient is in comfortable position.	10		
11. Apply the water bag for the prescribed time, refilling the bag with hot water as needed to maintain proper temperature and checking patient.	10		
12. Sanitize the hands.	5		
13. Provide verbal and written follow-up instructions.	5		
14. Document the procedure.	10		
15. Care for the hot water bag and store properly.	5		

Total Points Possible   100

Comments: Total Points Earned _____ Divided by _____ Total Possible Points = _____ % Score

Instructor's Signature _____

Student Name _____ **Date** _____

PROCEDURE 35-10: APPLY A HEATING PAD

TASK: Apply a heating pad to an affected area.
CONDITIONS: Given the proper equipment and supplies, the student will be required to apply a heating pad to prescribed area.

EQUIPMENT AND SUPPLIES
- Heating pad
- Protective covering
- Patient's medical record

STANDARDS: Complete the procedure within _____ minutes and achieve a minimum score of _____ %.

Time began _____   **Time ended** _____

Steps	Possible Points	First Attempt	Second Attempt
1. Sanitize hands.	5		
2. Assemble equipment and supplies. Inspect the heating pad to ensure it is in proper working order. Place the heating pad in the protective covering.	15		
3. Obtain the patient's medical record.	5		
4. Greet and identify the patient. Escort the patient to the examination room and explain the procedure to the patient.	10		
5. Connect the heating pad to the electrical outlet and set controls to proper setting as prescribed by physician.	5		
6. Place the patient in a position of comfort. Apply the heating pad to the affected area and check on patient during the prescribed time.	10		
7. Sanitize the hands.	5		
8. Provide verbal and written follow-up instructions. Allow for questions.	5		
9. Document the procedure.	10		
10. Store the equipment appropriately.	5		

Total Points Possible   75

Comments: Total Points Earned _____ Divided by _____ Total Possible Points = _____ % Score

Instructor's Signature _____

Student Name _____ **Date** _____

PROCEDURE 35-11: APPLY A HOT COMPRESS

TASK: Apply a hot compress to an affected area according to physician's order.

CONDITIONS: Given the proper equipment and supplies, the student will be required to apply a hot compress to an affected area to increase circulation.

EQUIPMENT AND SUPPLIES
- Solution ordered by physician or commercially prepared hot, moist heat packs.
- Bath thermometer
- Washcloths or gauze squares
- Basin
- Towel
- Patient's medical record

STANDARDS: Complete the procedure within _____ minutes and achieve a minimum score of _____ %.

Time began _____   **Time ended** _____

Steps	Possible Points	First Attempt	Second Attempt
1. Sanitize hands.	5		
2. Assemble equipment and supplies.	5		
3. Obtain the patient's medical record.	5		
4. Greet and identify the patient. Escort the patient to the examination room, and explain the procedure.	10		
5. Fill the basin with ordered solution and check temperature.	10		
6. Place the patient in a comfortable position, cover the compress with a waterproof cover, and apply the compress to the affected area.	15		
7. Ask the patient if the temperature is tolerable.	10		
8. Prepare additional compresses as needed and reapply the compress; periodically check the patient's comfort and replace the cooled water if necessary.	10		
9. After the prescribed time has elapsed, gently dry the area.	5		
10. Sanitize the hands.	5		
11. Provide verbal and written follow-up instructions.	5		
12. Document the procedure.	10		
13. Care for the equipment and return it to its storage place.	5		

Total Points Possible   100

Comments: Total Points Earned _____ Divided by _____ Total Possible Points = _____ % Score

Instructor's Signature _____

Student Name _____ Date _____

PROCEDURE 35-12: APPLY A HOT SOAK

TASK: Apply a hot soak to an affected area as prescribed by physician.
CONDITIONS: Given the proper equipment and supplies, the student will be required to apply a hot soak to an affected area.

EQUIPMENT AND SUPPLIES
- Soaking solution ordered by physician
- Bath thermometer
- Basin
- Towels
- Patient's medical record

STANDARDS: Complete the procedure within _____ minutes and achieve a minimum score of _____ %.

Time began _____   **Time ended** _____

Steps	Possible Points	First Attempt	Second Attempt
1. Sanitize hands.	5		
2. Assemble equipment and supplies.	5		
3. Obtain the patient's medical record.	5		
4. Greet and identify the patient. Escort the patient to the examination room and explain the procedure.	10		
5. Fill the basin with ordered solution and check temperature.	5		
6. Place the patient in a comfortable position and gently and slowly immerse the appropriate patient's affected body part into the solution.	15		
7. Ask the patient if the temperature is tolerable.	5		
8. Apply the soak for the appropriate amount of time as ordered. Periodically check the patient and temperature of the water, replacing the cooled water with hot water as appropriate.	15		
9. After the prescribed time has elapsed, gently dry the area.	10		
10. Sanitize the hands.	5		
11. Provide verbal and written follow-up instructions. Allow for questions.	5		
12. Document the procedure.	10		
13. Properly care for the equipment and return it to storage place.	5		

Total Points Possible   100

Comments: Total Points Earned _____ Divided by _____ Total Possible Points = _____ % Score

*Instructor's Signature*_____

Student Name _____ Date _____

PROCEDURE 35-13: ADMINISTER AN ULTRASOUND TREATMENT

TASK: Administer an ultrasound treatment according to physician's order.

CONDITIONS: Given the proper equipment and supplies, the student will be required to administer an ultrasound treatment.

EQUIPMENT AND SUPPLIES
- Ultrasound machine
- Coupling agent
- Paper towels or tissues
- Patient's medical record

STANDARDS: Complete the procedure within _____ minutes and achieve a minimum score of _____ %.

Time began _____   Time ended _____

Steps	Possible Points	First Attempt	Second Attempt
1. Sanitize hands.	5		
2. Assemble equipment and supplies.	5		
3. Obtain the patient's medical record.	5		
4. Greet and identify the patient, escort the patient to the examination room, and explain the procedure.	10		
5. According to physician, place the patient in a comfortable position.	5		
6. Apply coupling gel to completely cover the treatment area.	10		
7. Use the ultrasound applicator head to spread the coupling agent evenly over the treatment area before turning on machine.	10		
8. Set ultrasound machine to "On" and place to the intensity level and time ordered by physician.	10		
9. Increase the intensity level to the level ordered.	10		
10. Place the applicator head at a right angle into the coupling agent on the patient's skin.	10		
11. Depending on the area of the body being treated, move the applicator in either a continuous back-and-forth motion or a circular motion.	10		
12. If the patient complains of any pain, burning, or discomfort, stop the procedure immediately and notify the physician.	10		
13. Continue ultrasound treatment until the prescribed time has expired.	5		
14. Remove the applicator head from the patient's skin and turn the intensity control to the minimum position.	10		
15. Wipe excessive coupling agent from the patient's skin and applicator head.	5		

Steps	Possible Points	First Attempt	Second Attempt
16. Instruct the patient to dress; assist as needed.	5		
17. Sanitize the hands.	5		
18. Document the procedure.	10		
19. Properly care for the equipment and return it to its appropriate storage place.	10		

Total Points Possible   150

Comments: Total Points Earned _____ Divided by _____ Total Possible Points = _____ % Score

Instructor's Signature _____

Student Name _____ Date _____

PROCEDURE 35-14: MEASURE FOR AXILLARY CRUTCHES

TASK: Measure a patient for axillary crutches.
CONDITIONS: Given the proper equipment and supplies, the student will be required to measure properly a patient for crutches.

EQUIPMENT AND SUPPLIES
- Crutches
- Goniometer
- Patient's medical record

STANDARDS: Complete the procedure within _____ minutes and achieve a minimum score of _____ %.

Time began _____   **Time ended** _____

Steps	Possible Points	First Attempt	Second Attempt
1. Sanitize hands.	5		
2. Assemble equipment and supplies.	5		
3. Obtain the patient's medical record.	5		
4. Greet and identify the patient, escort to the examination room, and explain the procedure to the patient.	10		
5. Position the patient in the standing position. Place crutch in axillary area and position the crutch tips to create an appropriate triangle.	15		
6. Ask the patient to stand erect with a crutch beneath each axilla and to support his or her weight on the handgrips.	5		
7. To avoid pressure on axillary area, adjust the crutches.	5		
8. Adjust the handgrip so elbows are at 15-degree angle.	10		
9. Perform a final check of the crutch measurement so no damage to body will occur.	15		

Total Points Possible   75

Comments: Total Points Earned _____ Divided by _____ Total Possible Points = _____ % Score

*Instructor's Signature*_____

Student Name _____ **Date** _____

PROCEDURE 35-15: INSTRUCT THE PATIENT IN CRUTCH GAITS

TASK: Provide proper instructions for the appropriate crutch gait, depending on the injury or condition.
CONDITIONS: Given the proper equipment and supplies, the student will be required to instruct a patient on the proper crutch gait.

EQUIPMENT AND SUPPLIES
- Properly adjusted crutches
- Patient's medical record

STANDARDS: Complete the procedure within _____ minutes and achieve a minimum score of _____ %.

Time began _____   **Time ended** _____

Steps	Possible Points	First Attempt	Second Attempt
1. Sanitize hands.	5		
2. Assemble equipment and supplies as necessary.	5		
3. Obtain the patient's medical record as necessary.	5		
4. Greet and identify the patient as necessary.	5		
5. Explain the procedure to the patient.	10		
6. Ask the patient to stand erect and face straight ahead.	5		
7. Position the crutches.	5		
8. Instruct the patient in the four-point gait and obtain verbal and practical feedback.	10		
9. Instruct the patient in the three-point gait and obtain verbal and practical feedback.	10		
10. Instruct the patient in the two-point gait and obtain verbal and practical feedback.	10		
11. Instruct the patient in the swing gaits and obtain verbal and practical feedback.	10		
12. Provide patient with appropriate written instruction.	5		
13. Sanitize the hands.	5		
14. Document the instructions.	10		

Total Points Possible   100

Comments: Total Points Earned _____ Divided by _____ Total Possible Points = _____ % Score

Instructor's Signature _____

Student Name _____ Date _____

PROCEDURE 35-16: INSTRUCT THE PATIENT IN THE USE OF A WALKER

TASK: Accurately measure and provide patient instructions for proper use of a walker.
CONDITIONS: Given the proper equipment and supplies, the student will be required measure and provide instructions for proper use of a walker.

EQUIPMENT AND SUPPLIES
- Walker
- Patient's medical record

STANDARDS: Complete the procedure within _____ minutes and achieve a minimum score of _____ %.

Time began _____   **Time ended** _____

Steps	Possible Points	First Attempt	Second Attempt
1. Sanitize hands.	5		
2. Provide a walker for instructional purposes.	5		
3. Obtain the patient's medical record.	5		
4. Greet and identify the patient, and explain the procedure to the patient.	5		
5. Adjust the walker to the proper height.	5		
6. Instruct the patient to pick up the walker and move it 6 inches forward.	5		
7. Have the patient move the dominant foot and then the nondominant foot into the "cage" of the walker.	10		
8. Caution the patient to be sure he or she has good balance before moving the walker ahead again.	10		
9. Repeat steps 9 and 10 as appropriate.	5		
10. Observe the patient for several repetitions until the patient understands instructions and can safely have mobility with the walker.	10		
11. If the walker folds for storage or transport, instruct the patient on the appropriate method of folding the walker. Demonstrate and practice as needed.	10		
12. Provide written instructions for use of the walker.	5		
13. Sanitize the hands.	5		
14. Document the instructions.	10		
15. If using facility's equipment, return to proper storage.	5		

Total Points Possible 100

Comments: Total Points Earned _____ Divided by _____ Total Possible Points = _____ % Score

Instructor's Signature _____

Student Name _____ Date _____

PROCEDURE 35-17: INSTRUCT THE PATIENT IN THE USE OF A CANE

TASK: Measure and provide instructions for proper use of cane.
CONDITIONS: Given the proper equipment and supplies, the student will be required measure and provide instruction on cane use.

EQUIPMENT AND SUPPLIES
- Cane
- Patient's medical record

STANDARDS: Complete the procedure within _____ minutes and achieve a minimum score of _____ %.

Time began _____   **Time ended** _____

Steps	Possible Points	First Attempt	Second Attempt
1. Sanitize hands.	5		
2. Obtain cane if applicable.	5		
3. Obtain the patient's medical record.	5		
4. Greet and identify the patient, and explain the procedure.	10		
5. Measure cane to correct height on the unaffected side.	10		
6. Position the cane.	5		
7. Instruct the patient to move the cane and affected leg forward at the same time.	10		
8. Repeat steps to ensure the patient understands the use of and can manage the cane.	5		
9. Sanitize the hands.	5		
10. Provide written instructions for use at home.	5		
11. Document the instructions.	10		
12. As appropriate, return equipment to proper storage.	5		

Total Points Possible   80

Comments: Total Points Earned _____ Divided by _____ Total Possible Points = _____ % Score

Instructor's Signature _____

Student Name _____ Date _____

PROCEDURE 35-18: ASSIST IN PLASTER-OF-PARIS OR FIBERGLASS CAST APPLICATION

TASK: Provide supplies and assistance during cast application, and instruct the patient in cast care.

CONDITIONS: Given the proper equipment and supplies, the student will be required to assist with the application of a plaster or fiberglass cast.

EQUIPMENT AND SUPPLIES
- Cast material
- Stockinette to fit extremity
- Sheet wadding (cast padding)
- Basin or bucket to hold warm water
- Scissors
- Disposable glove
- Hand cream
- Patient's medical record

STANDARDS: Complete the procedure within _____ minutes and achieve a minimum score of _____ %.

Time began _____   Time ended _____

Steps	Possible Points	First Attempt	Second Attempt
1. Sanitize hands.	5		
2. Assemble equipment and supplies.	5		
3. Obtain the patient's medical record.	5		
4. Greet and identify the patient, and explain the procedure.	10		
5. Place the patient in a comfortable position to allow access for the type of cast being applied.	5		
6. Clean and dry the area to be cast. Observe the area for any broken skin, redness, and bruising.	10		
7. Prepare the area by appropriately applying stockinette.	10		
8. Prepare the area by wrapping area in cast padding.	10		
9. Apply disposable gloves at proper time to assist with cast application.	10		
10. Prepare the plaster or fiberglass roll.	10		
11. Assist as needed by holding the body part in the position requested by the physician. Reassure the patient as needed.	15		
12. Repeat steps 10 and 11 as needed.	10		
13. Assist with folding the stockinette down over the edge of casting material as appropriate.	5		
14. Provide scissors or a plastic knife to the physician to trim areas around thumb, fingers, or toes as necessary.	10		
15. Provide appropriate verbal and written instructions and isometric exercise instructions as prescribed by the physician.	5		

Steps	Possible Points	First Attempt	Second Attempt
16. Clean the equipment room of supplies. Return unused supplies to proper storage.	5		
17. Remove glove and sanitize the hands.	5		
18. Provide patient with written instructions for possible danger signs and symptoms.	5		
19. Document the procedure.	10		

Total Points Possible   150

Comments: Total Points Earned _____ Divided by _____ Total Possible Points = _____ % Score

Instructor's Signature _____

CHAPTER QUIZ

Multiple Choice

Identify the letter of the choice that best completes the statement or answers the question.

1. The _____ bandage application is most commonly used to hold dressings in place or support a joint area.
   A. circular turn
   B. figure eight turn
   C. spiral reverse
   D. recurrent turn

2. Heat therapy is used when trying to reduce or prevent swelling.
   A. True
   B. False

3. Heat therapy cannot be used when _____ exists.
   A. damaged skin areas
   B. pregnancy
   C. major circulatory problems
   D. all of the above

4. The top of the crutch pads should be _____ inches from the axillary areas.
   A. 1
   B. 2
   C. 3
   D. 4

5. _____ bandages are used to mold around irregular areas and are most often used to support dressings.
   A. Elastic
   B. Fabric
   C. Kling
   D. Tubular

6. Overuse of hot or cold therapies can cause the opposite of the desired effect.
   A. True
   B. False

7. The _____ are used when more mobility and support are needed than a cane can provide.
   A. axillary crutches
   B. Lofstrand crutches
   C. platform crutches
   D. none of the above

8. _____ is a typical sign of circulation impairment.
   A. Lack of pain sensation
   B. Tingling
   C. Red coloration
   D. Warm to the touch

9. A hot soak requires a body part to be totally immersed in a water bath.
   A. True
   B. False

10. A chemical hot/cold pack will last with desired effect for about _____.
    A. 10 minutes
    B. 20 to 30 minutes
    C. 30 to 45 minutes
    D. 30 to 60 minutes

11. The _____ bandage is most often used for a stump area.
    A. figure eight
    B. recurrent
    C. spiral
    D. spiral reverse

12. When performing an eye irrigation, the medical assistant _____.
    A. irrigates from the back of the patient with the patient's head tilted back toward you
    B. has patient tilt head away from affected eye
    C. has patient tilt head away from the unaffected eye
    D. uses slightly warm tap water for irrigation

13. _____ is normally used for more complicated fractures.
    A. Air cast
    B. Plaster cast
    C. Splint
    D. Synthetic cast

14. A cast will usually dry within _____ hours.
    A. 8
    B. 12
    C. 48
    D. 72

15. When applying heat to an area, you are _____.
    A. promoting growth of new cells
    B. removing waste from the area
    C. increasing nutrients to the area
    D. all of the above

CHAPTER THIRTY-SIX

Specialty Diagnostic Testing

VOCABULARY REVIEWS

Matching

Match each term with the correct definition.

A. abstinence

B. Apgar score

C. barrier method

D. Bethesda System

E. blood chemistry

F. candidiasis

G. colposcopy

H. conduction

I. corpus luteum

J. culture and sensitivity

K. dysplasia

L. endocervical curettage

M. estimated date of delivery

N. forced vital capacity

O. *Gardnerella*

P. guaiac test

Q. hearing acuity tests

R. human chorionic gonadotropin

_____ 1. Slide preparation used to observe for fungal or bacterial growth

_____ 2. Process or action of giving birth

_____ 3. Laboratory test that reveals the levels of chemicals in the blood

_____ 4. Measurement of the maximum volume of air that can be expired when the patient exhales forcefully

_____ 5. Instrument used to view the sigmoid region of the colon

_____ 6. Hormone found during pregnancy that maintains the corpus luteum during pregnancy

_____ 7. Laboratory test ordered to identify a microorganism and its susceptibility to antibiotics

_____ 8. Small endocrine tissue located on the surface of the ovary following the release of an egg; secretes the progesterone required to maintain the endometrium during implantation and pregnancy

_____ 9. Contraceptive method that prohibits sexual contact between partners

_____ 10. Tests used to check for hearing loss

S. morning-after pill

T. Nägele's rule

U. oximetry sensor

V. parturition

W. photodetector

X. protozoa

Y. puerperium

Z. pulmonary function tests

AA. pulse oximetry

BB. serum pregnancy test

CC. sigmoidoscope

DD. specimen adequacy

EE. spirometry

FF. titer

GG. trichomoniasis

HH. vaginal irrigation

II. vital capacity

JJ. wet mount

_____ 11. Tests done to assess lung function

_____ 12. Infection with *Trichomonas* protozoa spread through sexual contact, making it an STD

_____ 13. Birth control method that places a physical barrier between the egg and the sperm

_____ 14. Removal of endocervical tissue by scraping

_____ 15. Method used to calculate a woman's due date by adding 7 days to the first day of the LMP, subtracting 3 months and adding 1 year

_____ 16. Term that refers to the condition of a specimen

_____ 17. Device that records the percentage of oxygen in the blood after a light source passes through arterial blood

_____ 18. Examination of vaginal and cervical tissue with a colposcope

_____ 19. Test for hidden (occult) blood in the stool or other body secretions

_____ 20. Oral contraceptive that uses large doses of hormones to prevent conception following sexual intercourse

_____ 21. Method to measure the amount of oxygen in a patient's blood

_____ 22. System of measurement used to evaluate an infant at birth

_____ 23. Abnormal development of tissue

_____ 24. Single-celled parasitic organisms that have the ability to move

_____ 25. Measurement of the volume of air that can be expired when the patient exhales completely

_____ 26. Fungal infection affecting vaginal mucosa, skin, and other areas

_____ 27. A mother's probable due date for birth based on her last menstrual period

_____ 28. Device attached to a patient's finger that detects oxygen content in arterial blood

_____ 29. Type of test that measures lung volume and capacity over time

_____ 30. Ability to move from one area to another, as in hearing with transmission of sound through nervous tissue

_____ 31. Genus of bacteria that exists in the vagina and can cause infection if pH is not balanced

_____ 32. Blood test to detect the presence of human chorionic gonadotropin

_____ 33. Time period after childbirth; postpartum

_____ 34. Measurement of the amount of a substance in a specimen

_____ 35. Grading system used for a Pap smear

_____ 36. Instillation of large amounts of solution into the vagina as a method of cleansing

THEORY RECALL

True/False

Indicate whether the sentence or statement is true or false.

_____ 1. The American Cancer Society strongly recommends that at age 30, besides performing monthly BSE, you should have a clinical breast exam performed by a physician.

_____ 2. A cytology laboratory requisition must accompany all specimens to the laboratory for microscopic examination and evaluation.

_____ 3. A fecal occult test can identify the cause of rectal bleeding.

_____ 4. Bacteria is a single-celled parasitic organism that has the ability to move.

_____ 5. It is highly recommended that another female be present when a male doctor performs a pelvic exam.

Multiple Choice

Identify the letter of the choice that best completes the statement or answers the question.

1. Trichomoniasis is an infection caused by _____.
   A. bacteria
   B. fungi
   C. protozoa
   D. yeast

2. A(n) _____ is a procedure performed to examine and treat a portion of the digestive system.
   A. endoscope
   B. proctology
   C. sigmoidoscopy
   D. none of the above

3. An initial prenatal exam consists of _____.
   A. blood chemistry panel
   B. glucose testing
   C. measurement of fetal heart tones
   D. ultrasound

4. _____ is a screening to measure the volume of air that can be expired when the patient exhales completely.
   A. Forced vital capacity
   B. Vital capacity
   C. Pulse oximetry
   D. PFT

5. An _____ is a record produced by an audiometer.
   A. audiogram
   B. audiologist
   C. audiometry
   D. none of the above

6. _____ care is the care a pregnant women receives before the birth of a child.
   A. Postpartum
   B. Prenatal
   C. Puerperium
   D. Obstetrics

7. A BSE should be performed _____.
   A. every time you shower
   B. at least once a week
   C. at least once a month
   D. twice a year

8. A patient should be instructed to not douche or insert any medications for at least _____ hours before a Pap test.
   A. 2
   B. 8
   C. 12
   D. 24

9. _____ is performed to detect the presence of lung dysfunction.
   A. Vital capacity
   B. Forced vital capacity
   C. Spirometry
   D. All of the above

10. Rinne and Weber tests are types of _____.
    A. blood tests
    B. hearing tests
    C. postpartum tests
    D. prenatal tests

11. A(n) _____ is an examination performed to establish the location of internal reproductive organs.
    A. colorectal exam
    B. obstetric exam
    C. pelvic exam
    D. Pap exam

12. _____ has symptoms of frothy discharge, dysuria, and itching.
    A. Candidiasis
    B. Trichomoniasis
    C. *Gardnerella*
    D. Vaginal infection

13. Contraceptive barrier methods include _____.
    A. condoms
    B. hormones
    C. IUD
    D. morning-after pill

14. Candidiasis may result from _____.
    A. antibiotic use
    B. chemicals
    C. fungus
    D. sexual activity

15. The Bethesda System has _____ main categories of reporting.
    A. two
    B. three
    C. four
    D. five

16. _____ is a condition that can occur during pregnancy when the effects of insulin are blocked by hormones produced in the placenta.
    A. Diabetes type 2
    B. Diabetes type 1
    C. Gestational diabetes
    D. All of the above

17. The _____ is a small endocrine gland located on the surface of the ovary following the release of an egg.
    A. corpus christi
    B. corpus luteum
    C. pineal corpus
    D. chorionic gonadotropin

18. _____ rule is a method used to calculate a women's due date by adding 7 days to the first day of the LMP, subtracting 3 months, and adding 1 year (as necessary).
    A. Robert's
    B. Nägele's
    C. Frost's
    D. Weber's

19. A _____ is a slide preparation used to observe for fungal or bacterial growth.
    A. wet mount
    B. dry mount
    C. covered mount
    D. stained mount

20. _____ is the time period after childbirth.
    A. Prenatal
    B. Parturition
    C. Obstetrics
    D. Puerperium

Sentence Completion

Complete each sentence or statement.

1. _____ is a screening tool that evaluates the squamous epithelial tissue covering the

   visible part of the cervix.

2. _____ is an inflammation of the vaginal tissue caused by fungi, bacteria, protozoa,

   or irritation from chemicals, or foreign objects.

3. Most frequent complaint of a patient with *Gardnerella* is _____ odor.

4. The _____ test assesses the hearing in both ears at once.

5. _____ is a noninvasive procedure used to measure the oxygen level of a patient's blood.

6. _____ is a birth control device that prevents a fertilized egg from implanting in the

   uterine wall.

7. _____ is a contraceptive method that does not allow the egg or sperm to travel the normal pathway in the body.

8. When having a pelvic exam, the patient is in the _____ position.

9. The _____ is special tissue that attaches to the uterus during pregnancy and provides nutrients and oxygen to the fetus.

10. An instrument used in a pelvic examination to view the cervix is called a(n) _____.

Short Answers

1. List the five items found in a postpartum visit.

_____

_____

_____

_____

2. List the four parts of a gynecologic exam.

_____

_____

_____

_____

3. Explain the patient preparation for a sigmoidoscopy.

_____

_____

_____

_____

4. Explain the method called "liquid prep."

_____

_____

_____

_____

5. Each slide prepared from each specimen must be labeled with the location from which the sample was taken. List the three labels that are placed on the slides.

_____

_____

_____

_____

CRITICAL THINKING

There is much controversy over the use of hormone replacement therapy and the role they play on breast cancer. Research several articles either in trade journals or online. Through your research, state your personal opinion and support your stand with documentation.

INTERNET RESEARCH

Keywords: Colorectal Cancer Prevention, Pulmonary Function Testing, Papanicolaou Test, Breast Cancer

Choose one of these topics to research: Colorectal cancer prevention; Pulmonary function testing; Papanicolaou test; Breast cancer. Write a one-page report. Cite your source. Be prepared to give a 2-minute oral presentation should your instructor assign you to do so.

WHAT WOULD YOU DO?

If you have accomplished the objectives in this chapter, you will be able to make better choices as a medical assistant. Take a look at this situation and decide what you would do.

Kari, age 20, is a new patient in the office of Dr. Berg, a gynecologist. Francine is the medical assistant for Dr. Berg and has only been on the job for about 2 weeks. Arriving for her appointment, Kari is given the history and physical paperwork to fill out because she is a new patient. When Francine calls Kari to the back to question her further on some specifics regarding her menstrual periods and sexual activity, four other patients are sitting close to Kari in the lab/workup area. Later, Francine is overheard discussing Kari's history with co-workers by yet more patients in the waiting room.

After taking Kari to the examination room, Francine tells her to get undressed without providing instructions for putting on the gown and drape. When Francine returns to see if Kari is undressed, she then places her into the lithotomy position for what turns out to be a 30-minute wait.

When Dr. Berg starts to examine Kari, Francine leaves the room and tells Dr. Berg to call her when he is ready to do the pelvic examination. During the breast examination, Kari asks Dr. Berg about birth control and tells him that she has been sexually active with a partner who has been diagnosed with a sexually transmitted disease (STD). Dr. Berg completes the pelvic examination, obtaining a Pap smear as well as cultures for STD and a wet prep. Dr. Berg takes the wet mount to the microscope for observation. He sees Francine in the hallway chatting with some co-workers and asks where she was when he needed her during the pelvic exam. She explains she never heard him call for assistance.

Dr. Berg returns to the examination room and begins discussing forms of birth control with Kari, asking if she would rather have a barrier method, an intrauterine device, or a hormonal method such as birth control pills. He also explains to her that she has trichomoniasis, an STD, as seen on the wet prep. Dr. Berg gives Kari a prescription to treat the trichomoniasis for herself and her sexual partner.

Would you be prepared to handle this situation better than Francine did?

1. **What was unethical about the way Francine took Kari's history? What HIPAA regulations did Francine not follow?**

2. **What are the issues concerning the privacy of Kari's medical record when Francine discussed the symptoms and patient history with co-workers?**

3. **How did Francine mishandle the preparation of the patient and the assistance with the physical examination?**

4. Why do you think that Kari did not tell Francine about the sexual partner with an STD? Would you have told Francine if you had been in Kari's situation? Why?

_____

_____

_____

_____

_____

_____

_____

5. What are the elements of a pelvic examination, and how should the medical assistant help with these?

_____

_____

_____

_____

_____

_____

6. Why would Dr. Berg do a gonorrhea and chlamydia culture? What other methods did Dr. Berg use to diagnose trichomoniasis?

_____

_____

_____

_____

_____

_____

7. **What medication would you expect Dr. Berg to prescribe for both sexual partners, and why do both need to be treated?**

_____

_____

_____

_____

_____

_____

_____

8. **What is included in barrier methods of birth control? What is included in hormonal methods? How is an IUD effective?**

_____

_____

_____

_____

_____

_____

_____

APPLICATION OF SKILLS

Procedure Check-off Sheets (*) and Assignments from MACC CD (see Procedure Check-off Sheets for which procedure from the MACC CD to perform).

Perform Procedure 36-1: Teach Breast Self-Examination.*

Perform Procedure 36-2: Assist with a Gynecologic Examination.*

Perform Procedure 36-3: Assist with a Follow-up Prenatal Examination.*

Perform Procedure 36-4: Instruct the Patient in Obtaining a Fecal Specimen.*

Perform Procedure 36-5: Test for Occult Blood.*

Perform Procedure 36-6: Assist with Sigmoidoscopy.*

Perform Procedure 36-7: Perform Spirometry Testing (Pulmonary Function Testing).*

Perform Procedure 36-8: Perform Pulse Oximetry.*

Student Name _____ Date _____

PROCEDURE 36-1: TEACH BREAST SELF-EXAMINATION

TASK: Instruct the patient to perform breast self-examination (BSE).

CONDITIONS: Given the proper equipment and supplies, the student will be required to provide instructions for performing a self-breast examination.

NOTE: The student should practice the procedure using the MACC CD in the back of the textbook and then practice and perform the task in the classroom: MACC CD MACC/Clinical skills/Patient care/Teaching breast self-examination.

EQUIPMENT AND SUPPLIES
- Small pillow or rolled towel
- Model of breast with known irregularities
- BSE instruction sheet
- Patient's medical record

STANDARDS: Complete the procedure within _____ minutes and achieve a minimum score of _____ %.

Time began _____   Time ended _____

Steps	Possible Points	First Attempt	Second Attempt
1. Sanitize hands.	5		
2. Assemble equipment and supplies.	5		
3. Obtain the patient's medical record.	5		
4. Greet and identify the patient, escort to the examination room, and ask her to have a seat on the end of the examination table.	10		
5. Explain the importance of performing the monthly BSE.	10		
6. Provide an instruction card and explain the steps for BSE.	5		
7. Instruct patient to visually inspect both breasts in a mirror for color, texture, and symmetry.	5		
8. Instruct patient to raise both arms at the same time and to check both breasts and nipples for reaction to movement.	5		
9. Instruct patient to rest palms on hips and press down firmly; and then to flex the chest and tighten the chest muscles while observing breast.	5		
10. Instruct patient to bend forward at the waist with hands on hips and to check for dimpling of the skin or nipples.	5		
11. Instruct patient to stand up and gently squeeze the nipple of each breast with the fingertips for any discharge.	5		
12. Instruct patient to use the pads of her index, middle, and ring fingers to palpate the model to determine abnormalities.	5		

Steps	Possible Points	First Attempt	Second Attempt
13. Using the model, instruct patient to use a small circular motion, in a systematic pattern, over all areas of the breast (about the size of a dime) and to apply continuous pressure while palpating both breasts for lumps or thickening of breast tissue.	15		
14. Palpate toward the nipple, keeping fingers on the breast to avoid missing a spot.	5		
15. Check the entire breast, from the armpit to breastbone and from the collarbone to the bra line.	10		
16. Position the patient for inspection of her own breasts and to follow a pattern while palpating her own breasts in a standing position.	10		
17. Instruct patient to place her right hand on her right shoulder and palpate her right breast with her left hand, checking for lumps, thickening, or hard knots.	10		
18. Instruct patient to repeat the process and to examine her left breast.	5		
19. After having adequately completed the return demonstration, assist patient with dressing as necessary.	5		
20. Provide the patient with an instruction card, and ask if there are any questions.	5		
21. Remind the patient that the health care provider will answer any questions she may have about any abnormalities found.	5		
22. Document the instructions in the patient's medical record.	10		

Total Points Possible　　　　　　　　　150

Comments: Total Points Earned _____ Divided by _____ Total Possible Points = _____ % Score

Instructor's Signature _____

Student Name _____ Date _____

PROCEDURE 36-2: ASSIST WITH A GYNECOLOGIC EXAMINATION

TASK: Prepare a patient for and assist the health care provider with a gynecologic examination, including Pap smear (direct smear method and "liquid prep" method).

CONDITIONS: Given the proper equipment and supplies, the student will be required to prepare a patient for and assist with a gynecologic examination, including a Pap smear

NOTE: The student should practice the procedure using the MACC CD in the back of the textbook and then practice and perform the task in the classroom: MACC CD MACC/Clinical skills/Patient care/Assisting with a gynecologic exam.

EQUIPMENT AND SUPPLIES
- Patient gown and drape
- Nonsterile disposable gloves
- Gauze squares
- Disposable vaginal speculum or sterilized stainless steel speculum
- Light source
- Lubricant (water based)
- Tissues
- Cytology requisition
- Transport media
- Urine specimen container
- Biohazardous waste container
- Patient's medical record

"Dry Prep" (Direct Smear) Method
- Wooden spatula
- Endocervical brush; cotton-tipped applicator
- Microscope slides with frosted edge
- Slide holder
- Cytology fixative

"Liquid Prep" Method
- Cervical broom
- Plastic spatula
- Transport medium vial

STANDARDS: Complete the procedure within _____ minutes and achieve a minimum score of _____ %.

Time began _____   Time ended _____

Steps	Possible Points	First Attempt	Second Attempt
1. Sanitize hands.	5		
2. Assemble equipment and supplies.	5		
3. Obtain the patient's record.	5		
4. Greet and identify the patient.	5		
5. Ask the patient if she needs to empty her bladder before the exam.	5		
6. Escort the patient to the examination room, and ask the patient to have a seat on the end of the examination table.	5		

Copyright © 2005 by Elsevier Inc.

Steps	Possible Points	First Attempt	Second Attempt
7. Obtain and record the following preliminary patient information.			
a. Vital signs	5		
b. Height and weight	5		
c. Menstrual and obstetric history	5		
d. Ask if she has any particular concerns or complaints.	5		
8. Complete the cytology requisition form.	10		
9. Ask the patient to undress completely and put on the gown with opening on back and to sit at the end of the examination table with the drape across her lap. Assistant leaves the room and knocks on door before entering.	5		
10. Position and drape the patient for a breast exam and assist physician as needed.	5		
11. Adjust the drape for the abdominal exam in supine position and assist physician as needed.	10		
12. Position and drape the patient into the lithotomy position for the pelvic exam.	10		
13. Apply disposable gloves.	5		
14. Fold back the corner of the drape to expose the perineal area; adjust and focus the light on the perineum for the physician.	5		
15. Warm the vaginal speculum using warm water.	5		
16. Assist the physician with the pelvic exam by encouraging the patient to breathe deeply and evenly.	5		
17. Prepare slides for the specimens with labeling as required by lab. Pass instruments and equipment as needed.	10		
18. Pass spatula for cervical specimen. Hold the glass slide marked "C" for the physician to apply the specimen. Discard the applicator in biohazardous waste container.	10		
19. Pass the endocervical brush. Hold out the slide with an "E" to receive the next specimen. Discard the endocervical brush in biohazardous waste container.	10		
20. Hand the physician a cotton-tipped applicator to collect a vaginal specimen. Discard the applicator in biohazardous waste container. Hold out the slide marked with a "V."	10		
21. Spray the Pap slides immediately with fixative (within 10 seconds).	10		
22. If performing "liquid prep" method, label the liquid-prep vial or slides as required by the laboratory and place the liquid-prep vial or slides in a biohazardous transport bag.	10		
23. Assist the physician with the bimanual pelvic examination including passing speculum and encouraging deep breathing. Assist with occult blood test including the developing of guaiac slide.	10		

Steps	Possible Points	First Attempt	Second Attempt
24. Dispose of disposable speculum, guaiac slide, and gloves in a biohazardous waste container.	5		
25. Assist the patient from the lithotomy position and down from the examination table.	5		
26. Instruct the patient to dress.	5		
27. Leave the room and complete the cytology requisition form.	5		
28. Attach the completed cytology form to either the microscope slide holder or the transport medium vial, and chart the transport to the laboratory.	5		
29. Clean the examination room in preparation for the next patient.	5		
30. Sanitize the hands.	5		
31. Document the procedure in the patient's medical record.	10		

Total Points Possible   225

Comments: Total Points Earned _____ Divided by _____ Total Possible Points = _____ % Score

Instructor's Signature _____

Student Name _____ Date _____

PROCEDURE 36-3: ASSIST WITH A FOLLOW-UP PRENATAL EXAMINATION

TASK: Assist the physician during a follow-up prenatal visit.
CONDITIONS: Given the proper equipment and supplies, the student will be required to assist the physician during a follow-up prenatal examination.

EQUIPMENT AND SUPPLIES
- Flexible, nonstretchable centimeter tape measure
- Nonsterile disposable gloves
- Doppler fetal pulse detector
- Lubricant (water based)
- Ultrasound coupling agent
- Vaginal speculum
- Examining gown and drape
- Biohazardous waste container
- Patient's medical record

STANDARDS: Complete the procedure within _____ minutes and achieve a minimum score of _____ %.

Time began _____   Time ended _____

Steps	Possible Points	First Attempt	Second Attempt
1. Sanitize hands.	5		
2. Assemble equipment and supplies.	5		
3. Obtain the patient's medical record.	5		
4. Greet and identify the patient.	5		
5. Collect the first morning urine specimen that the patient has brought from home.	5		
6. Weigh and document the results in the patient's medical record.	10		
7. Escort patient to the examination room and explain the procedure.	5		
8. Document problems, concerns, or complaints.	5		
9. Measure the patient's vital signs and document the results in the patient's medial record.	10		
10. Prepare the patient for the examination by applying drape and gown.	10		
11. Test the urine specimen using a reagent strip and document the results in the patient's medical record.	10		
12. Inform the physician that the patient is ready to be examined, and provide the physician with the medical record for review.	5		
13. Position and drape the patient, just prior to when the physician is ready to start the exam.	10		
14. Assist the physician as required for the prenatal examination, passing instruments and equipment as needed. Collect and prepare specimens as requested. Apply gloves as appropriate.	10		

Steps	Possible Points	First Attempt	Second Attempt
15. After the examination, assist the patient from the examination table.	10		
16. Remove gloves and dispose of disposable equipment in correct container as appropriate.	5		
17. Allow patient time to redress.	5		
18. Provide the patient education, and clarify any of the physician's instructions as appropriate.	10		
19. Apply gloves to clean the examination room in preparation for the next patient. Discard gloves in appropriate waste container.	10		
20. Sanitize hands.	5		
21. Document appropriately in the patient's medical record.	5		

Total Points Possible   150

Comments: Total Points Earned _____ Divided by _____ Total Possible Points = _____ % Score

Instructor's Signature _____

Student Name _____ **Date** _____

PROCEDURE 36-4: INSTRUCT THE PATIENT IN OBTAINING A FECAL SPECIMEN

TASK: Provide the patient with accurate and complete instructions on the preparation and collection of a stool sample for testing.

CONDITIONS: Given the proper equipment and supplies, the student will be required to provide the patient with instructions on the preparation and collection of a stool sample.

NOTE: The student should practice the procedure using the MACC CD in the back of the textbook and then practice and perform the task in the classroom: MACC CD MACC/Clinical skills/Diagnostic testing/Instructing how to obtain a fecal specimen and testing for occult blood.

EQUIPMENT AND SUPPLIES
- Hemoccult slide testing kit
  - 3 occult blood slides
  - 3 applicator sticks
  - Diet and collection instruction sheet
- Patient's medical record

STANDARDS: Complete the procedure within _____ minutes and achieve a minimum score of _____ %.

Time began _____   **Time ended** _____

Steps	Possible Points	First Attempt	Second Attempt
1. Sanitize hands.	5		
2. Assemble equipment and supplies.	5		
3. Greet and identify the patient.	5		
4. Explain the procedure to the patient. Escort the patient to the examination room.	5		
5. Explain the procedure to the patient.	5		
6. Provide the patient with verbal and written instructions including diet modification and other conditions that might affect the test results, such as menses.	10		
7. Provide the patient with the Hemoccult slide test kit.	5		
8. Instruct the patient to use a ballpoint pen to complete the required information on the front of the card.	5		
9. Inform the patient of the requirements for proper care and storage of the slides.	5		
10. Instruct patient to collect a stool specimen in the toilet from the first bowel movement after the 48-hour preparation period.	5		
11. Explain the stool collection procedure to the patient; include the manner of obtaining specimen and the means of placing specimen on slide.	10		
12. Instruct the patient to allow the slides to air dry minimally overnight.	5		

Steps	Possible Points	First Attempt	Second Attempt
13. Instruct the patient to repeat the process on the next two bowel movements, repeating the collection steps.	5		
14. Once all three specimens have been collected and allowed to air dry, instruct the patient to place the cardboard slides in the envelope, carefully seal, and return it as soon as possible to the medical office.	5		
15. Be certain that patient understands the instructions required for patient preparation, collection, and processing of the stool specimens and for storage of the slides.	5		
16. Document that instructions have been provided in the patient's medical record.	10		
17. Sanitize the hands.	5		

Total Points Possible   100

Comments: Total Points Earned _____ Divided by _____ Total Possible Points = _____ % Score

Instructor's Signature _____

Student Name _____ Date _____

PROCEDURE 36-5: TEST FOR OCCULT BLOOD

TASK: Accurately develop the occult blood slide test and document the results.

CONDITIONS: Given the proper equipment and supplies, the student will be required to demonstrate competency in developing an occult blood slide test and document the results.

NOTE: The student should practice the procedure using the MACC CD in the back of the textbook and then practice and perform the task in the classroom: MACC CD MACC/ Clinical skills/Diagnostic testing/Instructing how to obtain a fecal specimen and testing for occult blood.

EQUIPMENT AND SUPPLIES
- Prepared cardboard slides
- Reference card
- Developing solution
- Nonsterile disposable gloves
- Biohazardous waste container
- Patient's medical record

STANDARDS: Complete the procedure within _____ minutes and achieve a minimum score of _____ %.

Time began _____   Time ended _____

Steps	Possible Points	First Attempt	Second Attempt
1. Sanitize hands.	5		
2. Assemble supplies including test kit reference card.	5		
3. Check the expiration date on the developing solutionbottle.	10		
4. Obtain the patient's medical record.	5		
5. Apply nonsterile disposable gloves.	5		
6. Prepare the patient by removing clothes as appropriate; drape and gown the patient.	5		
7. Prepare the slides.	10		
8. Develop slides according to manufacturer's instructions.	10		
9. Read the results within 60 seconds.	10		
10. Perform quality control procedure on slide, and document the results in the quality control laboratory log book.	10		
11. Properly dispose of the Hemoccult slides in a biohazardous waste container.	10		
12. Remove gloves and sanitize hands.	5		
13. Document the results.	10		

Total Points Possible   100

Comments: Total Points Earned _____ Divided by _____ Total Possible Points = _____ % Score

Instructor's Signature _____

Student Name _____ Date _____

PROCEDURE 36-6: ASSIST WITH SIGMOIDOSCOPY

TASK: Assist the physician and the patient during sigmoidoscopy.
CONDITIONS: Given the proper equipment and supplies, the student will be required to assist the physician and patient during sigmoidoscopy.

EQUIPMENT AND SUPPLIES
- Nonsterile disposable gloves
- Sterile specimen container with preservative
- Flexible sigmoidoscope
- 4 × 4-inch gauze squares
- Water-soluble lubricant
- Tissue wipes
- Drape
- Biopsy forceps
- Biohazardous waste container
- Patient's medical record

STANDARDS: Complete the procedure within _____ minutes and achieve a minimum score of _____ %.

Time began _____   Time ended _____

Steps	Possible Points	First Attempt	Second Attempt
1. Sanitize hands.	5		
2. Assemble equipment and supplies.	5		
3. Obtain the patient's medical record.	5		
4. Greet and identify the patient, escort the patient to the examination room, and explain the procedure to the patient.	5		
5. Ask the patient if he or she needs to empty the bladder before the examination.	5		
6. Assist patient in preparing for exam by gowning, positioning, and draping the patient.	5		
7. Assist physician in application of disposable gloves. Lubricate the physician's gloved index finger.	10		
8. Lubricate the distal end of the sigmoidoscope for insertion into anus.	10		
9. Assist the physician with the suction equipment as required.	5		
10. On completion of the examination, apply clean gloves and clean the patient's anal area with tissues to remove excess lubricant.	5		
11. Remove gloves and sanitize hands.	5		
12. Assist the patient from the examination table; instruct the patient to dress.	5		
13. Provide for the patient a restroom to expel any air that was used to inflate the colon during the procedure.	5		

Steps	Possible Points	First Attempt	Second Attempt
14. Prepare the laboratory requisition form and accompanying specimens.	10		
15. Clean the examination room and clean equipment in preparation for the next patient.	5		
16. Document the procedure in the patient's medical record.	10		
Total Points Possible	100		

Comments: Total Points Earned _____ Divided by _____ Total Possible Points = _____ % Score

Instructor's Signature _____

Student Name _____ **Date** _____

PROCEDURE 36-7: PERFORM SPIROMETRY TESTING (PULMONARY FUNCTION TESTING)

TASK: Prepare and operate a simple spirometer to measure lung volume.

CONDITIONS: Given the proper equipment and supplies, the student will be required to demonstrate competency in performing spirometry.

NOTE: The student should practice the procedure using the MACC CD in the back of the textbook and then practice and perform the task in the classroom: Medical Assisting Competency Challenge CD MACC/ Clinical skills/Diagnostic testing/Performing a spirometry test.

EQUIPMENT AND SUPPLIES
- Spirometry machine
- Disposable mouthpiece
- Disposable tubing
- Nose clips
- Biohazardous waste container
- Patient's medical record

STANDARDS: Complete the procedure within _____ minutes and achieve a minimum score of _____ %.

Time began _____   **Time ended** _____

Steps	Possible Points	First Attempt	Second Attempt
1. Sanitize hands.	5		
2. Assemble equipment and supplies.	5		
3. Obtain the patient's medical record.	5		
4. Greet and identify the patient, escort the patient to the examination room, and explain the procedure to the patient.	10		
5. Measure the patient's height and weight.	5		
6. Enter the patient's information into the spirometer.	5		
7. Perform the spirometry test.	15		
8. Instruct the patient in breathing.	15		
9. Coach the patient into performing the task to the best of their ability.	10		
10. Allow rest periods for the patient, if needed.	5		
11. Ensure the physician reviews the spirometry test results.	10		
12. Before documenting the procedure, make the patient comfortable and put the equipment away.	10		
13. Discard the disposable components of the spirometry test in a biohazardous waste container.	10		

Steps	Possible Points	First Attempt	Second Attempt
14. Sanitize the hands.	5		
15. Document the test results.	10		

Total Points Possible 125

Comments: Total Points Earned _____ Divided by _____ Total Possible Points = _____ % Score

Instructor's Signature _____

Student Name _____ **Date** _____

PROCEDURE 36-8: PERFORM PULSE OXIMETRY

TASK: Accurately determine a patient's blood oxygen saturation using pulse oximetry.

CONDITIONS: Given the proper equipment and supplies, the student will be required to demonstrate the competency of performing pulse oximetry.

EQUIPMENT AND SUPPLIES
- Pulse oximeter
- Probe
- Alcohol prep pads
- Patient's medical record

STANDARDS: Complete the procedure within _____ minutes and achieve a minimum score of _____ %.

Time began _____   **Time ended** _____

Steps	Possible Points	First Attempt	Second Attempt
1. Sanitize hands.	5		
2. Assemble equipment and supplies.	5		
3. Obtain the patient's medical record.	5		
4. Greet and identify the patient; escort the patient to the examination room.	5		
5. Explain the procedure to the patient.	5		
6. Ask the patient to have a seat in a comfortable position with arms well supported.	5		
7. Connect the oximeter finger probe to the monitor.	10		
8. Turn on the power switch.	5		
9. Wipe the probe clean with the alcohol prep pad and let dry.	10		
10. Apply the oximeter probe to the patient's finger.	10		
11. Wait while the system stabilizes.	5		
12. Read the pulse rate and the arterial blood saturation on the digital display.	10		
13. Remove the sensor from the patient's finger.	5		
14. Sanitize hands.	5		
15. Document the pulse oximetry results in the patient's medical record.	10		

Total Points Possible   100

Comments: Total Points Earned _____ Divided by _____ Total Possible Points = _____ % Score

Instructor's Signature _____

CHAPTER QUIZ

Multiple Choice

Identify the letter of the choice that best completes the statement or answers the question.

1. According to the American Cancer Society, at age _____, in addition to the BSE and clinical breast exam, an annual mammogram is recommended.
   A. 20
   B. 30
   C. 40
   D. 50

2. Patient preparation for a sigmoidoscopy should include _____.
   A. an enema
   B. a high-fiber diet
   C. 16 ounces of water
   D. a mild sedative

3. Spirometry is performed when _____.
   A. lung assessment before major surgery is advised
   B. assessment of patient's response to treatment is required
   C. it is desired to screen a patient at risk because of smoking or the environment
   D. All of the above

4. _____ exam is an internal examination to evaluate the size and location of reproductive organs.
   A. Pelvic
   B. Prenatal
   C. Pap
   D. Obstetric

5. Candidiasis is an inflammation of the vaginal tissue caused by fungi, bacteria, protozoa, or chemical irritation.
   A. True
   B. False

6. The _____ secretes the progesterone required to maintain the endometrium during implantation and pregnancy.
   A. uterus
   B. vaginal walls
   C. corpus luteum
   D. placenta

7. _____ is a noninvasive test that measures the oxygen levels of the body.
   A. Forced vital capacity
   B. Pulse oximetry
   C. Vital capacity
   D. PFT

8. Pap smear results are recorded according to _____.
   A. Bethesda System
   B. office policy
   C. lab policy
   D. state policy

9. Gynecologic exams should include not only a bimanual examination but also a rectal exam.
   A. True
   B. False

10. _____ is an instrument used to visualize and inspect the internal genitalia.
    A. Goose neck lamp
    B. Spatula
    C. Speculum
    D. None of the above

11. BSE exam should be performed _____.
    A. every day
    B. once a week
    C. once a month
    D. once every 2 months

12. Barrier devices include _____.
    A. diaphragms
    B. hormones
    C. IUDs
    D. Morning-after pills

13. _____ has symptoms of yellowish green discharge; itching, and vaginal irritation.
    A. Candidiasis
    B. *Gardnerella*
    C. Trichomoniasis
    D. Pelvic infection

14. The first postpartum examination following a cesarean birth should take place _____ after birth.
    A. 12 hours
    B. 1 week
    C. 2 weeks
    D. 1 month

15. When testing for occult blood, a test card impregnated with guaiac reagent is used.
    A. True
    B. False

CHAPTER **THIRTY-SEVEN**

Introduction to the Physician Office Laboratory

VOCABULARY REVIEW

Matching

Match each term with the correct definition.

A. 24-hour urine specimen

B. bacteremia

C. blood bank

D. butterfly method

E. Center for Medicare and Medicaid Services

F. certificate of provider-performed microscopy procedures

G. certificate of waiver

H. chain of evidence

I. Clinical Laboratory Improvement Amendments of 1998

J. coagulation studies

K. compound

L. crossmatching

M. drug screening

N. evacuated tube

O. filter paper

_____ 1. Blood collection method using a syringe and sterile needle

_____ 2. Bacteria in the blood; sepsis

_____ 3. Tests performed to study microorganisms

_____ 4. Solutions used when testing specimens in the laboratory

_____ 5. Having two sets of lenses on a microscope

_____ 6. Part of the microscope that holds the objectives

_____ 7. Order or manner in which blood collection tubes are to be drawn

_____ 8. Blood collection method using a winged infusion set

_____ 9. Insufficient amount of a specimen for performing the desired test

_____ 10. Laboratory form showing the identification of a specimen and the lab test to be performed

_____ 11. Certificate that allows a physician office laboratory to perform low-complexity testing

P. first morning specimen

Q. heparin

R. laboratory requisition

S. microbiology

T. midstream clean-catch urine specimen

U. nosepiece

V. order of draw

W. phlebotomy

X. plasma

Y. quantity not sufficient

Z. reagents

AA. solutes

BB. sputum

CC. syringe method

DD. urinalysis

EE. venipuncture

FF. pipette

_____ 12. Materials suspended in liquid that are not dissolvable

_____ 13. Blood collection tube in which the internal atmosphere is a vacuum allowing blood to flow into the tube

_____ 14. Urine or blood collection to determine the presence or absence of specific substances

_____ 15. Liquid portion of the blood

_____ 16. Puncture of a vein to obtain a venous blood sample

_____ 17. Federal agency that oversees financial regulations of Medicare and Medicaid

_____ 18. Urine specimen that requires a strict cleaning procedure and collection during the middle of voiding

_____ 19. Collection of urine over a 24-hour period to test kidney function, checking for high levels of creatinine, uric acid, hormones, electrolytes, and medications

_____ 20. Lung secretions produced by the bronchi

_____ 21. Urine specimen taken when the patient first awakens; most concentrated specimen

_____ 22. Process of identifying blood compatibility by determining proteins on the red blood cells of the donor and recipient

_____ 23. Analysis of urine to include physical, chemical, and microscopic properties

_____ 24. Organization that conducts studies for ABO blood grouping and Rh typing

_____ 25. Process of drawing blood from a vein; venipuncture

_____ 26. Special paper used to pass a liquid through or to collect a blood specimen

_____ 27. Studies that evaluate the clotting process of blood

_____ 28. Natural substance that prevents clotting; a vacuum tube additive that prevents the clotting of blood in the tube

_____ 29. Collection routine for a specimen used as evidence

_____ 30. Certificate that allows a physician in the office laboratory to conduct both low-complexity and moderate-complexity tests

_____ 31. Legislation enacted to ensure the quality of laboratory results by setting performance standards

_____ 32. Narrow tube used for transferring liquids by suction

THEORY RECALL

True/False

Indicate whether the sentence or statement is true or false.

_____ 1. The "course" focus adjustment knob on a microscope is used to bring the specimen into sharper focus.

_____ 2. It is imperative that lancets, once used, be bleached and reused.

_____ 3. The medical assistant should always listen to the patients when they suggest where successful blood draws have been taken in the past.

_____ 4. There are five levels of CLIA tests.

_____ 5. All medical offices have a POL.

Multiple Choice

Identify the letter of the choice that best completes the statement or answers the question.

1. The oil immersion lens on a microscope is _____ power.
   A. ×4
   B. ×10
   C. ×40
   D. ×100

2. _____ tests are performed to study bacteria, fungi, viruses, and parasites in body fluids.
   A. Chemistry
   B. Hematology
   C. Microbiology
   D. Serology

3. _____ specimen is the most frequently collected urine from the patient.
   A. Clean-catch
   B. Midstream
   C. Timed
   D. Random

4. The syringe method of venipuncture is used when the patient _____.
   A. has a fear of needles
   B. has small, fragile veins
   C. is a young adult
   D. None of the above

5. A _____-gauge needle is used to draw a large sample of blood directly from a vein.
   A. 16- to 18
   B. 18- to 22
   C. 22- to 25
   D. 25- to 27

6. Medical laboratories are regulated by _____.
   A. the lab director
   B. state law and federal laws
   C. federal laws only
   D. state laws only

7. Urine collected must be processed within _____ or it must be refrigerated until the tests can be performed.
   A. 30 minutes
   B. 1 hour
   C. 6 hours
   D. 1 day

8. _____ is used when only a small amount of blood is needed.
   A. Butterfly draw
   B. Capillary puncture
   C. Syringe draw
   D. Venipuncture

9. _____ is the part of the microscope that connects the objectives and ocular lenses to the base.
   A. Arm
   B. Condenser
   C. Eyepieces
   D. Iris diaphragm

10. _____ tests require proficient testing, test management, and specialized training.
    A. CLIA-waived
    B. Minimal-complexity
    C. Moderate-complexity
    D. High-complexity

11. The _____ of the microscope is the platform that holds the slide for viewing.
    A. condenser
    B. nosepiece
    C. objective
    D. stage

12. The butterfly method of blood collection is used for _____.
    A. difficult to find veins
    B. infants
    C. small children
    D. all of the above

13. No more than _____ venipuncture attempts by the same medical assistant should be done on a patient.
    A. two
    B. three
    C. four
    D. five

14. When collecting a blood sample for serum, the specimen must sit for a minimum of _____ to allow a clot to form.
    A. 10 minutes
    B. 15 minutes
    C. 20 to 30 minutes
    D. 1 hour

15. A _____-top tube is used to collect specimens for plasma or whole blood for blood counts.
    A. blue
    B. gold
    C. lavender
    D. red

16. The _____ knob is used to bring the specimen into focus when a lower-power objective is used.
    A. coarse focus
    B. medium focus
    C. fine focus
    D. nonfocus

17. _____ is the secretion from the lungs produced in the bronchi and throat.
    A. Saliva
    B. Sputum
    C. Spit
    D. All of the above

18. Microhematocrit centrifuge is used to _____.
    A. process blood in a capillary tube
    B. process blood in a venipuncture tube
    C. process urine in a conical bottom tube
    D. process urine in a round bottom tube

19. _____ tests are performed to study the body's immune response by detecting antibodies in the serum.
    A. Chemistry
    B. Hematology
    C. Microbiology
    D. Serology

20. A cultures swab in transport media must be processed within _____.
    A. 8 hours
    B. 12 hours
    C. 24 hours
    D. 48 hours

Sentence Completion

Complete each sentence or statement.

1. A(n) _____ is a program for laboratory testing and is designed to monitor and evaluate

   the quality and accuracy of the test results.

2. A(n) _____ is a small, sterile, needle-like piece of metal used to make a small puncture

   in the skin.

3. _____ tests do not require personnel to have a high level of specific training.

4. A(n) _____ microscope has two eyepieces.

5. A(n) _____ urine specimen is testing for kidney function over a full day's collection rather

   than a random specimen.

6. The GTT is an example of a(n) _____ specimen.

7. _____ can be used to detect group A beta-hemolytic streptococci.

8. _____ is the end product of the digestive process.

9. _____ established the order of draw for quality control purposes.

10. _____ is the study that evaluates the clotting process of blood.

Short Answers

1. Explain the three different laboratory methods of obtaining a specimen.

_____

_____

_____

_____

2. Describe four poor capillary collection techniques that could render the results useless.

_____

_____

_____

_____

3. Explain the difference between multisample and single-sample needles.

_____

_____

_____

_____

4. Explain five quality control actions as it relates to the required accuracy of tests.

_____

_____

_____

_____

5. List six categories and types of tests performed in the POL.

_____

_____

_____

_____

CRITICAL THINKING

You have just started working at a community clinic, where your patients have a variety of ethnicity and ages. This afternoon you have a patient who speaks very little English and you need to provide him with instructions on how to collect a urine sample. An interpreter is not available. Describe how you would handle this situation.

INTERNET RESEARCH

Keyword: Laboratory Quality Assurance

Choose one of the following topics to research: Newborn screening; Cholesterol/lipids. Cite your source. Be prepared to give a 2-minute oral presentation should your instructor assign you to do so.

WHAT WOULD YOU DO?

If you have accomplished the objectives in this chapter, you will be able to make better choices as a medical assistant. Take a look at this situation and decide what you would do.

The full-time laboratory technician at Dr. Macinto's office is on sick leave for a week. Dr. Macinto asks Sherri, a medical assistant, to fill in for the sick technician. Sherri has just been hired from another office, where she was trained by the physician. She has not done laboratory tests and has not prepared patients for laboratory work.

On the first day, Dr. Macinto asks Sherri to collect a midstream urine sample on a patient for a culture and sensitivity and to send some of the urine to an outside laboratory for a drug screen. Sherri hands the urine collection container to the patient without any instructions and allows the patient to go to the bathroom alone to collect the specimen. When the specimen is collected, Sherri leaves the drug screen on the counter to await the arrival of the laboratory courier for transport to the outside laboratory. Neither Sherri nor the courier signs for the specimen. Furthermore, the laboratory form is not complete, and no documentation was made of the collection of the specimen.

Mrs. Gorchetzki, a postmastectomy patient, is seen next. Dr. Macinto has ordered a fasting blood sugar and a fasting blood chemistry test. Without talking to Mrs. Gorchetzki about the preparation she has made for the test, Sherri gathers the supplies for the testing. Mrs. Gorchetzki mentions that she had bacon and eggs for breakfast. Sherri draws the blood sugar using a capillary puncture. Sherri performs the testing before doing quality control for the day. When the specimen is drawn for the blood chemistry, the laboratory request form asks for serum. Sherri starts the process of drawing the venipuncture specimen from the side of the mastectomy in a heparinized tube. Mrs. Gorchetzki tries to tell Sherri to collect the specimen from the other arm because it is easier to draw blood from that arm, but Sherri does not listen.

When Sherri places the specimen in the centrifuge, she spins only one tube. She pipettes off the liquid and sends it to the laboratory. As it turns out, the liquid sent to the laboratory is plasma, but the laboratory had requested serum.

What things would you have done differently in this situation?

1. What instructions should Sherri have given the patient for preparation for a midstream urine specimen?

_____

_____

_____

2. **How should urine for a drug screen be collected? What was the problem with leaving the specimen on the counter for the laboratory courier to collect?**

_____

_____

_____

_____

_____

3. **Would the results of the test have been acceptable in a court case or to an employer who desired this information before hiring the person?**

_____

_____

_____

_____

4. **What is the difference between quality control and quality assurance? Is Dr. Macinto's office practicing quality assurance when Sherri is working in the laboratory?**

_____

_____

_____

_____

5. **Why is quality control so important when performing laboratory tests?**

_____

_____

_____

6. **What color tube should have been used for the blood chemistry? What is the common tube used for whole blood and plasma?**

_____

_____

_____

7. Why shouldn't Sherri have used the arm on the side of the mastectomy? What should she have done when Mrs. Gorchetzki told her that there was a vein that was usually used for venipuncture?

_____

_____

_____

_____

_____

8. Why is it important to close the cover of a centrifuge when it is operating?

_____

_____

_____

9. After Mrs. Gorchetzki stated that she had eaten breakfast, what should Sherri have done rather than collecting the blood specimens? What part of quality assurance was broken by Mrs. Gorchetzki's action of eating?

_____

_____

_____

_____

_____

10. What is Dr. Macinto's responsibility in regard to Sherri's actions?

_____

_____

_____

_____

APPLICATION OF SKILLS

Procedure Check-off Sheets (*) and assignments from MACC CD (**)

1. Perform Procedure 37-1: Use Methods of Quality Control.*
   A. MACC CD
      Clinical skills/Diagnostic testing/Specimen collection & testing/Instructing how to obtain a urine specimen & performing urinalysis.**

2. Perform Procedure 37-2: Focus the Microscope.*
   A. MACC CD
      Clinical skills/Diagnostic testing/Specimen collection & testing/Preparing a urine sediment &using a microscope.**

3. Perform Procedure 37-3: Complete a Laboratory Requisition Form.*
   A. MACC CD
      Clinical skills/Patient care/The physical exam/Assisting with a gynecologic exam.**
   B. MACC CD
      Clinical skills/Diagnostic testing/Specimen collection & testing/Obtaining a wound specimen & preparing for transport to an outside lab.**
   C. MACC CD
      Clinical skills/Diagnostic testing/Specimen collection & testing/Performing a venipuncture using the evacuated tube method.**
   D. MACC CD
      Clinical skills/Diagnostic testing/Specimen collection & testing/Performing a venipuncture using the butterfly & syringe method.**

4. Perform Procedure 37-4: Collect a Specimen for Transport to an Outside Laboratory.*
   A. MACC CD
      Clinical skills/Diagnostic testing/Specimen collection & testing/Obtaining a wound specimen & preparing for transport to an outside lab.**

5. Perform Procedure 37-5: Screen and Follow Up on Patient Test Results.*
   A. MACC CD
      Clinical skills/Diagnostic testing/Specimen collection & testing/Obtaining a wound specimen &and performing a rapid strep test.**

6. Perform Procedure 37-6: Collect a Specimen for CLIA-Waived Throat Culture and Rapid Strep Test.*
   A. MACC CD
      Clinical skills/Diagnostic testing/Specimen collection & testing/Obtaining a wound specimen &and performing a rapid strep test.**

7. Perform Procedure 37-7: Obtain a Urine Specimen from an Infant Using a Pediatric Urine Collector.*

8. Perform Procedure 37-8: Instruct Patient in Collection of a Midstream Clean-Catch Urine Specimen.*
   A. MACC CD
      Clinical skills/Diagnostic testing/Specimen collection & testing/Instructing how to obtain a urine specimen & performing urinalysis.

9. Perform Procedure 37-9: Instruct Patient in Collection of a 24-Hour Urine Specimen.*

10. Perform Procedure 37-10: Use a Sterile Disposable Microlancet for Skin Puncture.*
    A. MACC CD
       Clinical skills/Diagnostic testing/Specimen collection & testing/Performing a capillary puncture &spun microhematocrit.**

11. Perform Procedure 37-11: Collect a Blood Specimen for a Phenylketonuria (PKU) Screening Test.*

12. Perform Procedure 37-12: Perform Venipuncture Using the Evacuated Tube Method (Collection of Multiple Tubes).*
    A. MACC CD
       Clinical skills/Diagnostic testing/Specimen collection & testing/Performing a venipuncture using the evacuated tube method.**

13. Perform Procedure 37-13: Perform Venipuncture Using the Syringe Method.*
    A. MACC CD
       Clinical skills/Diagnostic testing/Specimen collection & testing/Performing a venipuncture using the butterfly & syringe method.**

14. Perform Procedure 37-14: Perform Venipuncture Using the Butterfly Method (Collection of Multiple Evacuated Tubes).*
    A. MACC CD
       Clinical skills/Diagnostic testing/Specimen collection & testing/Performing a venipuncture using the butterfly & syringe method.**

15. Perform Procedure 37-15: Separate Serum from Whole Blood.*

Student Name _____ **Date** _____

PROCEDURE 37-1: USE METHODS OF QUALITY CONTROL

TASK: Practice quality control procedures in the medical laboratory to ensure accuracy of test results through detection and elimination of errors.

CONDITIONS: Given the proper equipment and supplies, the student will demonstrate the proper methods of quality control.

EQUIPMENT AND SUPPLIES
- MACC CD/computer
- Quality control logbook
- Quality control samples (as provided in CLIA-waived prepackaged test kits)
- Patient sample
- Copy of CLIA 88 guidelines
- Copy of state regulation and guidelines
- Patient's medical record

STANDARDS: Complete the procedure within _____ minutes and achieve a minimum score of _____ %.

Time began _____   **Time ended** _____

Steps	Possible Points	First Attempt	Second Attempt
1. Sanitize hands.	5		
2. Assemble equipment and supplies.	5		
3. Obtain the quality control (QC) sample provided in a CLIA-waived prepackaged kit.	5		
4. Check the expiration date on the prepackaged test kit and on each QC specimen.	10		
5. Perform QC using the test kit supplied.	5		
6. Obtain the specimen from the patient, and identify the specimen as belonging to the patient.	15		
7. Perform testing of the specimen following the specific protocols outlined for the sample by the manufacturer.	20		
8. Perform QC testing as outlined by the manufacturer's protocols for the specimen being tested.	10		
9. Determine the results for both the patient's specimen and the QC sample.	10		
10. Sanitize the hands.	5		
11. Document the results in the QC logbook and the patient's medical record.	10		

Total Points Possible   100

Comments: Total Points Earned _____ Divided by _____ Total Possible Points = _____ % Score

Instructor's Signature _____

Student Name _____ **Date** _____

PROCEDURE 37-2: FOCUS THE MICROSCOPE

TASK: Focus the microscope on a prepared slide from low power to high power and oil immersion.
CONDITIONS: Given the proper equipment and supplies, the student will be required to demonstrate the proper method for focusing a microscope.

EQUIPMENT AND SUPPLIES
- MACC CD/computer
- Microscope with cover
- Lens paper
- Lens cleaner
- Specimen slide
- Soft cloth
- Tissue or gauze

STANDARDS: Complete the procedure within _____ minutes and achieve a minimum score of _____ %.

Time began _____   **Time ended** _____

Steps	Possible Points	First Attempt	Second Attempt
1. Sanitize hands.	5		
2. Assemble equipment and supplies.	5		
3. Clean the ocular and objective lenses of the microscope with lens paper and lens cleaner.	10		
4. Turn on the light source, and adjust the ocular lenses to fit your eye span.	5		
5. Place the slide on the stage and secure it in the slide clip.	10		
6. Rotate the nosepiece to the scanning objective (×4) or to the low-power objective (×10) if the scanning objective is not attached to your microscope.	10		
7. Adjust the coarse focus adjustment knob.	5		
8. Open the diaphragm to allow in the maximum amount of light.	10		
9. Focus the specimen.	5		
10. Further focus the specimen into finest detail by using the fine focus adjustment knob.	10		
11. Adjust the diaphragm and condenser to regulate and adjust the amount of light focused on the specimen to obtain the sharpest image.	10		
12. Rotate the nosepiece to high power and use fine adjustment as needed to bring specimen in focus.	10		
13. Examine the specimen by scanning the slide using the stage movement knob to move it in four directions.	10		
14. Examine the specimen as required for the procedure or test, and report the results.	10		

Steps	Possible Points	First Attempt	Second Attempt
15. Upon completion of the examination of the specimen, lower the stage or raise the objective, turn off the light, and remove the slide from the stage.	10		
16. Return objectives to highest placement and turn objective to lowest power.	10		
17. Clean the stage with lens paper or gauze.	5		
18. Once clean, cover the microscope with a dust cloth and return it to storage.	5		
19. Sanitize the hands.	5		

Total Points Possible 150

Comments: Total Points Earned _____ Divided by _____ Total Possible Points = _____ % Score

Instructor's Signature _____

Student Name _____ Date _____

PROCEDURE 37-3: COMPLETE A LABORATORY REQUISITION FORM

TASK: Accurately complete a laboratory requisition form for specimen testing.

CONDITIONS: Given the proper equipment and supplies, the student will be required to complete a laboratory requisition form.

EQUIPMENT AND SUPPLIES
- MACC CD/computer
- Physician's written order for laboratory tests
- Laboratory requisition form
- Patient's medical record
- Pen

STANDARDS: Complete the procedure within _____ minutes and achieve a minimum score of _____ %.

Time began _____   Time ended _____

Steps	Possible Points	First Attempt	Second Attempt
1. Obtain the patient's medical record, and confirm the physician's orders for laboratory test(s).	5		
2. Obtain the laboratory requisition form for the laboratory where the test will be performed; be sure the lab is acceptable for patient's insurance policy.	10		
3. Complete the section of the requisition requiring the physician's name and address.	5		
4. Complete the patient's demographic information.	5		
5. Complete the section of the requisition requiring the patient's insurance and billing information.	10		
6. Complete the desired laboratory test(s) information.	10		
7. Complete the section of the requisition requiring date and time of specimen collection.	10		
8. Enter the patient's diagnosis code on the requisition as required.	10		
9. Enter the type and amount of medication the patient is taking if appropriate for test to be performed.	10		
10. Complete the patient authorization to release and assign the benefits portion as applicable.	10		
11. Attach copy of insurance identification cards if required by lab.	5		

Steps	Possible Points	First Attempt	Second Attempt
12. Attach the laboratory requisition securely to the specimen before sending it to the laboratory.	5		
13. Document in the patient's medical record and in the laboratory logbook showing the lab where specimen was sent for testing.	5		

Total Points Possible 100

Comments: Total Points Earned _____ Divided by _____ Total Possible Points = _____ % Score

Instructor's Signature _____

Student Name _____ **Date** _____

PROCEDURE 37-4: COLLECT A SPECIMEN FOR TRANSPORT TO AN OUTSIDE LABORATORY

TASK: Collect a specimen to be sent to an outside laboratory.
CONDITIONS: Given the proper equipment and supplies, the student will be required to demonstrate the proper method of collecting a specimen for transport to an outside laboratory.

EQUIPMENT AND SUPPLIES
- MACC CD/computer
- Specimen and container
- Laboratory request form
- Patient's medical record
- Laboratory logbook
- Pen

STANDARDS: Complete the procedure within _____ minutes and achieve a minimum score of _____ %.

Time began _____   **Time ended** _____

Steps	Possible Points	First Attempt	Second Attempt
1. Be sure the patient has followed any advance preparation or special instructions necessary for test accuracy.	5		
2. Review the requirements in the laboratory directory for collection and handling of the specimen ordered by the physician.	5		
3. Complete the laboratory requisition form.	10		
4. Sanitize hands.	5		
5. Assemble equipment and supplies.	5		
6. Greet and identify the patient, and escort the patient to the examination room.	5		
7. Collect the specimen using OSHA standards. Be sure specimen has been collected according to laboratory specifications.	10		
8. Process the specimen further as required by the outside laboratory.	5		
9. Clearly label the tubes and specimen containers and prepare for transport to outside lab.	10		
10. Record information about the collection in the patient's medical record and the laboratory logbook.	10		
11. Properly handle and store the specimen, according to the laboratory's specifications.	10		
12. Remove gloves and sanitize the hands.	5		

Steps	Possible Points	First Attempt	Second Attempt
13. When the laboratory report is returned to the physician's office, screen the test results and place in location for review. Indicate abnormal results.	10		
14. File report after evaluation by proper personnel.	5		

Total Points Possible   100

Comments: Total Points Earned _____ Divided by _____ Total Possible Points = _____ % Score

Instructor's Signature _____

Student Name _____ **Date** _____

PROCEDURE 37-5: SCREEN AND FOLLOW UP ON PATIENT TEST RESULTS

TASK: Follow up with a patient who has abnormal test results.

CONDITIONS: Given the proper equipment and supplies, the student will screen and follow up with a patient's test results.

EQUIPMENT AND SUPPLIES
- MACC CD/computer
- Laboratory test results
- Tickler file (3 × 5-inch cards or computer software program) or laboratory log of patient results
- Follow-up reminder cards
- Pen
- Patient's medical record

STANDARDS: Complete the procedure within _____ minutes and achieve a minimum score of _____ %.

Time began _____   **Time ended** _____

Steps	Possible Points	First Attempt	Second Attempt
1. Review the test results as returned from the laboratory.	5		
2. Attach the laboratory report to the patient's medical record, and submit it to the physician for review.	5		
3. If the physician requests that you schedule the patient for a follow-up appointment, determine the most appropriate method of contact, using HIPAA guidelines.	10		
4. Contact the patient and schedule an appointment.	10		
Total Points Possible	30		

Comments: Total Points Earned _____ Divided by _____ Total Possible Points = _____ % Score

Instructor's Signature _____

Student Name _____ Date _____

PROCEDURE 37-6: COLLECT A SPECIMEN FOR CLIA-WAIVED THROAT CULTURE AND RAPID STREP TEST

TASK: Collect an uncontaminated throat specimen to test for group A beta-hemolytic streptococci, and perform a rapid strep test.

CONDITIONS: Given the proper equipment and supplies, the student will collect a specimen to perform a CLIA-waived throat culture and rapid strep.

EQUIPMENT AND SUPPLIES
- MACC CD/computer
- Nonsterile disposable gloves
- Sterile polyester (Dacron) swab
- Face mask
- Culture transport system
- Test tube rack
- Tongue depressor
- Gooseneck lamp
- Timer
- Biohazardous waste container
- Patient's medical record

STANDARDS: Complete the procedure within _____ minutes and achieve a minimum score of _____ %.

Time began _____   Time ended _____

Steps	Possible Points	First Attempt	Second Attempt
Specimen Collection for Throat Culture			
1. Sanitize hands.	5		
2. Assemble equipment and supplies.	5		
3. Obtain the patient's medical record.	5		
4. Greet and identify the patient, and escort the patient to the examination room.	5		
5. Instruct the patient to have a seat on the end of the examination table, and explain the procedure to the patient.	5		
6. Put on gloves and face mask.	5		
7. Prepare the culture transport system.	5		
8. Prepare the polyester (Dacron) swab.	5		
9. Visually inspect the patient's throat.	5		
10. Remove the culture transport system from the peel-apart package, being careful to prevent contamination caused by touching tip to any extraneous objects.	5		
11. Remove the Dacron swab from the paper wrapper, again being careful not to contaminate it by touching the tip.	5		
12. Place both swabs in your right hand with the tips close together, almost like one swab.	5		
13. Ask the patient to tilt the head back and open the mouth.	5		

Steps	Possible Points	First Attempt	Second Attempt
14. Use a tongue depressor to hold the tongue away from testing materials.	5		
15. Carefully insert the swabs into the patient's mouth without touching the inside of the mouth, tongue, or teeth.	10		
16. Ask the patient to say "Ahh...."	5		
17. Firmly swab the back of the throat (posterior pharynx) with a figure-eight motion between the tonsillar areas.	10		
18. Continue to hold down the tongue with the depressor, and carefully remove the swabs from the patient's mouth without touching the tongue, teeth, or inside of the cheeks.	10		
19. Discard the tongue depressor in a biohazardous waste container.	5		
20. Remove and discard the cap from the tube, and place the swab from the transport system firmly into the bottom of the tube so that it is dampened with the transport medium and secure tightly. Return the Dacron swab to the original wrapper.	10		
21. Label the transport tube and swab, with the patient's name.	10		
22. Once the specimens have been returned to their individual packaging, remove personal protective equipment (PPE) and sanitize the hands.	5		
Rapid Strep Test (Quickvue)			
23. Sanitize the hands.	5		
24. Put on PPE (if not already applied).	5		
25. Assemble equipment and supplies, being sure to have sufficient supplies for quality control.	5		
26. Unwrap each of the three cassettes that are wrapped in foil pouches.	5		
27. Record the lot number and expiration date of the kit on the log sheets.	10		
28. Label each cassette for the controls and the patient.	10		
29. Insert the swab into the swab chamber of the cassette.	5		
30. Make sure a glass ampule is inside. Break ampule.	5		
31. Shake the bottle vigorously five times to mix the solution.	5		
32. Fill the swab chamber to the rim with the extraction solution and remove the required amount.	10		
33. Set the timer for the required time, and do not move the cassette during that time.	5		
34. Examine the results window at the end of minutes. Check for positive or negative test results.	10		
35. Sanitize hands.	5		
36. Record the known controls on the quality control log sheet.	10		

Steps	Possible Points	First Attempt	Second Attempt
37. Record the results from the patient's cassette, including the internal quality assurance.	10		
38. Document the test results.	10		

Total Points Possible 250

Comments: Total Points Earned _____ Divided by _____ Total Possible Points = _____ % Score

Instructor's Signature _____

Student Name _____ Date _____

PROCEDURE 37-7: OBTAIN A URINE SPECIMEN FROM AN INFANT USING A PEDIATRIC URINE COLLECTOR

TASK: Collect an uncontaminated urine specimen from an infant.
CONDITIONS: Given the proper equipment and supplies, the student will role-play obtaining a urine specimen from an infant using a pediatric urine collector.

EQUIPMENT AND SUPPLIES
• Nonsterile disposable gloves
• Antiseptic wipes, or gauze squares and antiseptic solution
• Sterile water and sterile gauze squares
• Pediatric urine collector bag
• Sterile urine specimen container and label
• Patient's medical record

STANDARDS: Complete the procedure within _____ minutes and achieve a minimum score of _____ %.

Time began _____   Time ended _____

Steps	Possible Points	First Attempt	Second Attempt
1. Sanitize hands.	5		
2. Assemble equipment and supplies.	5		
3. Obtain the patient's medical record.	5		
4. Greet the infant's parent or guardian and identify the patient, and escort them to the examination room.	5		
5. Explain the procedure to the parent or guardian.	5		
6. Don disposable gloves.	5		
7. Position the infant in a supine position and remove diaper, asking parent or guardian to help spread the legs.	10		
8. Cleanse the child's genitalia thoroughly as with a clean-catch procedure.	10		
9. Prepare the urine collection bag by removing peel-off tab.	10		
10. Firmly attach the urine collection bag to the perineum of female and base of penis of male.	10		
11. Loosely diaper the child and, having the parent or guardian remain with the child, check the urine collection bag every 15 minutes until a urine specimen is obtained or provide instructions to parent/guardian to check for specimen and bring bag to office.	10		
12. Remove gloves and sanitize hands.	5		
13. When a sufficient volume of urine has been collected, apply new gloves and gently remove the urine collection bag.	10		
14. Clean the genital area and re-diaper the child.	10		

Steps	Possible Points	First Attempt	Second Attempt
15. Transfer the urine specimen into a sterile urine container, and tightly secure the lid.	10		
16. Label the specimen.	10		
17. Process the specimen based on the laboratory protocol.	10		
18. Remove gloves and sanitize the hands.	5		
19. Document the procedure.	10		

Total Points Possible 150

Comments: Total Points Earned _____ Divided by _____ Total Possible Points = _____ % Score

Instructor's Signature _____

Student Name _____ Date _____

PROCEDURE 37-8: INSTRUCT A PATIENT IN COLLECTION OF MIDSTREAM CLEAN-CATCH URINE SPECIMEN

TASK: Instruct a patient in the correct method for obtaining a midstream clean-catch urine specimen.

CONDITIONS: Given the proper equipment and supplies, the student will be required to demonstrate the proper method for instructing a patient in the collection of a midstream clean-catch urine specimen.

EQUIPMENT AND SUPPLIES
- MACC CD/computer
- Midstream urine collection kit OR
- Sterile specimen container with lid and three antiseptic towelettes

STANDARDS: Complete the procedure within _____ minutes and achieve a minimum score of _____ %.

Time began _____   Time ended _____

Steps	Possible Points	First Attempt	Second Attempt
1. Sanitize hands.	5		
2. Assemble equipment and supplies and verify the order.	5		
3. Greet and identify the patient, and escort the patient to the examination room.	5		
4. Label the container with the patient's name and clinic identification number.	10		
5. Instruct the patient to wash and dry his or her hands.	10		
6. Instruct the patient to loosen the top of the collection container and to not touch the inside of the container.	10		
7. Provide the patient with instructions.	5		

Total Points Possible   50

Comments: Total Points Earned _____ Divided by _____ Total Possible Points = _____ % Score

Instructor's Signature _____

Student Name _____ Date _____

PROCEDURE 37-9: INSTRUCT PATIENT IN COLLECTION OF A 24-HOUR URINE SPECIMEN

TASK: Instruct a patient in the correct method for obtaining a 24-hour urine specimen, and process the urine specimen.

CONDITIONS: Given the proper equipment and supplies, the student will be required to provide instructions to a patient in the collection of a 24-hour urine specimen.

EQUIPMENT AND SUPPLIES
• Large urine collection container
• Written instruction sheet
• Laboratory requisition
• Patient's medical record

STANDARDS: Complete the procedure within _____ minutes and achieve a minimum score of _____ %.

Time began _____   Time ended _____

Steps	Possible Points	First Attempt	Second Attempt
1. Sanitize hands.	5		
2. Assemble equipment and supplies.	5		
3. Greet and identify the patient, and escort the patient to the examination room.	5		
4. Explain the procedure to the patient, being sure patient drinks normal amounts of fluids and does not consume alcoholic beverages.	10		
5. Provide the patient with the collection container.	5		
6. Instruct the patient to empty bladder as usual on the first morning of the procedure and to collect the next specimen in a collection hat or other suitable container. Continue collecting all specimens, including the first morning specimen the second day.	30		
7. Keep the container refrigerated with lid on.	10		
8. When the patient returns the specimen, ask the patient whether he or she encountered any difficulties during the 24-hour collection process.	10		
9. Prepare the specimen for transport to the laboratory.	10		
10. Document the results.	10		

Total Points Possible   100

Comments: Total Points Earned _____ Divided by _____ Total Possible Points = _____ % Score

Instructor's Signature _____

Student Name _____ Date _____

PROCEDURE 37-10: USE A STERILE DISPOSABLE MICROLANCET FOR SKIN PUNCTURE

TASK: Obtain a capillary blood specimen acceptable for testing using the index or middle finger.

CONDITIONS: Given the proper equipment and supplies, the student will be required to use a sterile disposable microlancet for puncturing the skin to obtain a capillary sample.

EQUIPMENT AND SUPPLIES
- MACC CD/computer
- Nonsterile disposable gloves
- Alcohol wipes
- Sterile disposable microlancet with semiautomated lancet device or semiautomatic, one-use lancet system
- Sterile 2 × 2-inch gauze pads
- Sharps container
- Bandage and adhesive
- Patient's medical record

SUPPLIES FOR ORDERED TEST
Depending on the test ordered, the following supplies must be available
- Unopette
- Microhemtocrit capillary tubes
- Microcontainers
- Glass slides
- Glucometer or cholesterol device
- Clay sealant tray

STANDARDS: Complete the procedure within _____ minutes and achieve a minimum score of _____ %.

Time began _____   Time ended _____

Steps	Possible Points	First Attempt	Second Attempt
1. Sanitize hands.	5		
2. Assemble equipment and supplies, and verify order.	5		
3. Greet and identify the patient, and escort the patient to the examination room.	5		
4. Explain the procedure to the patient.	5		
5. Open the sterile gauze packet and place the gauze pad on the inside of its wrapper.	5		
6. Open the sterile lancet system.	5		
7. Position the patient comfortably either sitting or lying down with the palmer surface of the hand facing up and the arm supported.	10		
8. Select the appropriate puncture site.	10		
9. Warm the site to increase blood flow.	10		
10. Don gloves.	5		
11. Cleanse the puncture site with an alcohol wipe, and allow to air-dry.	10		

Steps	Possible Points	First Attempt	Second Attempt
12. Prepare the lancet as appropriate to perform the puncture.	5		
13. Dispose of the lancet in biohazardous sharps container.	5		
14. Wipe away the first drop of blood with dry gauze.	10		
15. If necessary, massage the finger by applying gentle, continuous pressure from the knuckles to the puncture site to increase the blood flow.	15		
16. Allow a second well-rounded drop of blood to form, and collect the specimen in the correct manner for the test ordered.	10		
17. Provide clean gauze square and apply pressure directly over the site upon completion of collection.	10		
18. Bandage the puncture site as appropriate.	10		
19. Remove the gloves and sanitize the hands before transporting the specimen to the laboratory for processing.	10		

Total Points Possible   150

Comments: Total Points Earned _____ Divided by _____ Total Possible Points = _____ % Score

Instructor's Signature _____

Student Name _____ Date _____

PROCEDURE 37-11: COLLECT A BLOOD SPECIMEN FOR A PHENYLKETONURIA (PKU) SCREENING TEST

TASK: Collect a capillary specimen for PKU screening.

CONDITIONS: Given the proper equipment and supplies, the student will be required to role-play the collection of a capillary blood specimen for PKU screening.

EQUIPMENT AND SUPPLIES
- Nonsterile disposable gloves
- Personal protective equipment (PPE)
- Sterile disposable microlancet with semiautomated lancet device or semiautomatic, one-use lancet system (lancet must be 2.4 mm in length)
- PKU test card and mailing envelope
- Alcohol wipe
- Sharps container
- Sterile 2 × 2-inch gauze pads
- Laboratory requisition form
- Patient's medical record

STANDARDS: Complete the procedure within _____ minutes and achieve a minimum score of _____ %.

Time began _____   Time ended _____

Steps	Possible Points	First Attempt	Second Attempt
1. Sanitize hands.	5		
2. Verify the order, and assemble equipment and supplies.	5		
3. Greet and identify the child and the child's parent or guardian, and escort them to the examination room.	5		
4. Explain the procedure to the parent or guardian.	5		
5. Open the sterile gauze packet and place the gauze pad on the inside of its wrapper.	5		
6. Open the sterile lancet system and assemble as needed.	5		
7. Position the child in a supine position or lying across the parent's or guardian's lap or positioned in the parent's or guardian's arms with the foot exposed.	10		
8. Don gloves.	5		
9. Select an appropriate puncture site and warm the puncture site.	10		
10. Cleanse the puncture site with an alcohol wipe, and allow to air-dry.	10		
11. Position the lancet and perform the puncture on the medial or lateral surface of heel.	10		
12. Dispose of the lancet in biohazardous sharps container.	5		
13. Wipe away the first drop of blood with the dry gauze.	10		

Steps	Possible Points	First Attempt	Second Attempt
14. Allow a second well-rounded drop of blood to form, and collect the specimen in using a microcollection container or filter paper test cards.	10		
15. After sample is collected, apply pressure with a clean gauze square directly over the puncture site. Do not place a bandage on an infant.	10		
16. Discard contaminated materials in the appropriate biohazardous waste container.	10		
17. If a PKU test card is used, complete the information section.	10		
18. Remove gloves and sanitize the hands before transporting the specimen to the laboratory for processing.	5		
19. Process the specimen for transport to lab.	5		
20. Document the procedure.	10		

Total Points Possible   150

Comments: Total Points Earned _____ Divided by _____ Total Possible Points = _____ % Score

Instructor's Signature _____

Student Name _____ Date _____

PROCEDURE 37-12: PERFORM VENIPUNCTURE USING THE EVACUATED TUBE METHOD (COLLECTION OF MULTIPLE TUBES)

TASK: Obtain a venous blood specimen acceptable for testing using the evacuated tube system.
CONDITIONS: Given the proper equipment and supplies, the student will be required to perform a venipuncture using the evacuated tube system method of collection.

EQUIPMENT AND SUPPLIES
- MACC CD/computer
- Nonsterile disposable gloves
- Personal protective equipment (PPE)
- Tourniquet
- Evacuated tube holder
- Evacuated tube multidraw needle (21 or 22 gauge, 1 or 1 1/2 inch) with safety guards
- Evacuated blood tubes for requested tests with labels (correct evacuated tube required for designated test ordered)
- Alcohol wipe
- Sterile 2 × 2-inch gauze pads
- Bandage or nonallergenic tape
- Sharps container
- Laboratory requisition form
- Patient's medical record

STANDARDS: Complete the procedure within _____ minutes and achieve a minimum score of _____ %.

Time began _____   Time ended _____

Steps	Possible Points	First Attempt	Second Attempt
1. Sanitize hands.	5		
2. Verify the order, and assemble equipment and supplies.	5		
3. Greet and identify the patient, and escort the patient to the proper room. Ask to sit in phlebotomy chair.	5		
4. Explain the procedure to the patient.	5		
5. Confirm that the patient has followed the needed preparation.	10		
6. Prepare the evacuated tube system.	5		
7. Open the sterile gauze packet and place the gauze pad on the inside of its wrapper, or obtain sterile gauze pads from a bulk package.	10		
8. Position the remaining needed supplies for ease of reaching with nondominant hand. Place tube loosely in holder with label facing downward.	10		
9. Position and examine the arm to be used in the venipuncture.	10		
10. Apply the tourniquet.	10		
11. Don gloves and PPE.	5		
12. Thoroughly palpate the selected vein.	5		
13. Release the tourniquet.	5		

Steps	Possible Points	First Attempt	Second Attempt
14. Prepare the puncture site using alcohol swabs.	10		
15. Reapply the tourniquet.	10		
16. Position the holder while keeping the needle covered, being certain to have control of holder. Uncover the needle.	10		
17. Position the needle so that it follows the line of the vein.	5		
18. Perform the venipuncture.	5		
19. Push the bottom of the tube with the thumb of you're the nondominant hand so that the needle inside the holder pierces the rubber stopper of the tube. Follow the direction of the vein.	10		
20. Change tubes (minimum of two tubes) as required by test orders.	10		
21. Gently invert tubes that contain additives to be mixed with the specimen.	10		
22. While the blood is filling the last tube, release the tourniquet and withdraw the needle. Cover the needle with the safety shield.	10		
23. Apply direct pressure on the venipuncture site, and instruct the patient to raise the arm straight above the head and maintain pressure on the site for 1 to 2 minutes.	10		
24. Discard the contaminated needle and holder into the sharps container.	10		
25. Label the tubes as appropriate for lab.	10		
26. Place the tube into the biohazard transport bag.	5		
27. Check for bleeding at puncture site and apply a pressure dressing.	5		
28. Remove and discard the alcohol wipe and gloves.	5		
29. Sanitize the hands.	5		
30. Record the collection date and time on the laboratory requisition form, and place the requisition in the proper place in the biohazard transport bag.	10		
31. Ask and observe how the patient feels. Escort to front office.	5		
32. Clean the work area using Standard Precautions.	5		
33. Document the procedure, indicating tests for which blood was drawn and the labs to which blood will be sent.	10		

Total Points Possible   250

Comments: Total Points Earned _____ Divided by _____ Total Possible Points = _____ % Score

Instructor's Signature _____

Student Name _____ **Date** _____

PROCEDURE 37-13: PERFORM VENIPUNCTURE USING THE SYRINGE METHOD

TASK: Obtain a venous blood specimen acceptable for testing using the syringe method.
CONDITIONS: Given the proper equipment and supplies, the student will be required to perform a
venipuncture using the syringe method of collection.

EQUIPMENT AND SUPPLIES
- MACC CD/computer
- Nonsterile disposable gloves
- Personal protective equipment (PPE)
- Tourniquet
- Test tube rack
- 10-cc (10-mL) syringe with 21- or 22-gauge needle and safety guards
- Proper evacuated blood tubes for tests ordered
- Alcohol wipe
- Sterile 2 × 2-inch gauze pads
- Bandage or nonallergenic tape
- Sharps container
- Laboratory requisition form
- Patient's medical record

STANDARDS: Complete the procedure within _____ minutes and achieve a minimum score of _____ %.

Time began _____   **Time ended** _____

Steps	Possible Points	First Attempt	Second Attempt
1. Sanitize hands.	5		
2. Verify the order. Assemble equipment and supplies.	5		
3. Greet and identify the patient, and escort the patient to the room for the blood draw. Position in phlebotomy chair or on exam table.	5		
4. Explain the procedure to the patient. Confirm any necessary preparation has been accomplished.	5		
5. Prepare the needle and syringe, maintaining syringe sterility. Break the seal on the syringe by moving the plunger back and forth several times. Loosen the cap on the needle and check to make sure that the hub is screwed tightly onto the syringe.	15		
6. Place the evacuated tubes to be filled in a test tube rack on a work surface in order of fill.	15		
7. Open the sterile gauze packet and place the gauze pad on the inside of its wrapper, or obtain sterile gauze pads from a bulk package.	5		
8. Position and examine the arm to be used in the venipuncture.	10		
9. Put on gloves and PPE.	5		
10. Thoroughly palpate the selected vein.	10		

Steps	Possible Points	First Attempt	Second Attempt
11. Release the tourniquet.	10		
12. Prepare the puncture site and reapply tourniquet.	10		
13. If drawing from the hand, ask the patient to make a fist or bend the fingers downward. Pull the skin taut with your thumb over the top of the patient's knuckles.	15		
14. Position the syringe and grasp the syringe firmly between the thumb and the underlying fingers.	10		
15. Follow the direction of the vein and insert the needle in one quick motion at about a 45-degree angle.	10		
16. If drawing from AC vein, with your nondominant hand pull the skin taut beneath the intended puncture site to anchor the vein. Thumb should be 1 to 2 inches below and to the side of the vein.	15		
17. Position the syringe and grasp the syringe firmly between the thumb and the underlying fingers.	10		
18. Follow the direction of the vein and insert the needle in one quick motion at about a 15-degree angle.	10		
19. Perform the venipuncture. If flash does not occur, gently pull back on the plunger. Do not move the needle. If blood still does not enter the syringe, slowly withdraw the needle, secure new supplies, and retry the draw.	10		
20. Anchor the syringe, and gently continue pulling back on the plunger until the required amount of blood is in the syringe.	10		
21. Release the tourniquet.	5		
22. Remove the needle and cover the needle with safety shield.	10		
23. Apply direct pressure on the venipuncture site, and instruct the patient to raise the arm straight above the head. Instruct the patient to maintain pressure on the site for 1 to 2 minutes.	5		
24. Transfer the blood to the evacuated tubes as soon as possible.	10		
25. Properly dispose of the syringe and needle.	10		
26. Label the tubes and place into biohazard transport bag.	10		
27. Check for bleeding at venipuncture site and place a pressure dressing.	10		
28. Remove and discard the alcohol wipe and gloves.	5		
29. Sanitize the hands.	5		
30. Record the collection date and time on the laboratory requisition form, and place the requisition in the biohazard transport bag.	10		

Steps	Possible Points	First Attempt	Second Attempt
31. Ask and observe how the patient feels. Escort to the front desk.	5		
32. Clean the work area using Standard Precautions.	5		
33. Document the procedure.	10		

Total Points Possible 255

NOTE: Awards points for Steps 13-14-15 OR 16-17-18, not both

Comments: Total Points Earned _____ Divided by _____ Total Possible Points = _____ % Score

Instructor's Signature _____

Student Name _____ Date _____

PROCEDURE 37-14: PERFORM VENIPUNCTURE USING THE BUTTERFLY METHOD (COLLECTION OF MULTIPLE EVACUATION TUBES)

TASK: Obtain a venous blood specimen acceptable for testing using the butterfly method.

CONDITIONS: Given the proper equipment and supplies, the student will perform a venipuncture using the butterfly method of collection.

EQUIPMENT AND SUPPLIES
- MACC CD/computer
- Nonsterile disposable gloves
- Personal protective equipment (PPE)
- Tourniquet
- Test tube rack
- Winged-infusion set with Luer adapter and safety guard
- Multidraw needle (22 to 25 gauge) and tube holder, or 10-cc (10-mL) syringe
- Evacuated blood tubes for requested tests with labels (correct evacuated tube required for designated test ordered)
- Alcohol wipe
- Sterile 2 × 2-inch gauze pads
- Bandage or nonallergenic tape
- Sharps container
- Laboratory requisition form
- Patient's medical record

STANDARDS: Complete the procedure within _____ minutes and achieve a minimum score of _____ %.

Time began _____   Time ended _____

Steps	Possible Points	First Attempt	Second Attempt
1. Sanitize hands.	5		
2. Verify the order. Assemble equipment and supplies.	5		
3. Greet and identify the patient, and escort the patient to the proper room for venipuncture.	5		
4. Ask the patient to have a seat in the phlebotomy chair or on exam table.	5		
5. Explain the procedure to the patient. Verify that any preparation has been followed.	10		
6. Prepare the winged infusion set. Attach the winged infusion set to either a syringe or an evacuated tube holder.	15		
7. Open the sterile gauze packet and place the gauze pad on the inside of its wrapper, or obtain sterile gauze pads from a bulk package.	5		
8. Position and examine the arm to be used in the venipuncture.	10		
9. Apply the tourniquet.	10		
10. Put on gloves and PPE.	5		
11. Thoroughly palpate the selected vein.	10		
12. Release the tourniquet.	10		
13. Prepare the puncture site and reapply the tourniquet.	5		

Steps	Possible Points	First Attempt	Second Attempt
14. If drawing from the hand, ask the patient to make a fist or bend the fingers downward. Pull the skin taut with your thumb over the top of the patient's knuckles.	10		
15. Remove the protective shield from the needle of the infusion set, being sure the bevel is facing up. Position needle over vein to be punctured.	10		
16. Perform the venipuncture. With your nondominant hand, pull the skin taut beneath the intended puncture site to anchor the vein. Thumb should be 1 to 2 inches below and to the side of the vein. Follow the direction of the vein and insert the needle in one quick motion at about a 15-degree angle.	20		
17. After penetrating the vein, decrease the angle of the needle to 5 degrees until a "flash" of blood appears in the tubing.	5		
18. Secure the needle for blood collection.	10		
19. Insert the evacuated tube into the tube holder or gently pull back on the plunger of the syringe. Change tubes as required by the test ordered.	10		
20. Release the tourniquet and remove the needle.	10		
21. Apply direct pressure on the venipuncture site, and instruct the patient to raise the arm straight above the head. Maintain pressure on the site for 1 to 2 minutes, with the arm raised straight above the head.	10		
22. If a syringe was used, transfer the blood to the evacuated tubes as soon as possible.	10		
23. Dispose of the winged infusion set.	5		
24. Label the tubes and place the tube into the biohazard transport bag.	5		
25. Check for bleeding and place a bandage over the gauze to create a pressure dressing.	5		
26. Remove and discard the alcohol wipe and gloves.	5		
27. Sanitize the hands.	5		
28. Record the collection date and time on the laboratory requisition form, and place the requisition in the biohazard transport bag.	10		
29. Ask and observe how the patient feels.	5		
30. Clean the work area using Standard Precautions.	5		
31. Document the procedure.	10		

Total Points Possible   250

Comments: Total Points Earned _____ Divided by _____ Total Possible Points = _____ % Score

Instructor's Signature _____

Student Name _____ **Date** _____

PROCEDURE 37-15: SEPARATE SERUM FROM WHOLE BLOOD

TASK: Transfer serum separated from whole blood through the process of centrifugation into a transfer tube.
CONDITIONS: Given the proper equipment and supplies, the student will transfer serum separated from whole blood through the process of centrifugation into a transfer tube.

EQUIPMENT AND SUPPLIES
• Nonsterile disposable gloves
• Personal protective equipment (PPE)
• Clotted blood specimen
• Laboratory requisition form

STANDARDS: Complete the procedure within _____ minutes and achieve a minimum score of _____ %.

Time began _____   **Time ended** _____

Steps	Possible Points	First Attempt	Second Attempt
1. Sanitize hands.	5		
2. Assemble equipment and supplies, and verify order.	5		
3. Put on gloves and other appropriate PPE.	5		
4. Verify orders against the laboratory requisition form and the specimen tube.	5		
5. Place two-stoppered red-top tubes in the centrifuge to balance the centrifuge, and close and latch the centrifuge lid securely.	10		
6. Set timer for 15 minutes.	10		
7. When the time has elapsed, allow the centrifuge to come to a complete stop before opening the lid and removing the tube.	10		
8. Properly remove the stopper or apply a transfer device.	10		
9. Separate the serum from the top of the tube into a transfer tube using the transfer device or a disposable pipette. If a red/gray (marbled), speckled, or Hemogard gold tube is used, the serum may be poured into a transfer tube.	10		
10. Label the tubes and attach the laboratory requisition form.	10		
11. Properly dispose of all waste material in the appropriate waste receptacle.	5		
12. Package the specimen for transport to the laboratory.	10		
13. Remove gloves and sanitize the hands.	5		

Total Points Possible   100

Comments: Total Points Earned _____ Divided by _____ Total Possible Points = _____ % Score

Instructor's Signature _____

CHAPTER QUIZ

Multiple Choice

Identify the letter of the choice that best completes the statement or answers the question.

1. _____ is the most common urine specimen collected.
   A. Clean catch
   B. A 24-hour
   C. Midstream
   D. Random

2. _____ is a small, sterile, needle-like piece of metal used to make a small puncture.
   A. Butterfly
   B. Lancet
   C. Syringe
   D. Vacutainer

3. A level of CLIA tests is _____.
   A. low complexity
   B. medium complexity
   C. middle complexity
   D. waived

4. Venipuncture is performed with a sterile _____-gauge needle to obtain a large venous specimen for diagnostic testing.
   A. 15- to 20
   B. 18- to 20
   C. 18- to 22
   D. 20- to 25

5. The scanning lens on a binocular microscope is _____ power.
   A. ×4
   B. ×10
   C. ×40
   D. ×100

6. The centrifuge is a piece of equipment that separates solid material from liquid through centrifugal force.
   A. True
   B. False

7. Urine must be processed _____ or refrigeration is required to maintain a quality specimen.
   A. immediately
   B. within 30 minutes
   C. within 1 hour
   D. within 2 hours

8. _____ tests assess the formed elements of whole blood.
   A. Chemistry
   B. Hematology
   C. Microbiology
   D. Serology

9. Cultures being transported in swab-transport media system should be processed within _____ hours.
   A. 8
   B. 10
   C. 12
   D. 24

10. If a wound is deep, an aerobic culture kit may be used.
    A. True
    B. False

11. A _____ requires the patient to follow a strict cleaning procedure.
    A. first-morning specimen
    B. midstream clean-catch specimen
    C. random specimen
    D. timed specimen

12. A 24-hour urine specimen _____.
    A. tests for glucose
    B. tests for drugs
    C. tests kidney function
    D. all of the above

13. _____ is used when a small amount of blood is needed.
    A. Butterfly
    B. Capillary
    C. Syringe
    D. Venipuncture

14. When doing a venipuncture, the needle should be _____ gauge.
    A. 15 to 18
    B. 18 to 22
    C. 22 to 24
    d 24 to 26

15. A _____-top tube is used for a CBC.
    A. red
    B. green
    C. lavender
    D. gold

16. The _____ method is used on small, fragile veins.
    A. butterfly
    B. lancet
    C. venipuncture
    D. syringe

17. The _____ method of blood drawing is the most comfortable for the patient.
    A. butterfly
    B. capillary
    C. venipuncture
    D. syringe

18. If serum is required for a test, it will be drawn in a _____-top tube
    A. red/gray marbled
    B. purple
    C. green
    D. light blue

19. Serum is transferred to the proper transport system by _____.
    A. pouring it into the transport container
    B. pipetting it into the transport container
    C. not putting it into the transport container
    D. None of the above

20. A certificate of waiver is issued to a physician office laboratory qualified to perform only medium-complexity tests.
    A. True
    B. False

CHAPTER THIRTY-EIGHT

Laboratory Testing in the Physician Office

VOCABULARY REVIEW

Matching

Match each term with the correct definition.

A. 2-hour postprandial test

B. acetone

C. agar

D. automated urine analyzer

E. bilirubin

F. bilirubinuria

G. C&S

H. casts

I. chemistry profile

J. complete blood count

K. crenated

L. culture plate

M. diaphoresis

N. EDTA

O. enzyme immunoassay

P. fatty cast

_____ 1. To inoculate or put specimen onto a culture plate in an established pattern

_____ 2. Hyaline cast with fatty cells

_____ 3. Chemical formed when fats are metabolized rather than glucose

_____ 4. Excessive sweating

_____ 5. Fat deposits on the inside wall of an artery

_____ 6. Opening in a vessel, intestines, or tube

_____ 7. Byproduct of hemoglobin breakdown; orange-yellow pigment of bile

_____ 8. Pregnancy test that uses a color change reaction

_____ 9. Hemoglobin A1; test that measures the amount of glucose attached to hemoglobin over a 3-month period

_____ 10. Amount of a substance able to be measured; actual amounts

_____ 11. Hardened protein material shaped like the lumen of the kidney tubule and washed out by urine

Q. galactosemia

R. glucose reagent strip

S. glycosylated hemoglobin

T. Gram stain

U. HDL

V. hemoglobinuria

W. hemolyzed

X. hyaline cast

Y. ketonuria

Z. lumen

AA. myoglobinuria

BB. plaque

CC. precipitates

DD. quantitative

EE. reagent strip

FF. renal epithelial cells

GG. serum cholesterol

HH. streak

II. total cholesterol

JJ. turbid

KK. urochrome

LL. Westergren method

_____ 12. Shrunken; formation of notches on the edges of red blood cells

_____ 13. High-density lipoprotein; "good" cholesterol

_____ 14. Epithelial cells released by the kidney indicating disease

_____ 15. Blood test that details the chemical composition of the blood

_____ 16. Method to measure ESR using a self-zeroing tube calibrated from 0 to 200

_____ 17. Damaged, burst cells; hemolyzed red blood cells are colorless and cannot be seen under magnification

_____ 18. Test measuring a patient's ability to metabolize food 2 hours after a meal

_____ 19. Globin from damaged muscle cells in the urine

_____ 20. Yellow pigment derived from urobilin that is left over when hemoglobin breaks down during red blood cell destruction

_____ 21. Equipment that uses light photometry to analyze a reagent test strip

_____ 22. Chemical pad on a dipstick that tests for the presence of sugar

_____ 23. White, fatlike substance made in the liver

_____ 24. Seaweed extract used to make media solid for bacterial cultures

_____ 25. Total count of each blood element

_____ 26. Common casts found in urine that are pale and transparent; appear in unchecked hypertension

_____ 27. Combined measurement of LDL and HDL cholesterol

_____ 28. Culture and sensitivity; test to determine which antibiotic is most effective against cultured organisms

_____ 29. Tablet that reacts to a specific substance, confirming its presence

_____ 30. Presence of ketones in the urine

_____ 31. Covered container with nutritional substances that support growth of bacteria

_____ 32. Red blood cell component that carries oxygen and gives blood its color

_____ 33. Not clear or transparent; particles floating within; cloudy

_____ 34. Appearance of bilirubin in the urine

_____ 35. Staining method used to identify the shape and pattern of microorganisms

_____ 36. Particles in a solution brought on by a chemical reaction

_____ 37. Galactose in the blood

_____ 38. Anticoagulant used for preserving blood for hematology studies

THEORY RECALL

True/False

Indicate whether the sentence or statement is true or false.

_____ 1. Cholesterol is only metabolized from foods that are eaten and is not produced by the body.

_____ 2. RBCs are larger than WBCs.

_____ 3. A hematocit reading can be performed with venous or capillary blood.

_____ 4. LDL is considered "good" cholesterol.

_____ 5. Finding casts in urine is not of any importance.

Multiple Choice

Identify the letter of the choice that best completes the statement or answers the question.

1. A patient must fast at least _____ hours to perform a fasting blood sugar test.
   A. 2
   B. 8
   C. 12
   D. 24

2. Gram staining separates bacteria into _____ groups.
   A. two
   B. three
   C. four
   D. five

3. Throat cultures are usually cultured on which one of the following?
   A. Blood agar
   B. Seaweed broth
   C. Chocolate agar
   D. None of the above

4. Colors that can describe normal urine are _____.
   A. brown
   B. red
   C. light straw
   D. green

5. _____ is(are) a waste product of fat metabolism.
   A. Bilirubin
   B. Ketones
   C. Glucose
   D. Nitrates

6. hGC levels are detectable as early as _____ days after fertilization.
   A. 2
   B. 5
   C. 10
   D. 14

7. _____ carry oxygen to the body.
   A. Leukocytes
   B. Platelets
   C. RBCs
   D. WBCs

8. When performing a Wintrobe ESR, the sample must sit in the sedimentation rack for _____ to obtain a valid reading.
   A. 30 minutes
   B. 45 minutes
   C. 1 hour
   D. 1½ hours

9. The chemical pad for blood on the reagent strip will react to _____.
   A. intact RBCs
   B. hemoglobin
   C. myoglobin
   D. All of the above

10. Bilirubin appearing in urine is a clear sign of liver and biliary tract dysfunction.
    A. True
    B. False

11. Normal 24-hour adult urine volume output is _____ mL.
    A. 500 to 750
    B. 750 to 2000
    C. 1000 to 2000
    D. 1500 to 2500

12. Proteinuria is an indication of all of the following EXCEPT_____.
    A. congestive heart failure
    B. heavy exercising
    C. UTI
    D. stroke

13. You would count _____ white blood cells when performing a differential blood cell count.
    A. 50
    B. 100
    C. 125
    D. 150

14. Normal range for urine specific gravity is _____.
    A. 1.00 to 1.125
    B. 1.01 to 1.020
    C. 1.01 to 1.025
    D. 1.01 to 1.015

15. The life of an RBC is _____ days.
    A. 80
    B. 100
    C. 110
    D. 120

16. Examination of a urine slide first takes place under _____ power.
    A. ×10
    B. ×20
    C. ×40
    D. ×100

17. _____ casts have a saw-tooth edge.
    A. Fatty
    B. Granular
    C. Hyaline
    D. Waxy

18. Emotional stress may present itself as _____ in the urine.
    A. fat
    B. glucose
    C. protein
    D. nitrates

19. _____ is the study of microorganisms, especially pathogenic organisms.
    A. Bacteriology
    B. Cytology
    C. Microbiology
    D. Pathology

20. _____ is(are) the end product of nitrate metabolism.
   A. Acetone
   B. Bacteria
   C. Nitrites
   D. Squamous epithelial cells

Sentence Completion

Complete each sentence or statement.

1. A(n) _____ is used to screen for diabetes mellitus and to monitor the effects of a

   patient's insulin regimen

2. Cultured microorganism must grow in an incubator for _____ hours.

3. _____ is the presence of intact RBCs in the urine.

4. _____ found in large numbers is an indication of kidney problems.

5. Rod-shaped organisms found in urine are known as _____.

6. Powder, fibers, and hair are known as _____ in urine.

7. _____ is(are) formed in bone marrow and in lymphoid tissue.

8. _____ involve(s) a test done in the physician office for immediate feedback.

9. _____ is the destruction of RBCs caused by an antibody-antigen response.

10. _____ are oval shaped, vary in size, and have small buds.

Short Answers

1. List five factors that can affect the quality of blood smear.

_____

_____

_____

2. List 10 tests routinely done during a urinalysis.

_____

_____

_____

_____

_____

3. Explain the purpose of a hemoglobin measurement.

_____

_____

_____

4. Explain the purpose and procedure of a glucose tolerance test.

_____

_____

_____

_____

CRITICAL THINKING

Ann is a new employee at Dr Paul's practice. In observing her trainer she discovers that this office does not perform all of the diagnostics tests that her last employer did. What might cause this difference, and how is it determined which office performs what tests?

INTERNET RESEARCH

Keyword: Point-of-Care Tests

Choose the topic above or one type of POC test to research. Cite your source. Be prepared to give a 2-minute oral presentation should your instructor assign you to do so.

WHAT WOULD YOU DO?

If you have accomplished the objectives in this chapter, you will be able to make better choices as a medical assistant. Take a look at this situation and decide what you would do.

Dr. Carlson does not have a medical lab technician. Instead, she depends on the medical assistant to provide the test results of lab specimens that are ordered. Because of his training in a medical assisting program, Jerry is aware of the importance of quality control and quality assurance and that both should be done on a daily basis.

As part of the daily routine, Jerry, the medical assistant, is expected to perform physical and chemical testing of urine using reagent strips. Dr. Carlson also allows Jerry to examine specimens using a microscope to identify the urine sediment. Jerry completes hemoglobin testing using HemoCue and uses a centrifuge to spin hematocrits. As Jerry reads the hematocrit, he finds that the anticoagulated blood has separated into three layers, each of which has a specific characteristic. Because CLIA-waived tests are often performed in a physician's office, Jerry and other medical assistants must be able to perform these tests on a daily basis.

Would you be capable of performing these tasks?

1. **What is meant by a "CLIA-waived" test?**

   _____

   _____

2. **What do reagent strips show? Are all reagent strips the same?**

   _____

   _____

   _____

3. **Why is it important for Jerry to wait for the designated amount of time before reading the results of a reagent strip?**

   _____

   _____

   _____

4. **When checking a urine specimen for physical properties, what is Jerry looking for?**

   _____

   _____

   _____

5. What influences the physical properties of urine?

_____

_____

_____

_____

6. Can Jerry perform a microscopic examination of urine under CLIA standards? If not, what part of the microscopic examination can he perform?

_____

_____

_____

_____

7. What type of pregnancy tests can Jerry perform in the physician's office? What are the indications of a positive pregnancy test in each test?

_____

_____

_____

_____

8. When should a urine specimen be collected for a pregnancy test?

_____

_____

_____

9. Can Jerry perform hemoglobin and hematocrit measurements? Why or why not?

_____

_____

_____

10. **What are the three layers found in centrifuged whole blood? How are these used to measure a microhematocrit?**

_____

_____

_____

_____

_____

APPLICATION OF SKILLS

Procedure Check-off Sheets (*) and Assignments from MACC CD (see Procedure Check-off Sheets for which procedure from the MACC CD to perform).

1. Perform Procedure 38-1: Urinalysis Using Reagent Strips.*

2. Perform Procedure 38-2: Prepare a Urine Specimen for Microscopic Examination.*

3. Perform Procedure 38-3: Perform a Urine Pregnancy Test.*

4. Perform Procedure 38-4: Determine a Hemoglobin Measurement Using a HemoCue.*

5. Perform Procedure 38-5: Perform a Microhematocrit Test.*

6. Perform Procedure 38-6: Determine Erythrocyte Sedimentation Rate (ESR, Non-Automated) Using the Westergren Method.*

7. Perform Procedure 38-7: Prepare a Blood Smear.*

8. Perform Procedure 38-8: Perform Cholesterol Testing.*

9. Perform Procedure 38-9: Perform Glucose Testing.*

10. Perform Procedure 38-10: Obtain a Bacterial Smear from a Wound Specimen.*

Student Name _____ Date _____

PROCEDURE 38-1: URINALYSIS USING REAGENT STRIPS

TASK: Observe, record, and report the physical and chemical properties of a urine sample using Mulitstix 10-SG.

CONDITIONS: Given the proper equipment and supplies, the student will perform a urinalysis using reagent strips.

NOTE: The student should practice the procedure using the MACC CD in the back of the textbook and then practice and perform the task in the classroom. MACC CD MACC/Clinical skills/Diagnostic testing/Specimen collection & testing/Instructing how to obtain a urine specimen & performing urinalysis.

EQUIPMENT AND SUPPLIES
- MACC CD/computer
- Nonsterile disposable gloves
- Personal protective equipment (PPE)
- Multistix 10-SG reagent strips
- Normal and abnormal quality control reagent strips
- Laboratory report form
- Quality control logsheet
- Urine specimen container
- Conical urine centrifuge tubes
- Digital timer or watch with second hand
- Paper towel
- 10% Bleach solution
- Biohazardous waste container
- Patient's medical record
- Laboratory log

STANDARDS: Complete the procedure within _____ minutes and achieve a minimum score of _____ %.

Time began _____   Time ended _____

Steps	Possible Points	First Attempt	Second Attempt
1. Sanitize hands.	5		
2. Verify the order. Assemble equipment and supplies.	5		
3. Greet and identify the patient, and escort the patient to the examination room or laboratory area. Explain the procedure to the patient.	5		
4. Ask the patient to collect a midstream clean-catch urine specimen.	10		
5. Apply gloves and other PPE as indicated.	5		
6. While waiting for the patient to collect the specimen, record the lot number and expiration date of Multistik 10-SG on the laboratory quality control log sheet.	5		
7. Place controls from the manufacturer's container into the urine centrifuge tubes and record the lot number and expiration date on the tubes if the first samples of the day.	10		

Steps	Possible Points	First Attempt	Second Attempt
8. Observe and record the physical properties of the control samples as appropriate.	10		
9. Remove one strip from container. Recap the bottle immediately.	5		
10. Dip the strip in the abnormal control specimen and draw it out, pulling along the edge of the tube top to remove excess urine.	5		
11. Read each test on the strip after the manufacturer's recommended time has elapsed.	5		
12. Check the second hand on a watch to read the results after the recommended time has elapsed.	5		
13. Once the reagent strip has been interpreted and documented on the log sheet, discard the reagent strip in the biohazardous waste container.	5		
14. Repeat the process for the normal control specimen.	10		
15. Check controls to be sure recommended ranges have been achieved.	10		
16. After the reagent strip has been read interpreted and documented on the log sheet, discard the reagent strip in the biohazardous waste container.	10		
17. Prepare the patient specimen for testing.	5		
18. Perform steps 9 through 16 on the patient sample and record the result on the laboratory report form.	10		
19. Clean and disinfect the work area with a 10% bleach solution.	5		
20. Remove gloves and dispose of in a biohazardous waste container.	10		
21. Sanitize the hands.	10		
22. Document the results and provide to the physician.	10		
23. Document the procedure.	10		
24. After the physician has reviewed the results, place the laboratory report form if applicable in the patient's medical record.	5		

Total Points Possible   175

Comments: Total Points Earned _____ Divided by _____ Total Possible Points = _____ % Score

Instructor's Signature _____

Student Name _____ Date _____

PROCEDURE 38-2: PREPARE A URINE SPECIMEN FOR MICROSCOPIC EXAMINATION

TASK: Prepare a urine sample for examination using a microscope.

CONDITIONS: Given the proper equipment and supplies, the student will prepare a urine specimen for microscopic examination.

NOTE: The student should practice the procedure using the MACC CD in the back of the textbook and then practice and perform the task in the classroom: MACC CD MACC/Clinical skills/Diagnostic testing/Specimen collection & testing/Preparing urine sediment and using the microscope.

EQUIPMENT AND SUPPLIES
- MACC CD/computer
- Nonsterile disposable gloves
- Personal protective equipment (PPE)
- Urine specimen container
- Comical urine centrifuge tubes with caps
- Disposable pipette
- Microscope slide and coverslip
- Centrifuge
- Paper towel
- Biohazardous waste container
- Laboratory logbook

NOTE: Perform Procedure 37-8 and then Procedure 38-1 in preparation for a microscopic urinalysis.

STANDARDS: Complete the procedure within _____ minutes and achieve a minimum score of _____ %.

Time began _____   Time ended _____

Steps	Possible Points	First Attempt	Second Attempt
1. Sanitize the hands.	5		
2. Assemble equipment and supplies, and verify the order.	5		
3. Put on gloves and other PPE as indicated.	5		
4. Prepare a urine sediment sample by centrifuging. Properly fill tube and centrifuge prior to starting centrifuge.	10		
5. When the centrifuge stops, remove the cap from the specimen and discard it in the biohazardous waste container. Decant the supernatant fluid.	10		
6. Mix sediment with remaining urine in the bottom of the tube.	10		
7. Place a microscope slide on a paper towel, and pipette a drop of the mixed urine sediment in the center of the slide. Place coverslip on slide.	10		
8. Mount the slide on the microscope stage and adjust the coarse focus.	10		
9. Remove gloves and dispose of in a biohazardous waste container.	5		
10. Sanitize the hands.	5		

Steps	Possible Points	First Attempt	Second Attempt
11. Inform the physician that the slide is ready for viewing.	10		
12. Record the results in the laboratory logbook and medical record as reported by the physician and as office policy.	15		

Total Points Possible   100

Comments: Total Points Earned _____ Divided by _____ Total Possible Points = _____ % Score

Instructor's Signature _____

Student Name _____ Date _____

PROCEDURE 38-3: PERFORM A URINE PREGNANCY TEST

TASK: Perform a urine pregnancy test using a commercially prepared CLIA-waived test (Quick Vue).
CONDITIONS: Given the proper equipment and supplies, the student will be required to properly
perform a urine pregnancy test.

EQUIPMENT AND SUPPLIES
- Nonsterile disposable gloves
- Personal protective equipment (PPE)
- Urine specimen (preferably first morning specimen)
- Urine pregnancy testing kit (Quick Vue)
- Biohazardous waste container
- Laboratory logbook
- Patient's medical record

STANDARDS: Complete the procedure within _____ minutes and achieve a minimum score of _____ %.

Time began _____   **Time ended** _____

Steps	Possible Points	First Attempt	Second Attempt
1. Sanitize hands.	5		
2. Verify the order. Assemble equipment and supplies.	5		
3. Perform the quality control test as recommended by the manufacturer and document results in the laboratory log book.	10		
4. Greet and identify the patient, and escort the patient to the examination room.	5		
5. If a urine specimen is to be collected in the office, explain the procedure to the patient.	10		
6. Provide the patient with the collection container and instructions as needed.	5		
7. Put on gloves and other PPE as indicated.	5		
8. Obtain a pregnancy test and prepare for testing according to manufacturer's directions.	5		
9. Time the test according to manufacturer's direction.	15		
10. Interpret the test results, and dispose of the test cassette in a biohazardous waste container.	10		
11 Remove gloves and dispose of in a biohazardous waste container.	10		
12. Sanitize the hands.	5		
13. Document the results in the patient's medical record and the laboratory logbook.	10		

Total Points Possible   100

Comments: Total Points Earned _____ Divided by _____ Total Possible Points = _____ % Score

Instructor's Signature _____

Student Name _____ **Date** _____

PROCEDURE 38-4: DETERMINE A HEMOGLOBIN MEASUREMENT USING A HEMOCUE

TASK: Accurately measure the hemoglobin using a HemoCue analyzer.

CONDITIONS: Given the proper equipment and supplies, the student will determine a hemoglobin measurement using a HemoCue analyzer.

EQUIPMENT AND SUPPLIES
- Nonsterile disposable gloves
- Personal protective equipment (PPE)
- Alcohol wipes
- Sterile disposable microlancet
- Sterile 2 × 2-inch gauze squares
- HemoCue Analyzer
- Control cuvette—normal and abnormal
- Microcuvettes
- 10% Bleach solution
- Sharps container
- Biohazardous waste container
- Patient's medical record
- Laboratory quality control logsheet

STANDARDS: Complete the procedure within _____ minutes and achieve a minimum score of _____ %.

Time began _____   **Time ended** _____

Steps	Possible Points	First Attempt	Second Attempt
1. Sanitize hands.	5		
2. Verify the order, and assemble equipment and supplies.	5		
3. Perform the quality control test as recommended by the manufacturer and document in the laboratory quality control log sheet if first test of the day or new container of microcassettes.	10		
4. Prepare the HemoCue analyzers for testing.	5		
5. Place the control cuvette into the holder and push into the photometer to validate the control values. Perform testing using controls and read and record results.	10		
6. Greet and identify the patient, and escort the patient to the examination room.	10		
7. Explain the procedure to the patient.	5		
8. Sanitize the hands and apply gloves and PPE as indicated.	10		
9. Perform capillary puncture and dispose of the lancet in a sharps container. Wipe away the first drop of blood with a gauze pad.	10		
10. Collect the specimen.	15		
11. Wipe away excess blood from the tip of the cuvette.	10		

Steps	Possible Points	First Attempt	Second Attempt
12. Place the cuvette in its holder and push into the photometer.	10		
13. Read and record the hemoglobin value from LED screen.	10		
14. Discard the cuvette into the rigid biohazardous container.	5		
15. Turn the equipment "off" as appropriate. Clean the equipment with a mild soap and water.	10		
16. Disinfect the work area with 10% bleach solution.	10		
17. Remove gloves and sanitize the hands.	5		
18. Document the results in the patient's medical record and the laboratory logbook.	5		

Total Points Possible   150

Comments: Total Points Earned _____ Divided by _____ Total Possible Points = _____ % Score

Instructor's Signature _____

Student Name _____   **Date** _____

PROCEDURE 38-5: PERFORM A MICROHEMATOCRIT TEST

TASK: Collect a capillary blood sample for performing a microhematocrit.

CONDITIONS: Given the proper equipment and supplies, the student will perform a microhematocrit.

NOTE: The student should practice the procedure using the MACC CD in the back of the textbook and then practice and perform the task in the classroom: MACC CD MACC/Clinical skills/Diagnostic testing/Specimen collection & testing/Performing a capillary puncture & spun microhematocrit.

EQUIPMENT AND SUPPLIES
- MACC CD/computer
- Nonsterile disposable gloves
- Personal protective equipment (PPE), as indicated
- Microhematocrit capillary tubes (heparinized)
- Sealing compound
- Alcohol wipe
- Sterile disposable microlancet
- Sterile 2 × 2-inch gauze squares
- 10% Bleach solution
- Microhematocrit centrifuge or centrifuge with microhematocrit reading
- Microhematocrit reader
- Rigid biohazardous container
- Patient's medical record
- Laboratory logbook

STANDARDS: Complete the procedure within _____ minutes and achieve a minimum score of _____ %.

Time began _____   **Time ended** _____

Steps	Possible Points	First Attempt	Second Attempt
1. Sanitize hands.	5		
2. Verify the order, and assemble equipment and supplies.	5		
3. Greet and identify the patient, escort the patient to the examination room or laboratory, and explain the procedure to the patient.	5		
4. Put on gloves and PPE as indicated.	5		
Collecting the Specimen			
5. Perform a capillary puncture and dispose of the lancet in a ridged biohazardous container.	10		
6. Wipe away the first drop of blood with a gauze pad.	5		
7. After the samples have been collected, instruct the patient to press a clean gauze square to provide direct pressure to the puncture site.	5		
8. Seal the dry end of the capillary tubes with sealing clay.	10		
9. Leave the capillary tubes embedded in the sealing clay to prevent damage.	10		

Steps	Possible Points	First Attempt	Second Attempt
10. Check the puncture site.	5		
11. Remove gloves, and sanitize hands.	10		
Testing the Specimen			
12. Place the specimen in the centrifuge after donning gloves. Be sure to keep centrifuge balanced. The sealed end should be placed toward the outer edge. Record placement to prevent errors in identifying specimens.	10		
13. Secure the locking top by placing it over the threaded bolt on the centrifuge head and turning the fastener until tight.	5		
14. Spin for 5 minutes at 2500 rpm or use the high setting. If required by centrifuge being used, lock the high speed.	10		
15. When the centrifuge comes to a complete stop, unlatch the lid, and remove the locking top if appropriate.	10		
16. Position one of the tubes in the microhematocrit reader and adjust as necessary for reading the results.	10		
17. Determine the results of spun microhematocrit.	15		
18. Record the microhematocrit results.	10		
19. Discard the capillary tube in a rigid biohazardous container.	5		
20. Repeat the reading for the second capillary tube.	10		
21. Average the two results, and record the average value as the reading for the patient.	15		
22. Disinfect the work area with 10% bleach solution.	10		
23. Remove gloves and sanitize hands.	5		
24. Document the results in the patient's medical record.	10		

Total Points Possible   200

Comments: Total Points Earned _____ Divided by _____ Total Possible Points = _____ % Score

Instructor's Signature _____

Student Name _____ Date _____

PROCEDURE 38-6: DETERMINE ERYTHROCYTE SEDIMENTATION RATE (ESR, NON-AUTOMATED) USING THE WESTERGREN METHOD

TASK: Properly fill a Westergren tube and observe and report ESR results accurately.

CONDITIONS: Given the proper equipment and supplies, the student will be required to fill a Westergren tube and accurately report the results of a Westergren ESR.

EQUIPMENT AND SUPPLIES
- Nonsterile disposable gloves
- Personal protection equipment (PPE) as indicated
- Supplies to perform venipuncture
- EDTA-anticoagulated blood specimen (lavender-top tube)
- Sed-Pac ESR system (reservoir, diluents, Dispette tube) with rack
- Transfer pipette
- Timer
- 10% bleach solution
- Biohazardous waste container
- Patient's medical record
- Laboratory logbook

STANDARDS: Complete the procedure within _____ minutes and achieve a minimum score of _____ %.

Time began _____   Time ended _____

Steps	Possible Points	First Attempt	Second Attempt
1. Sanitize hands.	5		
2. Verify the order, and assemble equipment and supplies.	10		
3. Explain the procedure to the patient.	10		
4. Apply gloves and PPE as appropriate.	10		
5. Perform a venipuncture.	10		
6. Transport the specimen to laboratory.	5		
7. Transfer the specimen.	5		
8. Insert the Dispette tube into the reservoir, and push down until the tube touches the bottom of the reservoir. The Dispette tube will autozero the blood and any excess will flow into the closed reservoir compartment.	10		
9. Place ESR tube in a rack, making certain it remains vertical.	10		
10. Set the timer for 1 hour.	10		
11. Read the results.	10		
12. Properly dispose of the ESR tube in a rigid biohazardous container.	10		
13. Disinfect the work area with 10% bleach solution.	5		

Steps	Possible Points	First Attempt	Second Attempt
14. Remove gloves and sanitize the hands.	5		
15. Document the results in the patient's medical record and the laboratory logbook.	10		
Total Points Possible	125		

Comments: Total Points Earned _____ Divided by _____ Total Possible Points = _____ % Score

Instructor's Signature _____

Student Name _____ Date _____

PROCEDURE 38-7: PREPARE A BLOOD SMEAR

TASK: Prepare a blood smear.
CONDITIONS: Given the proper equipment and supplies, the student will prepare a blood smear.

EQUIPMENT AND SUPPLIES
- Nonsterile disposable gloves
- Personal protective equipment (PPE)
- Supplies to perform capillary puncture or venipuncture
- Glass slides (frosted end)
- Pipette or Diff-Safe
- Slide holder
- Pencil
- Sharps container

STANDARDS: Complete the procedure within _____ minutes and achieve a minimum score of _____ %.

Time began _____   **Time ended** _____

Steps	Possible Points	First Attempt	Second Attempt
1. Sanitize hands.	5		
2. Verify the order, and assemble equipment and supplies.	5		
3. Greet and identify the patient, escort the patient to the examination room or lab, and explain the procedure to the patient.	5		
4. Apply gloves and PPE as appropriate.	5		
5. Label two slides on the frosted end, using a pencil, with the patient's name and the date.	10		
6. Perform a venipuncture or capillary puncture.	10		
7. Place a well-rounded medium-sized drop (1 to 2 mm) of fresh whole blood on each slide.	10		
8. Pull back the drop of blood.	10		
9. Spread forward the drop of blood.	10		
10. Evaluate the slide.	10		
11. Repeat Steps 9 through 11 for the second glass slide.	10		
12. Allow both slides to air-dry standing at an angle, with the frosted end of the slide or blood end down.	10		
13. Dispose of the spreader slide in a sharps container; dispose of all other contaminated or regular waste appropriately.	5		
14. Once the slides are completely dry (a minimum of 20 minutes), both slides can be placed in slide holders and transported to the laboratory.	5		

Steps	Possible Points	First Attempt	Second Attempt
15. Disinfect the work area using 10% bleach solution.	5		
16. Remove gloves and sanitize the hands.	5		

Total Points Possible 120

Comments: Total Points Earned _____ Divided by _____ Total Possible Points = _____ % Score

Instructor's Signature _____

Student Name _____ **Date** _____

PROCEDURE 38-8: PERFORM CHOLESTEROL TESTING

TASK: Collect and process a blood specimen accurately for cholesterol testing using a CLIA-waived test such as Cholestech LDX.

CONDITIONS: Given the proper equipment and supplies, the student will perform a cholesterol test.

EQUIPMENT AND SUPPLIES
- Nonsterile disposable gloves
- Personal protective equipment (PPE) as indicated
- Capillary puncture supplies
- Cholesterol testing device (Cholestech LDX)
- Cholesterol testing kit (capillary tube with plunger, test cassette)
- 10% Bleach solution
- Sharps container
- Biohazardous waste container
- Quality control logsheet
- Patient's medical record
- Laboratory logbook

STANDARDS: Complete the procedure within _____ minutes and achieve a minimum score of _____ %.

Time began _____   **Time ended** _____

Steps	Possible Points	First Attempt	Second Attempt
1. Sanitize hands.	5		
2. Verify the order, and assemble equipment and supplies.	5		
3. Prepare the test supplies and analyzer.	5		
4. Perform a quality control test as recommended by the manufacturer, and document in the laboratory quality control logsheet.	10		
5. Greet and identify the patient, escort the patient to the examination room or lab, and explain the procedure to the patient.	5		
6. Apply gloves and PPE as indicated.	5		
7. Perform the capillary puncture.	10		
8. Put on disposable gloves. Wipe away the first drop of blood.	5		
9. Collect blood specimen in a capillary tube.	10		
10. Prepare the specimen as necessary for testing.	5		
11. Insert the cassette into the Cholestech LDX analyzer and activate the timer.	10		
12 When the timer stops, read the results.	10		
13. Discard the cassette, capillary tube, and plunger into a rigid biohazardous container.	5		
14. Turn off the analyzer and wipe with a damp cloth.	5		
15. Disinfect the work area using 10% bleach solution.	10		

Steps	Possible Points	First Attempt	Second Attempt
16. Remove gloves and sanitize hands.	5		
17. Document results.	10		

Total Points Possible   125

Comments: Total Points Earned _____ Divided by _____ Total Possible Points = _____ % Score

Instructor's Signature _____

Student Name _____ Date _____

PROCEDURE 38-9: PERFORM GLUCOSE TESTING

TASK: Collect and process a blood specimen for glucose testing using AccuCheck.

CONDITIONS: Given the proper equipment and supplies, the student will perform a glucose test.

NOTE: The student should practice the procedure using the MACC CD in the back of the textbook and then practice and perform the task in the classroom: MACC CD MACC/Clinical skills/Diagnostic testing/Specimen collection & testing/Performing glucose testing using AccuCheck.

EQUIPMENT AND SUPPLIES
- MACC CD/computer
- Nonsterile disposable gloves
- Personal protection equipments (PPE), as indicated
- Supplies for capillary puncture
- Glucose testing equipment (AccuCheck)
- AccuCheck supplies
- Control test solution
- 10% Bleach solution
- Sharps container
- Biohazardous waste container
- Patient's medical records
- Laboratory quality control logsheet
- Laboratory logbook

STANDARDS: Complete the procedure within _____ minutes and achieve a minimum score of _____%.

Time began _____   Time ended _____

Steps	Possible Points	First Attempt	Second Attempt
1. Sanitize hands.	5		
2. Verify the order, and assemble equipment and supplies.	5		
3. Prepare the analyzer according to the manufacture's instructions.	5		
4. Perform a quality control test as recommended by the manufacturer, and document in the laboratory quality control logsheet.	10		
5. Greet and identify the patient, and escort the patient to the examination room or laboratory. Explain the procedure to the patient. Determine when last food was ingested.	10		
6. Perform a capillary puncture.	10		
7. Insert a test strip into the test strip slot.	10		
8. Apply a rounded drop of blood from the capillary puncture to the test strip. Start the timer for testing.	10		
9. Discard the test strip into the biohazardous container.	5		
10. Turn off the glucometer and wipe it with a damp cloth	10		

Copyright © 2005 by Elsevier Inc.

Steps	Possible Points	First Attempt	Second Attempt
11. Disinfect the work area using 10% bleach solution.	5		
12. Remove gloves and sanitize the hands.	5		
13. Document the results in the patient's medical record and the laboratory logbook.	10		
Total Points Possible	100		

Comments: Total Points Earned _____ Divided by _____ Total Possible Points = _____ % Score

Instructor's Signature _____

Student Name _____ Date _____

PROCEDURE 38-10: OBTAIN A BACTERIAL SMEAR FROM A WOUND SPECIMEN

TASK: Collect a sample of wound exudates, using sterile collection supplies, and prepare the specimen for transport to laboratory.

CONDITIONS: Given the proper equipment and supplies, the student will role-play obtaining a bacterial smear from a wound specimen.

NOTE: The student should practice the procedure using the MACC CD in the back of the textbook and then practice and perform the task in the classroom: Medical Assisting Competency Challenge CD MACC/Clinical skills/Diagnostic testing/Specimen collection & testing/Obtaining a wound specimen & preparing for transport to an outside lab.

EQUIPMENT AND SUPPLIES
- MACC CD/computer
- Nonsterile disposable gloves
- Personal protective equipment (PPE), as indicated
- Laboratory requisition form
- Plastic –backed small drape
- Sterile gauze (4 × 4 inch)
- Bottle of 10% antiseptic solution
- Surgical tape
- Bandage roll
- Marking pen
- Agar-gel transport system (sterile tube with sterile swab and semisolid solution in the bottom)
- 10% Bleach solution
- Biohazardous waste container
- Patient's medical record

STANDARDS: Complete the procedure within _____ minutes and achieve a minimum score of _____ %.

Time began _____   Time ended _____

Steps	Possible Points	First Attempt	Second Attempt
1. Sanitize hands.	5		
2. Verify the order. Assemble equipment and supplies.	5		
3. Prepare a laboratory requisition form for microbiology department.	5		
4. Greet and identify the patient and escort the patient to the examination room.	5		
5. Explain the procedure to the patient.	5		
6. Apply gloves and PPE as indicated.	5		
7. Position the patient for easy access to the area for specimen collection.	5		
8. Remove dressing and dispose in a biohazardous waste container. Inspect wound for odor, color, amount of drainage, and depth.	15		
9. Open transport system and obtain sterile swab, being careful to prevent contamination when removing from kit.	10		
10. Change gloves.	5		

Steps	Possible Points	First Attempt	Second Attempt
11. Obtain the specimen from area with greatest amount of exudates by moving the swab from side to side.	10		
12. Carefully return the swab to the tube, taking care to prevent contamination by extraneous microorganisms.	10		
13. Label the specimen.	10		
14. Place the agar-gel transport tube in a biohazard transport bag and seal the bag.	10		
15. Cleanse the wound using medical aseptic technique.	10		
16. Apply a clean bandage to the wound site using sterile technique.	5		
17. Dispose of all waste material appropriately, and disinfect the work area using 10% bleach solution.	5		
18. Remove gloves and sanitize the hands.	5		
19. Complete the laboratory requisition form and transport the specimen to lab as soon as possible.	10		
20. Document the procedure.	10		

Total Points Possible   150

Comments: Total Points Earned _____ Divided by _____ Total Possible Points = _____ % Score

Instructor's Signature _____

CHAPTER QUIZ

Multiple Choice

Identify the letter of the choice that best completes the statement or answers the question.

1. _____ are produced in the red bone marrow.
   A. Leukocytes
   B. Platelets
   C. RBCs
   D. WBCs

2. Glucose in the urine may indicate _____.
   A. heavy meal
   B. emotional stress
   C. high doses of vitamin C
   D. all of the above

3. Normal range for specific gravity is _____.
   A. 1.00 to 1.010
   B. 1.01 to 1.015
   C. 1.01 to 1.025
   D. 1.01 to 1.125

4. _____ casts are commonly found in urine and are pale and transparent.
   A. Fatty
   B. Granular
   C. Hyaline
   D. Waxy

5. Myoglobinuria is the result of severe muscle injury caused by trauma.
   A. True
   B. False

6. _____ is the chemical formed when fats are metabolized.
   A. Hemoglobin
   B. Ketone
   C. Glucose
   D. Yeast

7. When bilirubin is broken down by the intestinal bacteria, it is known as _____.
   A. nitrates
   B. nitrites
   C. urobiligen
   D. urochrome

8. _____ is the measurement of the percentage of packed RBCs in a volume of whole blood.
   A. CBC
   B. ESR
   C. Hematocrit
   D. Hemoglobin

9. The Westergren method of ESR requires that the tube set upright for _____.
   A. 30 minutes
   B. 1 hour
   C. 1½ hours
   D. 2 hours

10. _____ cholesterol is known as the "good cholesterol."
    A. Low density lipoprotein
    B. High density lipoprotein
    C. Total cholesterol
    D. All of the above

11. _____ is the most sensitive test of the patient's ability to metabolize glucose.
    A. Fasting blood sugar
    B. The 2-hour postprandial test
    C. Glucose tolerance test
    D. Multistik 10 reagent strip test

12. _____ carry oxygen to the body.
    A. Leukocytes
    B. Platelets
    C. RBCs
    D. WBCs

13. Sediment is the top, liquid of a specimen that has been centrifuged to remove solid particles.
    A. True
    B. False

14. Increased WBCs in urine is an indication of _____.
    A. arthritis
    B. kidney disease
    C. transplant rejection
    D. All of the above

15. The appearance of urine can be described as _____.
    A. dark
    B. light
    C. turbid
    D. transparent

16. The normal volume of urine an adult can excrete is _____mL in a 24-hour period.
    A. 500 to 1000
    B. 750 to 1000
    C. 750 to 1500
    D. 750 to 2000

17. Hemoglobin is the component that gives WBCs their color.
    A. True
    B. False

18. _____ is a culture media used to support growth of microorganisms.
    A. Agar
    B. Broth
    C. Semisolid media
    D. All of the above

19. Petri dishes need to be placed in an incubator for _____ hours to promote microorganism growth.
    A. 12
    B. 24
    C. 48
    D. 72

20. The life span of an RBC is _____ days.
    A. 30
    B. 60
    C. 100
    D. 120

CHAPTER THIRTY-NINE

Understanding Medications

VOCABULARY REVIEW

Matching

Match each term with the correct definition.

A. adverse reaction

B. booster dose

C. caplet

D. contraindications

E. controlled substances

F. cumulative dose

G. curative dose

H. diagnostic drug

I. divided dose

J. elixirs

K. emulsion

L. enteric-coated tablet

M. initial dose

N. inscription

O. layered tablet

P. lethal dose

Q. maintenance dose

R. nomogram

_____ 1. Capsule that contains time-released beads of medication

_____ 2. Rod-shaped, compressed powdered drug form

_____ 3. Amount of medication that proves deadly to a patient

_____ 4. Lozenges

_____ 5. Undesirable and unexpected effects of medications that may be harmful

_____ 6. Total amount of medication that is administered in separate doses

_____ 7. Semisolid mixture of medications that has an oil base for external use

_____ 8. Solution that has undissolved particles and must be shaken to distribute evenly before administration

_____ 9. Route for medication given under the skin or other than the digestive system

_____ 10. Drugs that have a potential for abuse, misuse, and addiction

_____ 11. Tablet with a special coating that dissolves in the small intestine

_____ 12. Liquid medications mixed with an alcohol base

S. ointment

T. parenteral

U. percutaneous

V. prophylactic drug

W. scored tablet

X. seven rights

Y. spansule

Z. suspension

AA. therapeutic drug

BB. tinctures

CC. toxicity

DD. troches

_____ 13. Medication that lessens or prevents the effect of a disease

_____ 14. Drug that heals from disease or cures from infection

_____ 15. First dose of medication administered

_____ 16. Guidelines for drug administration: right patient, drug, dose, route, time, technique, and documentation

_____ 17. Solutions containing alcohol, water, sugar, and a drug or combination of drugs

_____ 18. Harmful effects of drugs on body

_____ 19. Route for medication given through the skin

_____ 20. Medication given to increase chances for long-term immunity, as with immunizations

_____ 21. Chart that shows the relationship of body surface area to height and weight in calculating drug dosage, usually for a child or an infant, but may be used with adults

_____ 22. Tablet with indentations across the middle that allows it to be broken in half

_____ 23. Substance in an oil-based liquid that must be shaken before use

_____ 24. Factors that indicate a medication should not be prescribed because potential risks outweigh potential benefits

_____ 25. Amount of medication needed by the body to maintain its desired effect

_____ 26. Medication that restores the body to its presymptom state

_____ 27. Total amount of medication in the body after repeated doses; medication that accumulates in the body one time

_____ 28. Drug that assists with diagnosing a disease during a procedure, such as radiopaque dye with x-rays

_____ 29. Section of a prescription where the name of the medication is entered

_____ 30. Tablet containing two or more ingredients layered to dissolve and be absorbed at different times

THEORY RECALL

True/False

Indicate whether the sentence or statement is true or false.

_____ 1. Prescriptions are legal documents.

_____ 2. Pharmacokinetics is the study of the biochemical and physiological effects of a drug within the body.

_____ 3. When documenting an immunization injection, the serum manufacturer's name must be noted in the patient's medical record.

_____ 4. Drug samples need to be documented in the patient's chart.

_____ 5. The physician's DEA number does not need to be written on a prescription for controlled substances.

Multiple Choice

Identify the letter of the choice that best completes the statement or answers the question.

1. Most drugs can be identified by _____.
   A. chemical name
   B. generic name
   C. trade name
   D. all of the above

2. The recommended adult dose is based on an age range between _____ years.
   1. 20 to 40
   2. 20 to 30
   3. 20 to 50
   4. 20 to 60

3. The _____ is the agency responsible for enforcing the Controlled Substance Act.
   A. AAMA
   B. AMA
   C. DEA
   D. FDA

4. Medication exists in _____ forms.
   A. two
   B. three
   C. four
   D. five

5. Schedule _____ drugs have no acceptable medical use.
   A. I
   B. II
   C. III
   D. IV

6. Which one of the following is not a solid form of medications?
   A. Spansules
   B. Powders
   C. Sublingual tablets
   D. Elixirs

7. _____ can be an oil-, water-, alcohol-, or soap-based medication intended to be rubbed into the skin.
   A. Cream
   B. Liniment
   C. Lotion
   D. Ointment

8. _____ is a liquid with dissolved particles.
   A. Solute
   B. Solution
   C. Solvent
   D. Tincture

9. _____ is a drug used to lessen or prevent the effects of a disease.
   A. Curative
   B. Prophylactic
   C. Replacement
   D. Therapeutic

10. Section 2 of the *PDR* _____.
    A. includes all participating drug companies
    B. lists each product alphabetically
    C. provides generic and brand name products by page number
    D. provides photographs of various drug forms and products

11. Medication dosage is prescribed for a patient based on _____.
    A. height
    B. nationality
    C. weight
    D. past history

12. Records concerning the dispensing of drugs must be kept for a minimum of _____ year(s).
    A. 1
    B. 2
    C. 5
    D. 10

13. The *Physicians' Desk Reference* is published _____ in conjunction with the pharmaceutical companies whose products are represented.
    A. annually
    B. biannually
    C. every 2 years
    D. only as changes occur

14. Package inserts are included with samples as well as prescription drugs from the pharmacy.
   A. True
   B. False

15. The *United States Pharmacopoeia/National Formulary* is published every _____ by the Council on Pharmacology of the American Medical Association.
   A. annually
   B. every 2 years
   C. every 5 years
   D. every 10 years

16. Dosages for _____ are most frequently calculated according to body weight.
   A. children
   B. the elderly
   C. young adults
   D. middle-aged adults

17. Solvents consist of one or more medications dissolved in _____.
   A. alcohol
   B. normal saline
   C. water
   D. any of the above

18. _____ are solutions of sugar and water that contain drugs.
   A. Aerosols
   B. Suspension
   C. Syrups
   D. Tincture

19. A _____ is the amount of medication that proves deadly to a patient.
   A. curative dose
   B. lethal dose
   C. maintenance dose
   D. all of the above

20. A(n) _____ is a hard candy–like tablet that dissolves in the mouth and releases medication.
   A. elixir
   B. suppository
   C. lozenge
   D. none of the above

Sentence Completion

Complete each sentence or statement.

1. _____ is the study of drugs and how they affect the body.

2. The _____ is legislation whose purpose is to control the manufacture, free offering, and selling of drugs that have potential for abuse.

3. Schedule _____ drugs do not have to be ordered on a special form, but records

must be kept.

4. _____ is a substance suspended in an oil-based liquid into which it does not mix.

5. The _____ is the line on a prescription that provides for the name of the medication

ordered, its strength, and the drug's form.

6. _____ is the study of what happens to a drug from the time it enters the body until it leaves.

7. _____ is medication that replaces substances normally found in the body.

8. _____ is a tablet that dissolves when placed between cheek and gum.

9. A(n) _____ or medicine is any substance that produces a chemical change in the body.

10. _____ must be locked, separate from other drugs, in a locked cabinet.

Short Answers

1. List the seven rights and give the reason for each.

_____

_____

_____

_____

_____

_____

_____

_____

_____

2. Explain the three rules for discarding a controlled substance.

_____

_____

_____

_____

_____

3. List the three basic considerations when administrating an immunization.

_____

_____

_____

_____

_____

CRITICAL THINKING

1. Calculate the following drug orders, make the necessary conversions.
   A. The physician orders 30 mg of Lasix IM. You have Lasix 40 mg/mL on hand. How many mL will be given to an adult patient?
   B. The physician orders 3 mg of Ativan IM. You have a 10-mL vial of Ativan 2 mg/mL on hand. How many mL will be given to an adult patient?
   C. The physician orders 7.5 mg of Compazine IM q3-4h for nausea and vomiting. You have a 10-mL vial of Compazine 5 mg/mL on hand. How many mL will be given to an adult patient?
   D. The physician orders 60 mg of Demerol IM q4h. You have Demerol 75 mg/1.5 mL on hand. How many mL will you give an adult patient?
   E. The physician orders ¼ gr of codeine SC q4h PRN for pain. You have a 20-mL vial of codeine 30 mg/mL on hand. How many mL will you give an adult patient?
   F. The physician orders digoxin 600 mcg IM stat. You have digoxin 0.5 mg/2 mL on hand. How many mL will you give an adult patient?
   G. The physician orders Bicillin 2,400,000 U, IM stat. You have a 10-mL vial of Bicillin containing 600,000 U/mL on hand. How many mL will you give an adult patient?
   H. The physician orders atropine gr 1:100 IM at least 3 hours, preferably 4 hours. You have 0.4 mg/mL of atropine on hand. How many mL will you give an adult patient?
   I. The physician orders hydrochlorothiazide 12.5 mg PO. You have 25-mg tablets available. How many tablets will you give an adult patient?

2. Convert the following measurements:
    A. 1 mg is _____ g.
    B. There are _____ mL in a liter.
    C. 10 mL = _____ cc.
    D. Which is largest: kilogram, gram, or milligram?
    E. Which is smallest: kilogram, gram, or milligram?
    F. 1 liter = _____ cc.
    G. 1000 mcg = _____ mg.
    H. 1 kg = _____ lb.
    I. 1 cm = _____ mm.

3. Select the correct notation
    A. .3 g, 0.3 gm, 0.3 g, .3 gm, 0.30 g _____
    B. 1 1/3 ml, 1.33 mL, 1.33 ML, 1 1/3 ML, 1.330 mL _____
    C. 5 Kg, 5.0 kg, kg 05, 5 kg, 5 kG _____
    D. 1.5 mm, 11/2 mm, 1.5 Mm, 1.50 MM, 1½ MM _____
    E. mg 10, 10 mG, 10.0 mg, 10 mg, 10 MG _____

4. Interpret these metric abbreviations.
    A. mcg _____
    B. mm _____
    C. mL _____
    D. kg _____
    E. cc _____
    F. cm _____
    G. g _____

5. Convert the following:
    A. 100 mg = _____ g
    B. 150 mcg = _____ mg
    C. 30 mg = _____ g
    D. 0.9 mg = _____ mcg
    E. 1500 mg = _____ g
    F. 250 mcg = _____ mg
    G. 4 mg = _____ g
    H. 450 mcg = _____ mg
    I. 0.065 gm = _____ mg
    J. 800 mcg = _____ mg
    K. 3.62 g = _____ mg
    L. 1000 mcg = _____ mg

6. Convert the following:
    A. gr ss = _____ mg
    B. oz 45 = _____ cc
    C. gr ¼ = _____ mg
    D. gr 15 = _____ g
    E. gr 1/6 = _____ g
    F. 0.3 gm = _____ gr
    G. gr 1/150 = _____ mg
    H. 60 mg = _____ gr
    I. 15 mg = _____ gr
    J. 5 mg = _____ gr

INTERNET RESEARCH

Keywords: Immunizations, Routes of Administration for Medication, Drug Interactions, Overmedicated Americans

Choose one of these topics to research: Immunizations; Routes of administration for medication; Drug interactions; Overmedicated Americans. Write a one-page paper. Cite your source. Be prepared to give a 2-minute oral presentation should your instructor assign you to do so.

WHAT WOULD YOU DO?

If you have accomplished the objectives in this chapter, you will be able to make better choices as a medical assistant. Take a look at this situation and decide what you would do.

Glenn is a medical assistant in an office of a family physician. His employer, Dr. Carbello, sees patients of all ages. Because Glenn lives in a state where medical assistants are allowed to call in prescriptions to the pharmacy, one of his regular duties is to call in prescriptions. Glenn is also responsible for performing the inventory on scheduled medications. Today, Dr. Carbello has asked Glenn to call a pharmacy with a prescription for meperidine for a patient who has a severe pain in her back.

After examining another patient, Mrs. Vouch, Dr. Carbello orders an antihistamine for itching, to be given by injection, and an antipyretic. Dr. Carbello tells Glenn to be sure that he tells Mrs. Vouch the side effects of the medications. Mrs. Vouch is also given a prescription for the antihistamine and antipyretic to take at home. The antihistamine is a capsule and the antipyretic is a tablet. Both these medications have systemic effects, and both can have indications of a toxic effect. As Mrs. Vouch leaves the office, Glenn asks her to call in the next week to tell him how the medications are helping with the itching.

If you were Glenn, would you be able to explain the side effects of the medications to Mrs. Vouch?

1. **What is the importance of doing an inventory of Schedule II medications in the medical office?**

2. **Can Glenn call in a Schedule II medication? Why or why not?**

3. **What type of illness would you expect to be treated with an antihistamine?**

4. What is the purpose of an antipyretic? What are some of the common antipyretics?

_____

_____

_____

_____

_____

5. What are the "seven rights" that Glenn must follow when giving medications?

_____

_____

_____

_____

_____

_____

_____

6. If Glenn does not know the interactions and the side effects of the antihistamine, what resource can he use to obtain this information?

_____

_____

_____

7. What is the difference between a side effect and an adverse reaction?

_____

_____

_____

_____

8. What is the difference between a capsule and a tablet?

_____

_____

_____

_____

9. What is the difference between a systemic effect and a local effect? Give an example of each.

_____

_____

_____

_____

_____

10. Why is it important for Glenn to explain "toxic effect" when the patient will be taking the medication at home on a regular basis?

_____

_____

_____

_____

11. What should Glenn document in the medical record at the office visit? What should he document when Mrs. Vouch calls in the next week?

_____

_____

_____

_____

_____

_____

12. **Why is it important for Glenn to understand a drug's actions before giving the drug?**

_____

_____

_____

_____

_____

13. **How are administering, prescribing, and dispensing a medication different?**

_____

_____

_____

_____

_____

_____

14. **How are the chemical name, generic name, and trade name of a medication different?**

_____

_____

_____

_____

_____

_____

APPLICATION OF SKILLS

1. Perform Procedure 39-1: Prepare and File an Immunization Record.

Student Name _____ Date _____

PROCEDURE 39-1: PREPARE AND FILE AN IMMUNIZATION RECORD

TASK: Prepare and file and immunization record
CONDITIONS: Given the proper equipment and supplies, the student will prepare and document an immunization in the medical record and then file the medical record.

EQUIPMENT AND SUPPLIES
- Medication container
- Patient immunization form
- Physician's orders for immunization
- Patient's medical record

STANDARDS: Complete the procedure within _____ minutes and achieve a minimum score of _____ %.

Time began _____   Time ended _____

Steps	Possible Points	First Attempt	Second Attempt
1. Obtain the patient's medical record.	5		
2. Confirm the date the previous immunization was ordered and administered.	10		
3. Verify that the immunization will be given within the required time frame.	5		
4. Enter the correct date into the patient's medical record and on the patient's immunization form.	10		
5. After the physician has examined the patient's ear, verify the physician's order and obtain the correct solution as ordered.	5		
6. Enter the required information into the patient's immunization record.	50		
7. Sign the entry.	10		
8. Return the patient's record to the filing system.	5		

Total Points Possible   100

Comments: Total Points Earned _____ Divided by _____ Total Possible Points = _____ % Score

Instructor's Signature _____

CHAPTER QUIZ

Multiple Choice

Identify the letter of the choice that best completes the statement or answers the question.

1. _____ is the study of drugs and how they affect the body.
   A. Pharmacology
   B. Pharmocodynamics
   C. Pharmacokinetics
   D. None of the above

2. _____ is a drug used to lessen or prevent the effects of a disease.
   A. Curative
   B. Prophylactic
   C. Replacement
   D. Therapeutic

3. The recommended adult dose is based on an age range of _____ years.
   A. 20 to 40
   B. 20 to 50
   C. 20 to 60
   D. 20 to 70

4. _____ is the nonproprietary name of a drug.
   A. Chemical name
   B. Generic name
   C. Trade name
   D. Over-the-counter

5. DEA tests and approves food, drug, and cosmetic products for the marketplace.
   A. True
   B. False

6. Schedule _____ drugs have a use, but severe restrictions apply.
   A. I
   B. II
   C. III
   D. IV

7. The *Physicians' Desk Reference* is published _____.
   A. annually
   B. biannually
   C. every 2 years
   D. every 3 years

8. Medication is prescribed for a patient based on _____.
   A. age
   B. body weight
   C. gender
   D. all of the above

9. Documentation should be done _____.
   A. immediately after the procedure
   B. just before the procedure
   C. at the end of the day
   D. when you have the time

10. _____ is a medication that is evenly distributed within the solution after shaking but not dissolved.
   A. Emulsion
   B. Elixir
   C. Solution
   D. Suspension

11. _____ is a semisolid mixture of medication in a water-soluble base for external use.
   A. Cream
   B. Lotion
   C. Liniment
   D. Ointment

12. _____ is the section of a prescription with instructions to the patient about how to take the medication.
   A. Inscription
   B. Signature
   C. Subscription
   D. Superscription

13. When dispensing drugs, the records must be kept for _____.
   A. 30 days
   B. 6 months
   C. 1 year
   D. 2 years

14. When a patient is given samples of drugs, the samples must be logged into the patient's chart.
   A. True
   B. False

15. _____ is a semisolid, cone-shaped medication that dissolves within a body cavity.
   A. Buccal tablet
   B. Sublingual tablet
   C. Spansule capsule
   D. Suppository

16. Most drugs are identified by _____.
   A. chemical name
   B. generic name
   C. trade name
   D. all of the above

17. The _____ is responsible for enforcing the Controlled Substance Act.
   A. DEA
   B. FDA
   C. AMA
   D. none of the above

18. The *United States Pharmacopoeia/National Formulary* is published every _____ year(s).
    A. 1
    B. 2
    C. 4
    D. 5

19. Package inserts are only included in prescription drugs received from a pharmacy.
    A. True
    B. False

20. The physician's DEA number must be on the prescription.
    A. True
    B. False

21. Convert the following:
    A. 10 cc = _____ oz
    B. gr 10 = _____ g
    C. 0.75 cc = _____ m
    D. m 25 = _____ mL
    E. 0.5 g = _____ mg
    F. gr 30 = _____ g
    G. gr iii = _____ mg
    H. oz i = _____ cc
    I. 0.5 cc = _____ m
    J. gr 1/100 = _____ mg
    K. 0.05 g = _____ mg
    L. 0.05 mg = _____ mcg
    M. 0.1 g = _____ mg
    N. 0.375 mg = _____ mcg
    O. 0.2 g = _____ mg
    P. 0.1 mg = _____ mcg

22. Interpret these metric abbreviations.
    A. kg   _____
    B. g   _____
    C. cc   _____
    D. mL   _____
    E. cm   _____
    F. mcg   _____
    G. mm   _____

23. Calculate the amount you will prepare for each dose.
    A. Order: Vit. B12 0.5 mg IM once/week
       Supply: Vit. B12 1 mg/mL 10-mL vial
    B. Order: Slow-K 16 mEq PO stat
       Supply: Slow-K 8 mEq tablets
    C. Order: Duricef 1 g PO QID. AC
       Supply: Duricef 500-mg capsules
    D. Order: Lanoxin 0.125 mg PO QD
       Supply: Lanoxin 0.25-mg tablets
    E. Order: Motrin 600 mg PO BID
       Supply: Motrin 300-mg tablets

CHAPTER **FORTY**

Administering Medications

VOCABULARY REVIEW

Matching

Match each term with the correct definition.

A. ampule

B. antipyretics

C. aspiration

D. beveled

E. bleb

F. dorsogluteal

G. enteral

H. hub

I. induration

J. isotonic solutions

K. lumen

L. Mantoux test

M. meniscus

N. nebulizer

O. parenteral

P. shaft

Q. spacer

R. subcutaneous

_____ 1. Hollow tube made of glass or plastic marked with specific measurements and with a tip that attaches to a needle

_____ 2. Fluid-filled raised area under the skin

_____ 3. Tuberculin test

_____ 4. Opening of a needle

_____ 5. Part of a needle that determines its length

_____ 6. Specially shaped single-dose glass container that contains a dose of medication and has been hermetically sealed

_____ 7. Intramuscular technique for administering medication that requires the pulling back or displacement of tissue using the injection to prevent discoloration of the skin

_____ 8. Area of hardened tissue that occurs as a result of sensitivity to an allergen

_____ 9. Air compressor unit that forces medication into the lungs

_____ 10. Taken through the digestive system

_____ 11. Vacuum-sealed bottle that contains a sterile solution with or without medication or a sterile oil-based substance

S. syringe

T. transdermal patch

U. vastus lateralis muscle

V. ventrogluteal

W. vial

X. wheal

Y. winged infusion set

Z. Z-track method

_____ 12. Pulling back, as in using suction to draw up blood in a syringe

_____ 13. Taken into the body through the skin by way of a needle

_____ 14. Solutions that contain the same salt concentration as a person's body fluids

_____ 15. Medications that reduce fever

_____ 16. Injection given into fatty layers of the skin beneath the dermis

_____ 17. Muscle area formed by the gluteus medius and gluteus minimus

_____ 18. Part of the needle that fits or locks onto a syringe

_____ 19. "Butterfly needles"; special needles with tabs that resemble butterfly wings used to grasp during insertion

_____ 20. Slanted; the slant of a needle that makes piercing the skin easier

_____ 21. Attachment added to a metered-dose inhaler that acts as a reservoir and changes the characteristics of the medication

_____ 22. Area of gluteus muscle in upper outer portion of the buttocks

_____ 23. Adhesive-backed patch that contains a premeasured dose of medication that is absorbed through the skin

_____ 24. Thigh muscle located between the greater trochanter of the femur and the knee

_____ 25. Fluid-filled bump; raised hive-like bump on the surface of skin seen after a properly placed intradermal injection

_____ 26. Concave level where air and a liquid come together; the surface of fluid when placed in a column or container

THEORY RECALL

True/False

Indicate whether the sentence or statement is true or false.

_____ 1. Vaginal medication usually works within 15 to 30 minutes of application.

_____ 2. Aspiration is performed on all injections.

_____ 3. The advantage of parenteral administration of a drug is that it has low absorption.

_____ 4. Oral medications come in either solid or liquid.

_____ 5. A medical assistant must be very careful not to allow medication to spill out when inverting an ampule.

Multiple Choice

Identify the letter of the choice that best completes the statement or answers the question.

1. _____ is the most frequently used route of administration.
   A. Inhalation
   B. Oral
   C. Parenteral
   D. Topical

2. When administering an intradermal injection, usually _____ mL of medication is given.
   A. 0.01 or less
   B. 0.1 or less
   C. 1.0 or less
   D. 2.0 or less

3. _____ is a solution used to maintain adequate fluids in the body or to prevent dehydration.
   A. Hydrating solution
   B. Hypertonic solution
   C. Isotonic solution
   D. Maintenance solution

4. The _____ syringe is the most commonly used, and is calibrated in both tenths and millimeter and minims.
   A. 0.5-mL
   B. 1-mL
   C. 3-mL
   D. 5-mL

5. A(n) _____ injection is placed 1 to 2 inches below the acromion process and across from the axilla.
   A. intradermal
   B. deltoid
   C. subcutaneous
   D. ventrogluteal

6. As a medical assistant, you should have a patient who has just received an injection wait for _____ minutes for observation of any adverse reactions.
   A. 5 to 10
   B. 10 to 15
   C. 15 to 30
   D. 30 to 60

7. Typically, the action of an oral medication will take _____ to take effect.
   A. 15 to 30 minutes
   B. 30 to 60 minutes
   C. 1 to 11/2 hours
   D. 1 to 2 hours

8. A(n) _____-gauge needle is used when administering a subcutaneous injection.
   A. 18- to 23
   B. 23- to 25
   C. 25- to 28
   D. 28- to 30

9. _____ is the fastest route of absorption when administering medication.
   A. Oral
   B. Intradermal
   C. Intravenous
   D. Subcutaneous

10. The preferred site for the administration of an intradermal injection is _____.
    A. forearm
    B. calf
    C. lower abdomen
    D. all of the above

11. When pouring liquid into a cup, always _____.
    A. pour with cup on the table
    B. read amount from the highest point of curvature
    C. rinse cup with water before pouring
    D. pour liquid at eye level

12. Which one of the following is the best method for administering medication to a patient with nausea and vomiting when the chance for further GI upset is possible?
    A. Liquids
    B. Vaginal suppositories
    C. Rectal suppositories
    D. Tablets

13. When performing an intradermal, a _____ angle is used.
    A. 0- to 10-degree
    B. 5- to 10-degree
    C. 10- to 15-degree
    D. 15- to 20-degree

14. The most common IM injection site is the _____.
    A. deltoid muscle
    B. fatty area on the back of the arm
    C. forearm
    D. stomach

15. Topical drug reactions occur within _____ after being administered.
    A. 10 minutes
    B. 30 minutes
    C. 45 minutes
    D. 1 hour

16. The _____ injection area is free of nerves and major blood vessels.
    A. mid-deltoid
    B. dorsogluteal
    C. vastus lateralis
    D. ventrogluteal

17. An intramuscular injection is administered at a _____ angle.
    A. 10- to 15-degree
    B. 45-degree
    C. 90-degree
    D. none of the above

18. Winged butterfly infusion sets are most commonly used when _____.
    A. patient is receiving multiple therapies
    B. patient has small veins
    C. patient is undergoing long-term therapies
    D. patient has good veins

19. When withdrawing medications from a vial, a _____ needle should be used.
    A. filter
    B. big-bore
    C. short-length
    D. small-bore

20. Topical medications include _____.
    A. creams
    B. lotions
    C. transdermal patches
    D. all of the above

Sentence Completion

Complete each sentence or statement.

1. _____ is a single-dose glass container that has been hermetically sealed.

2. The _____ of the needle describes the lumen of the needle.

3. A(n) _____ injection is placed into the fatty layer beneath the dermis.

4. _____ are absorbed into the bloodstream through capillary action.

5. _____ is the muscle of choice when giving an infant or a child an injection.

6. _____ injection prevents leakage of irritating medication to the skin level.

7. A(n) _____ provides a mist of medication.

8. _____ are sterile metal objects constructed to fit on the tip of a syringe.

9. Needles used most frequently range from _____ (thickest) to 30 (thinnest) and are color coded for easier identification.

10. A(n) _____ contains a single-dose of medication for injection.

Short Answers

1. Give four guidelines for preparing and administering oral medications.

_____

_____

_____

_____

2. Give four functions performed by body fluids.

_____

_____

_____

_____

3. List and explain the four categories of IV solutions.

_____

_____

_____

_____

CRITICAL THINKING

Edith, the medical assistant for Dr Wade, is asked to administer a tuberculin test and an antibiotic injection to a patient. When drawing the medications up, she placed them in 3-cc syringes with 25-gauge needles. While taking them to the patient, she forgets which medications were which. Because she is in a hurry, she chooses to give them both via an IM route.

Was Edith correct in giving both injections IM? Explain why or why not.

INTERNET RESEARCH

Keyword: Accidental Needlesticks

Choose one of the following topics to research: Hazardous exposures—Emergency procedures. Cite your source. Be prepared to give a 2-minute oral presentation should your instructor assign you to do so.

WHAT WOULD YOU DO?

If you have accomplished the objectives in this chapter, you will be able to make better choices as a medical assistant. Take a look at this situation and decide what you would do.

Sue, a medical assistant with no formal training, has been asked by her employer, Dr. Kenyon, to give Dylan, age 3 years, a single dose of acetaminophen 250 mg. Dylan's record shows that he is allergic to penicillin and has had a severe rash in the past. Sue goes to the medicine cabinet and removes amoxicillin, 250-mg tablets, and takes a single tablet to Dylan. Sue does not bother to read the label except when taking the medication from the shelf. Dylan's mother tells Sue that her child is unable to swallow the tablet, but Sue continues to give the tablet, telling the mother that at age 3, Dylan should be able to swallow a tablet.

Sue leaves Dylan and his mother with the tablet. Margie, the other medical assistant in the office, asks Sue to prepare a medication for Mrs. Abbott, who needs a 1-mL estrogen injection. Margie tells Sue that this aqueous medication will be given intramuscularly and that she will be back to give the medication. In preparing the estrogen medication from a vial, Sue shakes the medicine and then draws it into a 5-mL syringe with a 25-gauge 5/8-inch needle. Margie returns and gives the medication that Sue prepared.

In the meantime, Dylan has choked on the tablet and is having difficulty breathing. Because Sue left the room, she is unaware of the situation. When Dr. Kenyon arrives in the room, he immediately recognizes a problem and calls in both Sue and Margie to help remove the tablet from Dylan's throat.

What would you have done differently as a medical assistant?

1. **When should Sue have checked the medication to be sure she had the correct medication?**

    _____

2. **Does it make any difference that the medication ordered was acetaminophen and the medication given was amoxicillin? What are the specific dangers in this case?**

    _____

    _____

    _____

    _____

3. **Was the ordered dosage of the acetaminophen correct for a 3-year-old child? What should Sue have done to be sure the dosage was correct?**

    _____

    _____

    _____

    _____

4. **Why is it important for Sue to know the correct dosage of a medication rather than assuming that the physician is correct?**

    _____

    _____

    _____

    _____

5. **Why is oral administration of acetaminophen the correct route for a 3-year-old child?**

    _____

    _____

    _____

6. **If Dylan was unable to swallow a tablet, what form of medication could Sue have given him?**

    _____

    _____

    _____

7. What are the dangers of giving a tablet to a child who is unable to swallow that form of solid medication?

_____

_____

_____

_____

8. If Dr. Kenyon had prescribed an injection of antibiotic for Dylan, where would the appropriate site have been for administration?

_____

_____

_____

_____

9. What mistake did Sue make while removing the medication from the vial? What mistake did she make in the selection of the syringe and the needle?

_____

_____

_____

_____

10. Because Sue prepared the medication for administration and Margie administered the injection and documented the procedure, who is responsible if a mistake is made? Explain your answer.

_____

_____

_____

_____

APPLICATION OF SKILLS

Procedure Check-off Sheets (*) and Assignments from MACC CD (see Procedure Check-off Sheets for which procedure for the MACC CD to perform).

1. Perform Procedure 40-1: Administer Oral Medication.*

2. Perform Procedure 40-2: Apply a Transdermal Patch.*

3. Perform Procedure 40-3: Instruct the Patient in Administrating Medication Using a Metered-Dose Inhaler With the Closed Mouth Technique.*

4. Perform Procedure 40-4: Reconstitute a Powdered Drug.*

5. Perform Procedure 40-5: Prepare a Parenteral Medication From a Vial.*

6. Perform Procedure 40-6: Prepare a Parenteral Medication From an Ampule.*

7. Perform Procedure 40-7: Administer an Intradermal Injection.*

8. Perform Procedure 40-8: Administer a Subcutaneous Injection.*

9. Perform Procedure 40-9: Administer an Intramuscular Injection to a Pediatric Patient.*

10. Perform Procedure 40-10: Administer an Intramuscular Injection to an Adult.*

11. Perform Procedure 40-11: Administer an Intramuscular Injection Using the Z-Track Technique.*

Student Name _____ Date _____

PROCEDURE 40-1: ADMINISTER ORAL MEDICATION

TASK:
• Interpret the physician's orders for administering oral medication.
• Calculate the required dose of the prescribed medication.
• Pour and measure an accurate dose of the prescribed medication.
• Document the medication administration in the patient's medical chart.

CONDITIONS: Given the proper equipment and supplies, the student will be required to demonstrate the proper method of interrupting a physician's order and of preparing and administering an oral medication.

NOTE: The student should practice the procedure using the MACC CD in the back of the textbook and then practice and perform the task in the classroom: MACC CD MACC/Clinical skills/Patient care/ Medications/Pouring an oral liquid medication.

EQUIPMENT AND SUPPLIES
• MACC CD/computer
• Medication ordered by physician (liquid or solid)
• Medication cup (calibrated)
• Water, as appropriate
• Patient's medical record

STANDARDS: Complete the procedure within _____ minutes and achieve a minimum score of _____%.

Time began _____   Time ended _____

Steps	Possible Points	First Attempt	Second Attempt
1. Sanitize hands.	5		
2. Verify the order, and assemble equipment and supplies.	5		
3. Follow the "seven rights" of medication administration.	5		
4. Select the right drug.	10		
5. Perform the first of the three checks of medication. Verify that the medication name on the label matches the medication name in the written orders.	15		
6. Check the expiration date of the medication.	5		
7. Read the dosage information on the label, compare it with the physician's order, and calculate the right dose using the conversion formula as needed.	15		
8. Perform the second check of the medication against the written order.	10		
9. Prepare the right dose and perform the third check before returning the medication to the storage.	10		
10. Correctly open container, palm label, and pour medication to correct level by placing thumb at line to be administered.	15		

Steps	Possible Points	First Attempt	Second Attempt
11. Place the cup on a flat surface, and recheck the meniscus.	10		
12. Before returning the bottle to the cabinet, perform the third check against the written order.	10		
13. Carry medicine cup carefully to avoid spilling, and administer the medication.	10		
14. Offer water to the patient if appropriate.	5		
15. Remain with the patient until the medication has been swallowed.	5		
16. Sanitize hands.	5		
17. Document the administration of the medication, completing the seven rights.	10		

Total Points Possible   150

Comments: Total Points Earned _____ Divided by _____ Total Possible Points = _____ % Score

Instructor's Signature _____

Student Name _____ Date _____

PROCEDURE 40-2: APPLY A TRANSDERMAL PATCH

TASK: Apply a transdermal patch and provide the patient with instructions for accurate application and safe removal.

CONDITIONS: Given the proper equipment and supplies, the student will role-play the preparation and application of a transdermal patch.

EQUIPMENT AND SUPPLIES
- Medicated transdermal patch, as ordered by the physician
- Nonsterile disposable gloves
- Patient instruction sheet
- Patient's medical record

STANDARDS: Complete the procedure within _____ minutes and achieve a minimum score of _____%.

Time began _____   **Time ended** _____

Steps	Possible Points	First Attempt	Second Attempt
1. Sanitize hands.	5		
2. Verify the order, and assemble equipment and supplies.	5		
3. Follow the "seven rights" of medication administration.	10		
4. Select the right drug.	5		
5. Perform the first of the three checks of the medication.	10		
6. Check the expiration date of the medication.	10		
7. Read the dosage information on the label and compare it with the physician's order.	10		
8. Perform the second check of the medication against the written order.	10		
9. Return the package to storage, checking the medication for the third time.	10		
10. Identify the patient and explain the procedure to the patient.	10		
11. Instruct the patient that the location of the patch should be rotated to different sites at each application.	10		
12. Apply the transdermal patch, dispose of all waste materials appropriately, and disinfect the work area.	15		
13. Remove gloves. Sanitize hands.	5		
14. Instruct the patient on safe removal of the patch, its proper disposal, and the application of a new patch at the same time as per physician's orders.	10		

Steps	Possible Points	First Attempt	Second Attempt
15. Provide written instructions to the patient.	10		
16. Document the procedure.	15		

Total Points Possible 150

Comments: Total Points Earned _____ Divided by _____ Total Possible Points = _____ % Score

Instructor's Signature _____

Student Name _____ Date _____

PROCEDURE 40-3: INSTRUCT THE PATIENT IN ADMINISTERING MEDICATION USING A METERED-DOSE INHALER WITH THE CLOSED-MOUTH TECHNIQUE

TASK: Provide patient instruction for the use of a metered-dose inhaler.

CONDITIONS: Given the proper equipment and supplies, the student will provide patient instruction for the use of a metered-dose inhaler.

EQUIPMENT AND SUPPLIES
Medication ordered by the physician
Metered-dose inhaler (MDI)
Spacer, if required
Patient's medical record

STANDARDS: Complete the procedure within _____ minutes and achieve a minimum score of _____%.

Time began _____   Time ended _____

Steps	Possible Points	First Attempt	Second Attempt
1. Sanitize hands.	5		
2. Verify the order, and assemble equipment and supplies.	5		
3. Follow the "seven rights" of medication administration.	5		
4. Select the right dose.	10		
5. Check the expiration date of the medication.	5		
6. Read the dosage information on the label and compare it with the physician's order.	10		
7. Perform the second check of the medication against the written order.	10		
8. Return the package to storage, checking the medication for the third time.	10		
9. Identify the *right patient*.	10		
10. Prepare the medication as ordered by physician.	10		
11. Instruct the patient to inhale deeply and then gently expel as much air as the patient can comfortably do so.	10		
12. Instruct the patient to place the mouthpiece in the mouth, holding the inhaler upright and closing the lips around it.	10		
13. Instruct the patient to inhale slowly through the mouth, depress the medication canister fully while breathing in, and then hold breath for 10 seconds.	10		
14. Instruct the patient to exhale slowly.	10		
15. Repeat steps 13 through 16 as appropriate.	10		
16. Instruct the patient to clean the mouthpiece after each use.	10		

Steps	Possible Points	First Attempt	Second Attempt
17. Instruct the patient to wash and dry the hands.	5		
18. Document the procedure.	5		

Total Points Possible   150

Comments: Total Points Earned _____ Divided by _____ Total Possible Points = _____ % Score

Instructor's Signature _____

Student Name _____ Date _____

PROCEDURE 40-4: RECONSTITUTE A POWDERED DRUG

TASK: Reconstitute a powdered medication to its liquid dosage form.
CONDITIONS: Given the proper equipment and supplies, the student will reconstitute a powdered drug.

EQUIPMENT AND SUPPLIES
• Vial of powdered medication as ordered by physician
• 70% isopropyl alcohol wipes
• Reconstituting liquid: as indicated by manufacturer
• Appropriate needle and syringe
• Rigid biohazardous container

STANDARDS: Complete the procedure within _____ minutes and achieve a minimum score of _____%.

Time began _____   **Time ended** _____

Steps	Possible Points	First Attempt	Second Attempt
1. Sanitize hands.	5		
2. Verify the order, and assemble equipment and supplies.	5		
3. Follow the "seven rights" of medication administration.	5		
4. Check the medication against the physician's order three times before administration.	5		
5. Check the patient's medical record for drug allergies or conditions that may contraindicate the injection. Check expiration date of the medication.	10		
6. Select the correct medication powder and diluent from cabinet.	10		
7. Check expiration date of the medication.	10		
8. Follow the manufacturer's instructions for reconstituting the powder to correct strength.	10		
9. Prepare the needle and syringe.	5		
10. Fill the syringe and remove the needle from the vial stopper by pulling both hands away from each other.	10		
11. Insert diluent into the medication vial. Remove needle after filling vial.	5		

Steps	Possible Points	First Attempt	Second Attempt
12. Mix the powder and diluent thoroughly by rolling the vial between the flattened palms until all powder has been dissolved. Label the vial with the date and time of reconstitution and your initials.	10		
13. Sanitize hands.	10		

Total Points Possible 100

Comments: Total Points Earned _____ Divided by _____ Total Possible Points = _____ % Score

Instructor's Signature _____

Student Name _____ Date _____

PROCEDURE 40-5: PREPARE A PARENTERAL MEDICATION FROM A VIAL

TASK: From a vial, measure the ordered medication dosage into a 3-mL hypodermic syringe for injection.

CONDITIONS: Given the proper equipment and supplies, the student will prepare a parenteral medication from a vial in a 3-mL syringe.

NOTE: The student should practice the procedure using the MACC CD in the back of the textbook and then practice and perform the task in the classroom: MACC CD MACC/Clinical skills/Patient care/ Medications/Preparing parenteral medications from a vial & ampule.

EQUIPMENT AND SUPPLIES
- MACC CD/computer
- Vial of medication as ordered by physician
- 70% isopropyl alcohol wipes
- 3-mL syringe for ordered dose
- Needle with safety device appropriate for site of injection
- 2 × 2-inch gauze squares
- Rigid biohazardous container

STANDARDS: Complete the procedure within _____ minutes and achieve a minimum score of _____%.

Time began _____   Time ended _____

Steps	Possible Points	First Attempt	Second Attempt
1. Sanitize hands.	5		
2. Verify the order, and assemble equipment and supplies.	5		
3. Follow the "seven rights" of medication administration.	10		
4. Check the medication against the physician's order three times before administration.	10		
5. Check expiration date of the medication.	10		
6. Check the patient's medical record for drug allergies or conditions that may contraindicate the injection.	10		
7. Calculate the correct dose to be given, as necessary.	10		
8. Prepare the vial, needle, and syringe.	5		
9. Draw the amount of air into the syringe for the amount of medication to be administered.	5		
10. Remove the cover from the needle and insert the needle into the vial.	10		
11. Inject the air into vial and fill the syringe with the medication.	10		
12. Remove any air bubbles and recap the needle as necessary.	10		

Steps	Possible Points	First Attempt	Second Attempt
13. Compare the medication to the vial label, and return the medication to its proper storage.	5		
14. Sanitize hands.	10		

Total Points Possible 115

Comments: Total Points Earned _____ Divided by _____ Total Possible Points = _____ % Score

Instructor's Signature _____

Student Name _____ Date _____

PROCEDURE 40-6: PREPARE A PARENTERAL MEDICATION FROM AN AMPULE

TASK: From an ampule, measure the correct medication dosage in a 1-mL hypodermic syringe for injection.

CONDITIONS: Given the proper equipment and supplies, the student will prepare a parenteral medication from an ampule.

NOTE: The student should practice the procedure using the MACC CD in the back of the textbook and then practice and perform the task in the classroom: MACC CD MACC/Clinical skills/Patient care/ Medications/Preparing parenteral medications from a vial & ampule.

EQUIPMENT AND SUPPLIES
- MACC CD/computer
- Ampule of medication ordered by physician
- Ampule breaker or 2×2-inch gauze squares
- 70% isopropyl alcohol wipes
- Appropriate syringe for ordered dose
- Needle with safety device
- Filter needle (used for ampule only)
- Rigid biohazardous container

STANDARDS: Complete the procedure within _____ minutes and achieve a minimum score of _____%.

Time began _____   Time ended _____

Steps	Possible Points	First Attempt	Second Attempt
1. Sanitize hands.	5		
2. Verify the order, and assemble equipment and supplies.	5		
3. Follow the "seven rights" of medication administration.	10		
4. Check the medication against the physician's order three times before administration.	10		
5. Check expiration date of the medication.	10		
6. Check the patient's medical record for drug allergies or conditions that may contraindicate the injection.	10		
7. Calculate the correct dose to be given, as ordered by the physician.	10		
8. Clean neck of ampule.	5		
9. Prepare the syringe with a filter needle.	5		
10. Be sure liquid from the top of the ampule is in hollow reservoir and break the ampule.	10		
11. Remove the cover from the filter needle and insert filter needle into the ampule. Fill syringe.	15		
12. Remove filter needle and recap.	5		
13. Remove any air bubbles and check medication.	10		

Steps	Possible Points	First Attempt	Second Attempt
14. Check the medication label. Keep the medication ampule and syringe together until ready to administer.	10		
15. Sanitize hands.	5		

Total Points Possible   125

Comments: Total Points Earned _____ Divided by _____ Total Possible Points = _____ % Score

Instructor's Signature _____

Student Name _____ Date _____

PROCEDURE 40-7: ADMINISTER AN INTRADERMAL INJECTION

TASK:
- Identify the correct syringe, needle gauge, and length for an intradermal injection.
- Select and prepare an appropriate site for an intradermal injection.
- Demonstrate the correct technique to administer an intradermal injection.
- Document an intradermal injection correctly in the medical record.

CONDITIONS: Given the proper equipment and supplies, the student will prepare and administer an intradermal injection.

NOTE: The student should practice the procedure using the MACC CD in the back of the textbook and then practice and perform the task in the classroom: MACC CD MACC/Clinical skills/Patient care/Medications/Performing intradermal injections.

EQUIPMENT AND SUPPLIES
- MACC CD/computer
- Nonsterile disposable gloves
- Medication as ordered by physician
- Tuberculin syringe for ordered dose
- Needle with safety device (26 or 27 gauge, 3/8 inch to 1/2 inch)
- 2 × 2-inch sterile gauze
- 70% isopropyl alcohol wipes
- Written patient instructions for post testing as appropriate
- Rigid biohazardous container
- Patient's medical record

STANDARDS: Complete the procedure within _____ minutes and achieve a minimum score of _____%.

Time began _____   Time ended _____

Steps	Possible Points	First Attempt	Second Attempt
1. Sanitize hands.	5		
2. Verify the order, and assemble equipment and supplies.	5		
3. Check the patient's medical record for drug allergies or conditions that may contraindicate the injection.	10		
4. Follow the "seven rights" of medication administration.	10		
5. Check the medication against the physician's order three times before administration.	10		
6. Check expiration date of the medication.	10		
7. Calculate the dose to be given, if necessary.	15		
8. Follow the correct procedure for drawing the medication into syringe.	10		
9. Greet and identify the patient, and explain the procedure to the patient.	10		
10. Select an appropriate injection site and properly position the patient as necessary to expose the site adequately.	10		

Steps	Possible Points	First Attempt	Second Attempt
11. Apply gloves.	5		
12. Prepare the injection site.	10		
13. While the prepared site is drying, remove the cover from the needle.	10		
14. Pull the skin taut at the injection site.	10		
15. Inject the medication between the dermis and epidermis. Create a wheal.	10		
16. Withdraw the needle from the injection site at the same angle as it was inserted, and activate the safety device immediately.	10		
17. Dab the area with the gauze. Do not rub.	5		
18. Remove gloves and discard in a biohazardous container.	5		
19. Sanitize the hands.	5		
20. Check the patient.	5		
21. Read or discuss with the patient the test results.	10		
22. Sanitize hands.	5		
23. Document the procedure.	10		
Mantoux Test			
24. Check to be sure test was given 48 to 72 hours earlier.	10		
25. After sanitizing the hands and applying nonsterile gloves, gently rub the test site with a finger and lightly palpate for induration.	10		
26. Using the tape that comes with the medication, measure the diameter of the area of induration from edge to edge.	10		
27. Record the area of induration and notify the health care provider of the measurement if not within the negative range.	10		
28. Record the reading in the medical record.	10		

Total Points Possible   245

Comments: Total Points Earned _____ Divided by _____ Total Possible Points = _____ % Score

Instructor's Signature _____

Student Name _____ Date _____

PROCEDURE 40-8: ADMINISTER A SUBCUTANEOUS INJECTION

TASK:
- Identify the correct syringe, needle gauge, and length for a subcutaneous injection.
- Select and prepare an appropriate site for a subcutaneous injection.
- Demonstrate the correct technique to administer a subcutaneous injection.
- Document a subcutaneous injection correctly in the medical record.

CONDITIONS: Given the proper equipment and supplies, the student will prepare and administer a subcutaneous injection.

NOTE: The student should practice the procedure using the MACC CD in the back of the textbook and then practice and perform the task in the classroom: MACC CD MACC/Clinical skills/Patient care/Medications/Performing subcutaneous injections.

EQUIPMENT AND SUPPLIES
- MACC CD/computer
- Nonsterile disposable gloves
- Medication as ordered by physician
- Appropriate syringe for ordered dose of medication
- Appropriate needle with safety device
- 2 × 2-inch sterile gauze
- 70% Isopropyl alcohol wipes
- Sharps container
- Rigid biohazardous container
- Patient's medical record

STANDARDS: Complete the procedure within _____ minutes and achieve a minimum score of _____%.

Time began _____   Time ended _____

Steps	Possible Points	First Attempt	Second Attempt
1. Sanitize hands.	5		
2. Verify the order, and assemble equipment and supplies.	5		
3. Follow the "seven rights" of medication administration.	10		
4. Check the medication against the physician's order three times before administration.	10		
5. Check the patient's medical record for drug allergies or conditions that may contraindicate the injection.	10		
6. Check expiration date of the medication.	10		
7. Calculate the correct dose to be given, if necessary.	15		
8. Follow the procedure for drawing the medication into the syringe.	5		
9. Greet and identify the patient, and explain the procedure.	10		
10. Select an appropriate injection site and properly position the patient as necessary to expose the site.	10		

Steps	Possible Points	First Attempt	Second Attempt
11. Apply gloves.	5		
12. Prepare the injection site.	10		
13. While the prepared site is drying, remove the cover from the needle.	5		
14. Pinch the skin at the injection site and puncture the skin quickly and smoothly, making sure the needle is kept at a 45-degree angle.	10		
15. Aspirate the syringe to check for blood. If no blood is present, inject the medication.	10		
16. Place a gauze pad over the injection site and quickly withdraw the needle from the injection site at the same angle at which it was inserted.	10		
17. Massage the injection site, if appropriate.	5		
18. Discard the syringe and needle into a rigid biohazardous container.	5		
19. Remove gloves and discard in a biohazardous waste container.	5		
20. Sanitize the hands.	5		
21. Check on the patient.	5		
22. Document procedure.	10		

Total Points Possible 175

Comments: Total Points Earned _____ Divided by _____ Total Possible Points = _____ % Score

Instructor's Signature _____

Student Name _____ Date _____

PROCEDURE 40-9: ADMINISTER AN INTRAMUSCULAR INJECTION TO A PEDIATRIC PATIENT

TASK:
- Identify the correct syringe, needle gauge, and length for a pediatric intramuscular injection.
- Select and prepare an appropriate site for a pediatric intramuscular injection.
- Demonstrate the correct technique to administer an intramuscular injection to a pediatric patient.
- Document an intramuscular injection correctly in the medical record.

CONDITIONS: Given the proper equipment and supplies, the student will be required to demonstrate competency (through use of a pediatric mannequin) in the proper method of preparing and administering an intramuscular injection for a pediatric patient.

NOTE: The student should practice the procedure using the MACC CD in the back of the textbook and then practice and perform the task in the classroom: MACC CD MACC/Clinical skills/Patient Care/Medications/Administering intramuscular injections & recording immunizations.

EQUIPMENT AND SUPPLIES
- MACC CD/computer
- Nonsterile disposable gloves
- Medication order by physician
- Appropriate syringe for ordered dose
- Appropriate needle with safety device (25 or 27 gauge, 5/8 inch to 1 inch)
- 2 × 2-inch sterile gauze
- 70% isopropyl alcohol wipes
- Rigid biohazardous container
- Biohazardous waste container
- Patient's medical record

STANDARDS: Complete the procedure within _____ minutes and achieve a minimum score of _____%.

Time began _____   Time ended _____

Steps	Possible Points	First Attempt	Second Attempt
1. Sanitize hands.	5		
2. Verify the order, and assemble equipment and supplies.	5		
3. Follow the "seven rights" of medication administration.	10		
4. Check the medication against the physician's order three times before administration.	10		
5. Check the patient's medical record for drug allergies or conditions that may contraindicate the injection.	10		
6. Check expiration date of the medication.	10		
7. Calculate the correct dose to be given.	20		
8. Follow the procedure for drawing the medication into syringe.	10		

Steps	Possible Points	First Attempt	Second Attempt
9. Greet and identify the patient and the patient's parent or guardian, and explain the procedure to the patient or guardian, as appropriate.	15		
10. Select an appropriate injection site and properly position the patient as necessary.	10		
11. Apply disposable gloves.	10		
12. Secure the patient, asking help from parent or guardian as needed.	10		
13. Prepare the injection site.	10		
14. While the prepared site is drying, remove the cover from the needle.	10		
15. Secure the skin at the injection site.	10		
16. Puncture the skin quickly and smoothly, making sure the needle is kept at a 90-degree angle.	15		
17. Aspirate the syringe.	10		
18. Inject the medication appropriately for base of medication (oil, water, etc.).	10		
19. Place a gauze pad over the injection site and quickly withdraw the needle from the injection site at the same as insertion. Activate safety sheath over needle.	10		
20. Massage the injection site if appropriate.	5		
21. Dispose of the syringe and needle into a rigid biohazardous container.	5		
22. Remove gloves, and discard in a biohazardous waste container.	5		
23. Sanitize the hands.	5		
24. Check on the patient.	5		
25. Document procedure.	10		

Total Points Possible   235

Comments: Total Points Earned _____ Divided by _____ Total Possible Points = _____ % Score

Instructor's Signature _____

Student Name _____ Date _____

PROCEDURE 40-10: ADMINISTER AN INTRAMUSCULAR INJECTION TO AN ADULT

TASK:
- Identify the correct syringe, needle gauge, and length for an adult intramuscular injection.
- Select and prepare an appropriate site for a pediatric intramuscular injection.
- Demonstrate the correct technique to administer an intramuscular injection.
- Document an intramuscular injection correctly in the medical record.

CONDITIONS: Given the proper equipment and supplies, the student will prepare and administer an intramuscular injection to an adult patient.

NOTE: The student should practice the procedure using the MACC CD in the back of the textbook and then practice and perform the task in the classroom: MACC CD MACC/Clinical skills/Patient care/ Medications/Administering intramuscular injections & recording immunizations.

EQUIPMENT AND SUPPLIES
- MACC CD/computer
- Nonsterile disposable gloves
- Medication as ordered by physician
- Appropriate syringe for ordered medication dose
- Appropriate needle with safety device (21 or 25 gauge, 1 inch to 11/2 inch)
- 2 × 2-inch sterile gauze
- 70% isopropyl alcohol wipes
- sharps container
- Biohazardous waste container
- Patient's medical record

STANDARDS: Complete the procedure within _____ minutes and achieve a minimum score of _____%.

Time began _____   Time ended _____

Steps	Possible Points	First Attempt	Second Attempt
1. Sanitize hands.	5		
2. Verify the order, and assemble equipment and supplies.	5		
3. Follow the "seven rights" of medication administration.	10		
4. Check the medication against the physician's order three times before administration.	10		
5. Check the patient's medical record for drug allergies or conditions that may contraindicate the injection.	10		
6. Check expiration date of the medication.	10		
7. Calculate the correct dose to be given.	20		
8. Greet and identify the patient, and explain the procedure.	10		
9. Select an appropriate injection site by amount and density of medication. Properly position the patient as necessary to expose the site adequately.	10		
10. Apply gloves.	5		

Steps	Possible Points	First Attempt	Second Attempt
11. Prepare the injection site.	10		
12. While the prepared site is drying, remove the cover from the needle.	10		
13. Secure the skin at the injection site.	10		
14. Puncture the skin quickly and smoothly, making sure the needle is kept at a 90-degree angle.	10		
15. Aspirate the syringe.	10		
16. Inject medication using proper technique for density of medication.	10		
17. Place a gauze pad over the injection site and quickly withdraw the needle from the injection site at the same angle at which it was inserted. Activate the safety shield over the needle.	10		
18. Massage the injection site if appropriate for medication.	10		
19. Discard the syringe and needle into a sharps container.	5		
20. Remove gloves and discard in a biohazardous waste container.	5		
21. Sanitize the hands.	5		
22. Check on the patient.	10		
23. Document procedure.	10		

Total Points Possible   210

Comments: Total Points Earned _____ Divided by _____ Total Possible Points = _____ % Score

Instructor's Signature _____

Student Name _____ Date _____

PROCEDURE 40-11: ADMINISTER AN INTRAMUSCULAR INJECTION USING THE Z-TRACK TECHNIQUE

TASK: Demonstrate the correct technique to administer an intramuscular injection using the Z-track technique.

CONDITIONS: Given the proper equipment and supplies, the student will prepare and administer an intramuscular injection using the Z-track technique.

EQUIPMENT AND SUPPLIES
- Nonsterile disposable gloves
- Medication order by physician
- Appropriate syringe for ordered dose
- Appropriate needle with safety device
- 2 × 2-inch sterile gauze
- 70% isopropyl alcohol wipes
- Rigid biohazardous container
- Biohazardous waste container
- Patient's medical record

STANDARDS: Complete the procedure within _____ minutes and achieve a minimum score of _____%.

Time began _____   Time ended _____

Steps	Possible Points	First Attempt	Second Attempt
1. Sanitize hands.	5		
2. Verify the order, and assemble equipment and supplies.	5		
3. Follow the "seven rights" of medication administration.	10		
4. Check the medication against the physician's order three times before administration.	10		
5. Check the patient's medical record for drug allergies or conditions that may contraindicate the injection.	10		
6. Check expiration date of the medication.	10		
7. Calculate the correct dose to be given.	20		
8. Follow the correct procedure for drawing the medication into syringe.	10		
9. Greet and identify the patient, and explain the procedure to the patient.	15		
10. Select an appropriate injection site and properly position the patient.	5		
11. Apply disposable gloves.	5		
12. Prepare the injection site.	5		
13. While the prepared site is drying, remove the cover from the needle.	5		
14. Secure the skin at the injection site by pushing the skin away from the injection site.	10		
15. Puncture the skin quickly and smoothly, making sure the needle is kept at a 90-degree angle.	10		

Steps	Possible Points	First Attempt	Second Attempt
16. Continue to hold the tissue in place while aspirating and injecting the medication.	15		
17. Inject the medication.	10		
18. Withdraw the needle.	10		
19. Release the traction on the skin to seal the track as the needle is being removed. Activate safety shield over needle.	10		
20. Discard the syringe and needle into a rigid biohazardous container.	5		
21. Remove gloves and discard in a biohazardous waste container.	5		
22. Sanitize the hands.	5		
23. Check on the patient.	5		
24. Document the procedure.	5		
25. Clean the equipment and examination room.	10		

Total Points Possible   215

Comments: Total Points Earned _____ Divided by _____ Total Possible Points = _____ % Score

Instructor's Signature _____

CHAPTER QUIZ

Multiple Choice

Identify the letter of the choice that best completes the statement or answers the question.

1. The _____-mL syringe is the syringe most often used.
   A. 0.5
   B. 1
   C. 3
   D. 5

2. When administering an intradermal, the angle of insertion should be _____ degrees.
   A. 10 to 15
   B. 20
   C. 45
   D. 90

3. A(n) _____ injection is given in the fatty layer beneath the dermis.
   A. deltoid
   B. intradermal
   C. intramuscular
   D. subcutaneous

4. A mid-deltoid injection should be given in the upper outer quadrant of the hip.
   A. True
   B. False

5. The most common area to give an IM injection is _____.
   A. deltoid
   B. vastus lateralis
   C. gluteus muscles
   D. all of the above

6. The goal of IV fluid administration is to correct or replace fluid volume and restore electrolyte balance.
   A. True
   B. False

7. A dorsogluteal injection should be administered at a _____-degree angle.
   A. 10 to 15
   B. 20 to 30
   C. 45
   D. 90

8. The most frequently used route of medication administration is _____.
   A. oral
   B. parenteral
   C. injection
   D. topical

9. Administration of IV fluids allows for rapid absorption.
   A. True
   B. False

10. _____ are administered to replace electrolytes in severe cases of diarrhea and vomiting.
   A. Hydrating fluids
   B. Isotonic solutions
   C. Maintenance solutions
   D. Hypertonic solutions

11. _____ is an injection site used from infancy to adulthood because it lacks major nerves and blood vessels.
   A. Deltoid
   B. Forearm
   C. Vastus lateralis
   D. Ventrogluteal

12. _____ is a liquid preparation in a water base that is applied to the skin.
   A. Cream
   B. Lotion
   C. Ointment
   D. All of the above

13. _____ is a hand-held device that dispenses medication into the airway.
   A. Nebulizer
   B. Metered-dose inhaler
   C. Prefilled cartridge unit
   D. Spacer

14. Another name for the Mantoux test is the tuberculin test.
   A. True
   B. False

15. A(n) _____-gauge needle is used to administer a subQ injection.
   A. 18- to 21
   B. 21- to 23
   C. 23- to 25
   D. 25- to 28

16. Oral medication action usually takes _____ minutes.
   A. 10 to 15
   B. 20 to 30
   C. 30 to 60
   D. 40 to 60

17. When pouring liquid medications, you should _____.
   A. read the highest curvature of the liquid
   B. pour medication at eye level
   C. pour it on a level surface
   D. none of the above

18. Topical medication drug actions usually occur within _____.
    A. 10 minutes
    B. 20 minutes
    C. 30 minutes
    D. 1 hour

19. Rectal medications may be used because they cause less GI upset.
    A. True
    B. False

20. The medical assistant should check the medication against the physician's order _____.
    A. once
    B. twice
    C. three times
    D. four times

CHAPTER **FORTY-ONE**

Minor Office Surgery

VOCABULARY REVIEW

Matching

Match each term with the correct definition.

A. ambulatory surgery setting

B. approximate

C. box lock

D. cicatrix

E. closed wound

F. curette

G. debridement

H. dilating

I. dissecting

J. exudates

K. general anesthetic

L. hemostatic forceps

M. jaws

N. ligate

O. open technique

P. pick-ups

Q. purulent

R. retracting

_____ 1. Wound drainage that consists of serum or clear fluid

_____ 2. Instrument with serrated tips, ratchets, and a box lock used to clamp off blood vessels or to grasp materials

_____ 3. Area where an instrument is hinged

_____ 4. Sterile technique; used to prevent the spread of microorganisms when skin or mucous membranes have been broken

_____ 5. Long-handled instrument with a metal loop on one end that is used to scrape inside a cavity

_____ 6. Wound drainage that consists of pus

_____ 7. Break in the skin or soft tissue

_____ 8. Wound drainage such as oozing pus or serum

_____ 9. Application of only sterile gloves for performing a sterile procedure

_____ 10. Sterile material, such as gauze, used to cover a wound

_____ 11. Making wider or larger, as in a dilating instrument used to increase the diameter of an opening

_____ 12. Holding part of a clamp

S. sanguineous

T. serous

U. skin lesion removal

V. sterile dressing

W. surgical asepsis

X. surgical hand washing

Y. towel clamps

Z. wound

_____ 13. Special handwashing technique that decreases the total number of pathogens present; surgical scrub

_____ 14. Nonhospital setting where surgery is performed and the patient is not hospitalized

_____ 15. Pulling back tissue, as in a *retracting instrument* used to hold tissue away from a surgical area

_____ 16. Scar tissue

_____ 17. Common name for thumb forceps; also used by some physicians as another name for transfer forceps or sponge forceps

_____ 18. Removal of warts or other skin lesions through the use of a freezing agent or surgery

_____ 19. Instrument with sharp points used to hold the edges of a sterile towel together, usually to form a drape

_____ 20. To bring together skin edges

_____ 21. Removal of foreign or dead material from a wound

_____ 22. To tie off

_____ 23. Wound drainage that consists of blood

_____ 24. Tissues that are injured, such as a bruise, but the skin is not broken

_____ 25. Medication that produces unconsciousness by depressing the central nervous system

_____ 26. Cutting apart or separating tissue, as in *dissecting instrument* used to cut between tissue

THEORY RECALL

True/False

Indicate whether the sentence or statement is true or false.

_____ 1. Catgut sutures are used in areas that heal slower and when absorption of suture material needs to stay in place longer.

_____ 2. When sterile dressing is applied to a wound sterile technique must be used.

_____ 3. Surgical asepsis is the highest level of protection for patients.

_____ 4. The medical assistant should always wash a wound from the center outward.

_____ 5. Local anesthesia produces unconsciousness by depressing the central nervous system.

Multiple Choice

Identify the letter of the choice that best completes the statement or answers the question.

1. Scalpel blades range in size from _____.
   A. 5 to 10
   B. 10 to 15
   C. 5 to 25
   D. 10 to 30

2. _____ scalpels are used for growth removal.
   A. Concave
   B. Convex
   C. Straight
   D. Pointed

3. _____ is a break in the soft tissue of the body that does not extend beyond the subcutaneous tissue.
   A. Closed wound
   B. Open wound
   C. Deep wound
   D. Superficial wound

4. When charting the condition of a wound, the _____ must be charted in the patient's chart.
   A. amount of drainage
   B. appearance of drainage
   C. consistency of drainage
   D. all of the above

5. _____ have blunt ends with serrated tips used for removing or applying dressing materials.
   A. Dressing forceps
   B. Sponge forceps
   C. Tissue forceps
   D. Towel clamps

6. Scar tissue is made up of all of the following EXCEPT _____.
   A. connective tissue
   B. epithelial cells
   C. muscle tissue
   D. fibrous tissue

7. Before surgery, a patient must have _____.
   A. a second opinion
   B. given informed consent
   C. received a reimbursement check from the insurance company
   D. completed a living will

8. _____ have a sharp, pointed, slender tip and a spring mechanism used to grasp fine objects or particles.
   A. Hemostats
   B. Splinter forceps
   C. Thumb forceps
   D. Towel clamps

9. Scalpels and curettes are examples of _____ instruments.
   A. cutting
   B. dilating
   C. probing
   D. retracting

10. _____ drainage consists of blood from broken capillaries.
    A. Serous
    B. Sanguineous
    C. Serosanguineous
    D. Purulent

11. Patients who have had minor surgery usually return to the physician's office in approximately _____ to have their dressing changed.
    A. 2 to 4 days
    B. 6 to 8 days
    C. 5 to 10 days
    D. 2 weeks

12. Sebaceous cysts commonly occur on all of the following EXCEPT the _____.
    A. back
    B. ears
    C. face
    D. feet

13. _____ anesthesia is accomplished when an anesthetic is injected into and around a set of nerves.
    A. Local
    B. Topical
    C. Regional
    D. General

14. A(n) _____ for gloving ensures that the nonsterile hands never touch the outside of the gown or glove.
    A. closed technique
    B. open technique
    C. lateral technique
    D. all of the above

15. _____ have thick blades with a fine cutting edge used to dissect and cut muscle tissue.
    A. Dissecting scissors
    B. Operating scissors
    C. Suture scissors
    D. Littauer scissors

Sentence Completion

Complete each sentence or statement.

1. _____ is used when the skin surface is broken.

2. _____ are two-pronged instruments for grasping or holding body tissue.

3. _____ is the lack of feeling or absence of normal feeling caused by a substance, hypnosis, or traumatic injury.

4. _____ have serrated tips and a spring mechanism used to pickup or hold tissue.

5. _____ is a surgical procedure that cleans and debrides a wound with a suture closure.

6. A(n) _____ wound does not show a break in the skin.

7. _____ drainage consists of pus.

8. _____ are instruments used to hold back the edges of a wound.

9. _____ is a long-handled instrument with a metal loop on one end.

10. The _____ removes dead skin, oils, dirt, and pathogenic microorganisms.

Short Answers

1. List five guidelines that medical assistant should follow when handling and maintaining instruments.

_____

_____

_____

_____

_____

2. List the three classifications of wound healing.

_____

_____

_____

3. Explain the four factors that help in the healing process.

_____

_____

_____

_____

CRITICAL THINKING

Dr. Taylor has three minor office surgeries scheduled back-to-back today. He has asked for you to assist him in each procedure. Describe the general procedure guidelines that you will use for each procedure.

INTERNET RESEARCH

Keywords: Minor Surgery Instruments, Minor Surgery Suture Material, Alternative Skin Closures After Surgery

Choose one of these topics to research: Minor surgery instruments; Minor surgery suture material; Alternative skin closures after surgery. Write a one-page report. Cite your source. Be prepared to give a 2-minute oral presentation should your instructor assign you to do so.

WHAT WOULD YOU DO?

If you have accomplished the objectives in this chapter, you will be able to make better choices as a medical assistant. Take a look at this situation and decide what you would do.

Shirley, a patient of Dr. Jones, has arrived at the office for removal of a cyst on her face that has been present for about 2 months. Anna is the medical assistant at the front desk, and Lori is the clinical medical assistant for Dr. Jones. Shirley has been asked to cleanse the area around the lesion with an antiseptic wash for the past 2 days. Shirley wants to know exactly what will be done and if she has to sign papers. Anna tells her that these papers can be signed at any time before the actual opening of the wound. Anna also tells Shirley that Lori will explain what will be done after Shirley is taken to the room where minor surgery is done.

As Lori sets up the surgical tray, she uses surgical asepsis. She uses a sterile tray and peel-back wrappers to set up the needed instruments. On the tray are a scalpel, several hemostat forceps, a probe, a needle holder, scissors, and two retractors.

After the surgery, Lori is in a hurry and piles the instruments in the basin before sanitizing them. When she documents the procedure for Dr. Jones, she only documents the date and the type of surgery.

Would you be prepared to step into Anna's or Lori's shoes and perform the needed tasks correctly?

1. **What questions should Anna ask Shirley as she arrives at the office for the surgery?**

2. **Since Shirley is to receive a tranquilizer intravenously, what preparation should have been made for Shirley's safe return home?**

3. **Can Shirley wait to sign informed consent until after the incision has been made? Explain your answer.**

4. **Explain what role Lori can take in obtaining informed consent.**

_____

_____

_____

_____

5. **What is surgical asepsis? How does it differ from medical asepsis?**

_____

_____

_____

_____

_____

6. **What is the difference between a sterile tray and peel-wrapped instruments? What is the indication of the use of each of these?**

_____

_____

_____

_____

_____

_____

7. **What is the use of a scalpel? Forceps? Probe? Needle holder? Retractors?**

_____

_____

_____

_____

_____

_____

_____

_____

8. What did Lori miss in the correct documentation of the surgical procedure?

_____

_____

_____

_____

9. How did Lori mishandle the instruments after the procedure?

_____

_____

_____

_____

10. What instructions would you expect Lori to give to Shirley after the surgical procedure?

_____

_____

_____

_____

_____

11. How will the lack of correct documentation affect the coding of this surgical procedure for insurance reimbursement?

_____

_____

_____

_____

APPLICATION OF SKILLS

Procedure Check-off Sheets (*) and Assignments from MACC CD (see Procedure Check-off Sheets for which procedure for the MACC CD to perform).

1. Perform Procedure 41-1: Perform Handwashing for Surgical Asepsis.*

2. Perform Procedure 41-2: Apply a Sterile Gown and Gloves.*

3. Perform Procedure 41-3: Apply Sterile Gloves.*

4. Perform Procedure 41-4: Remove Contaminated Gloves.*

5. Perform Procedure 41-5: Open a Sterile Package.*

6. Perform Procedure 41-6: Pour a Sterile Solution.*

7. Perform Procedure 41-7: Assist with Minor Office Surgery.*

8. Perform Procedure 41-8: Remove Sutures or Staples and Change a Wound Dressing Using a Spiral Bandage.*

9. Perform Procedure 41-9: Apply and Remove Adhesive Skin Closures.*

Student Name _____ Date _____

PROCEDURE 41-1: PERFORM HANDWASHING FOR SURGICAL ASEPSIS

TASK: Performing a surgical handwashing (surgical scrub) following standard precautions.
CONDITIONS: Given the proper equipment and supplies, the student will perform a handwashing for surgical asepsis.

EQUIPMENT AND SUPPLIES
- Liquid antibacterial soap and nailbrush with orange stick, or prepackaged sterile scrub brush with antibacterial soap and orange stick
- Paper towels
- Warm running water
- Sterile towel pack
- Regular waste container and cloth hamper

STANDARDS: Complete the procedure within _____ minutes and achieve a minimum score of _____ %.

Time began _____   Time ended _____

Steps	Possible Points	First Attempt	Second Attempt
1. Remove jewelry.	5		
2. Open the sterile pack containing a scrub brush with an orange stick and sterile towel.	10		
3. Load the brush with liquid antibacterial soap or use prepackaged scrub.	5		
4. Turn on the faucets using correct methodology for facility.	10		
5. Use a paper towel to adjust the water temperature.	10		
6. Wet hands, wrists, and forearms.	10		
7. Clean nails with a nail brush or orange stick.	5		
8. Scrub hands, wrists, and forearms.	15		
9. Rinse hands, wrists, and forearms.	10		
10. Turn off the faucets using correct methodology for facility.	5		
11. Dry the hands and arms with sterile towel.	10		
12. Discard used towels in a regular waste container or soiled-linen container.	5		

Total Points Possible   100

Comments: Total Points Earned _____ Divided by _____ Total Possible Points = _____ % Score

Instructor's Signature _____

Student Name _____ Date _____

PROCEDURE 41-2: APPLY A STERILE GOWN AND GLOVES

TASK: Apply a sterile gown and gloves to maintain sterile technique.
CONDITIONS: Given the proper equipment and supplies, the student will apply a sterile gown and gloves to maintain sterile technique.

EQUIPMENT AND SUPPLIES
- Supplies for surgical handwashing
- Sterile gown
- Sterile gloves
- Hair cover
- Mask
- Goggles (as needed for standard precautions)
- Regular waste container and cloth hamper

STANDARDS: Complete the procedure within _____ minutes and achieve a minimum score of _____ %.

Time began _____   Time ended _____

Steps	Possible Points	First Attempt	Second Attempt
1. Remove jewelry (rings and watch).	5		
2. Sanitize hands.	5		
3. Open sterile package's outer wrappings for sterile gloves, sterile towels, and sterile gown.	10		
4. Open the inner packages.	10		
5. Apply hair cover, mask, and goggles.	10		
6. Unfold and apply sterile gown and secure.	10		
7. Apply sterile glove to the nondominant hand.	15		
8. Apply a sterile glove to the dominant hand.	15		
9. Adjust gloves and gown.	10		
10. Maintain sterile technique.	10		

Total Points Possible   100

Comments: Total Points Earned _____ Divided by _____ Total Possible Points = _____ % Score

Instructor's Signature _____

Student Name _____ Date _____

PROCEDURE 41-3: APPLY STERILE GLOVES

TASK: Apply sterile gloves to maintain sterile technique.

CONDITIONS: Given the proper equipment and supplies, the student will apply sterile gloves to maintain sterile technique.

NOTE: The student should practice the procedure using the MACC CD in the back of the textbook and then practice and perform the task in the classroom: MACC CD MACC/Clinical skills/Patient care/Minor office surgery/Donning sterile gloves.

EQUIPMENT AND SUPPLIES
- Supplies for surgical handwashing
- Sterile gloves
- Regular waste container

STANDARDS: Complete the procedure within _____ minutes and achieve a minimum score of _____ %.

Time began _____   Time ended _____

Steps	Possible Points	First Attempt	Second Attempt
1. Remove jewelry (rings and watch).	5		
2. Sanitize hands.	5		
3. Open the sterile glove package's outer wrapping.	10		
4. Open the inner package.	10		
5. Aseptically sanitize the hands.	15		
6. Pick up the sterile glove for the nondominant hand by the cuff.	10		
7. Lift the entire glove from the paper and pull it onto the nondominant hand	10		
8. Adjust the glove for the nondominant hand, being careful to not contaminate the gloved hand.	10		
9. Pick up the sterile glove for the dominant hand, being careful to not touch the fingers and palm of glove.	10		
10. Adjust the glove for the dominant hand.	5		
11. Inspect the gloves for tears.	10		

Total Points Possible   100

Comments: Total Points Earned _____ Divided by _____ Total Possible Points = _____ % Score

Instructor's Signature _____

Student Name _____ Date _____

PROCEDURE 41-4: REMOVE CONTAMINATED GLOVES

TASK: Remove contaminated gloves to avoid spreading contaminants.
CONDITIONS: Given the proper equipment and supplies, the student will properly remove contaminated gloves

EQUIPMENT AND SUPPLIES
- Gloves used in procedure
- Regular waste container
- Biohazardous waste container if gloves are contaminated with blood or body fluid

STANDARDS: Complete the procedure within _____ minutes and achieve a minimum score of _____ %.

Time began _____   **Time ended** _____

Steps	Possible Points	First Attempt	Second Attempt
1. Grasp the outside of dominant hand glove with the first three fingers of the nondominant hand 1 to 2 inches below the cuff.	10		
2. Remove the glove by pulling up to loosen glove.	5		
3. As the glove is pulled free from the hand, ball it in the palm of the gloved hand.	10		
4. Remove the second glove of nondominant hand by placing forefingers of dominant hand under the cuff and turning the glove as it is removed.	10		
5. Carefully dispose of the gloves in a regular or marked biohazardous waste container if the gloves are contaminated with blood or body fluids.	5		
6. Sanitize hands.	10		

Total Points Possible   50

Comments: Total Points Earned _____ Divided by _____ Total Possible Points = _____ % Score

Instructor's Signature _____

Student Name _____ Date _____

PROCEDURE 41-5: OPEN A STERILE PACKAGE

TASK: Open a sterile package, and establish a sterile field.

CONDITIONS: Given the proper equipment and supplies, the student will open a sterile package and create a sterile field.

NOTE: The student should practice the procedure using the MACC CD in the back of the textbook and then practice and perform the task in the classroom: Medical Assisting Competency Challenge CD MACC/Clinical skills/Patient care/Minor office surgery/Establishing sterile field & assisting with minor office surgery.

EQUIPMENT AND SUPPLIES
- MACC CD/computer
- Sterile package
- Mayo stand or other sturdy surface
- Regular waste container

STANDARDS: Complete the procedure within _____ minutes and achieve a minimum score of _____ %.

Time began _____   **Time ended** _____

Steps	Possible Points	First Attempt	Second Attempt
1. Sanitize hands.	5		
2. Verify order, and assemble equipment and supplies.	10		
3. Check the integrity of the sterile package.	10		
4. Position the sterile package.	10		
5. Remove the tape on the sterile package.	10		
6. Open the top flap.	10		
7. Open the side flaps.	10		
8. Do not contaminate the field by touching anything with ungloved or nonsterile hands.	10		
9. Maintain sterility of the inside of the pack and the supplies within the package.	10		

Total Points Possible   85

Comments: Total Points Earned _____ Divided by _____ Total Possible Points = _____ % Score

Instructor's Signature _____

Student Name _____ Date _____

PROCEDURE 41-6: POUR A STERILE SOLUTION

TASK: Add a sterile solution to a sterile field.

CONDITIONS: Given the proper equipment and supplies, the student will add a sterile solution to a sterile field without contaminating the field.

NOTE: The student should practice the procedure using the MACC CD in the back of the textbook and then practice and perform the task in the classroom: Medical Assisting Competency Challenge CD MACC/Clinical skills/Patient care/Minor office surgery/Establishing a sterile field & assisting with minor office surgery.

EQUIPMENT AND SUPPLIES
- MACC CD/computer
- Sterile solution
- Sterile container
- Sterile towel
- Regular waste container

STANDARDS: Complete the procedure within _____ minutes and achieve a minimum score of _____ %.

Time began _____   Time ended _____

Steps	Possible Points	First Attempt	Second Attempt
1. Sanitize hands.	5		
2. Verify orders, and assemble equipment and supplies.	5		
3. Read the label three times to make sure you have the correct solution as with any medication.	10		
4. Palm the label of the bottle.	10		
5. Remove the cap. Set the cap with the opening facing up.	15		
6. Pour a small amount of solution over the lip of the bottle into a waste receptacle for discarding, to wash away possible contaminants on the lip.	15		
7. Pour the solution from a height of 2 to 6 inches above the sterile container.	10		
8. Replace the cap on the bottle.	5		

Total Points Possible   75

Comments: Total Points Earned _____ Divided by _____ Total Possible Points = _____ % Score

Instructor's Signature _____

Student Name _____ Date _____

PROCEDURE 41-7: ASSIST WITH MINOR OFFICE SURGERY

TASK: To provide all equipment, supplies, and materials needed to perform a minor office surgery and assist with the procedure.

CONDITIONS: Given the proper equipment and supplies, the student will assist with preparing and performing in a minor office surgical procedure.

NOTE: The student should practice the procedure using the MACC CD in the back of the textbook and then practice and perform the task in the classroom: MACC CD MACC/Clinical skills/Patient care/Minor office surgery/Establishing a sterile field & assisting with minor office surgery.

EQUIPMENT AND SUPPLIES
- MACC CD/computer
- **Sterile Packs**

Sterile Skin Prep Pack
1 stainless steel bowl
Stack of 20 sterile 4 × 4-inch gauze squares
2 sterile towels

Sterile Drape Pack
1 fenestrated drape or 4 sterile drapes

Typical Sterile "Minor Surgery" Pack
2 tissue forceps
2 mosquito hemostats
2 kelly hemostats
Dressing forceps
Needle holder
Sponge forceps
Sharp/sharp operating scissors
Sharp/blunt operating scissors

Individual Sterile Items (as indicated)
Scalpel with blade appropriate for type of surgery
Fork retractor
3-cc syringe or 10-cc syringe depending on the type of surgery and amount of anesthesia
25-gauge, 5/8- to 1-inch needle or size appropriate for type of surgery
Sterile dressing
Package of suture or staples (physician's preference)
2 packages of sterile 4 × 4-inch gauze squares (20 squares per pack)

- **Additional Supplies**
Bottled sterile water
Bottle chorhexidine gluconate (Hibiclens)
Povidone-iodine (Betadine) swabs or other skin cleanser as preferred by physician
Anesthesia as ordered by physician
Bottle for specimen transport
Sterile gown for physician
Roll of surgical tape
Lister bandage scissors
Conforming bandages
2 packages of proper-sized sterile gloves

2 packages of sterile towels
2 plastic-backed underdrapes
Alcohol wipes
Disposable razor
Hair covers as indicated
Masks
Goggles
Biohazardous waste container
Rigid biohazardous container
Mayo stand
Waterproof waste bag
Signed consent form
Pathology request form
Biohazardous transport bag
Patient's medical record

- **Other Items That May Be Required Depending on Type of Surgery**

Urine specimen container (if a urine sample will be collected)
Patient gown and drapes
Intravenous (IV) equipment and supplies (medication as ordered by physician)
Blood pressure cuff and stethoscope
Tourniquets
Penrose drain
Sterile swabs
Venipuncture equipment (if a blood specimen is required)
Back-up sterile packs

STANDARDS: Complete the procedure within _____ minutes and achieve a minimum score of _____ %.

Time began _____   **Time ended** _____

Steps	Possible Points	First Attempt	Second Attempt
1. Sanitize hands.	5		
2. Verify orders, and assemble equipment and supplies.	5		
3. Greet and identify the patient, and escort the patient to the examination room.	5		
4. Explain the procedure to patient.	5		
5. Obtain written and informed consent for the procedure if not already obtained.	10		
6. Verify compliance of preoperative diet and medication instructions.	5		
7. Position the Mayo stand so that it is within easy reach of the procedure site.	5		
8. Create a sterile field, using a prepackaged sterile drape, and attach a temporary disposal bag to the edge of the Mayo stand.	10		
9. Open sterile packs for surgical hand scrubs and sterile towels in the staging area (not in the examination room).	10		
10. Open a scrub pack in the examination room.	10		
11. Position the patient for the procedure.	5		
12. Perform a surgical scrub of the incision site.	10		

Steps	Possible Points	First Attempt	Second Attempt
13. Drape the area with the fenestrated drape.	10		
14. Remove the contaminated supplies from the room after completing the scrub.	10		
15. Open the sterile packs including physician's gown and set up tray.	10		
16. Assist the physician with surgical gown and gloves.	10		
17. Prepare the anesthetic as ordered by the physician.	10		
18. Hand the physician the antiseptic skin cleanser (povidone-iodine swab) in preparation of the incision site. Ask the patient if he or she has an allergy to shellfish.	10		
19. Assist with sterile items as indicated.	10		
20. Collect the surgical specimen, as required and complete lab requisition form.	10		
21. Monitor the patient during the procedure.	10		
22. Cleanse the surgical site and apply a sterile dressing.	10		
23. Monitor the patient for the next 30 minutes.	10		
24. Clean the examination room by collecting surgical instruments and taking to the staging to rinse and place in soaking solution. Discard solutions as necessary.	15		
25. Any nonsharp disposable items are discarded in the biohazardous waste container.	15		
26. After the patient leaves, sanitize the room.	5		
27. Follow up with the patient.	10		
28. Document the procedure.	10		

Total Points Possible   250

Comments: Total Points Earned _____ Divided by _____ Total Possible Points = _____ % Score

Instructor's Signature _____

Student Name _____ Date _____

PROCEDURE 41-8: REMOVE SUTURES OR STAPLES AND CHANGE A WOUND DRESSING USING A SPIRAL BANDAGE

TASK: To remove sutures from a healed wound as ordered by the physician, apply a sterile dressing to a wound, and apply a bandage using a spiral turn.

CONDITIONS: Given the proper equipment and supplies, the student will role-play removing sutures from a healed wound, apply a sterile dressing to a wound, and apply a spiral turn bandage over a sterile dressing

NOTE: The student should practice the procedure using the MACC CD in the back of the textbook and then practice and perform the task in the classroom: MACC CD MACC/Clinical skills/Patient care/Minor office surgery/Removing sutures & changing a wound dressing using a spiral bandage.

EQUIPMENT AND SUPPLIES
- MACC CD/computer
- Nonsterile disposable gloves
- Sterile suture removal kit or staple removal kit
- Sterile gauze pads in appropriate size for size of wound
- Antiseptic or sterile swabs
- Sterile gloves
- Waterproof waste bag
- Surgical tape
- Scissors
- Biohazardous waste container
- Patient's medical record

STANDARDS: Complete the procedure within _____ minutes and achieve a minimum score of _____ %.

Time began _____   Time ended _____

Steps	Possible Points	First Attempt	Second Attempt
1. Sanitize hands.	5		
2. Verify orders, and assemble equipment and supplies and obtain the patient's medical record.	5		
3. Greet and identify the patient, escort the patient to the examination room, and explain the procedure to the patient.	10		
4. Position on exam table and expose area to be treated.	5		
5. Position the Mayo stand so that it is within easy reach of the procedure site.	5		
6. Create a sterile field, using a prepackaged sterile drape; attach a temporary disposal bag (waterproof waste bag) to the edge of the Mayo stand.	5		
7. Apply nonsterile gloves.	5		
8. Remove the soiled dressing.	10		
9. Check the incision line.	10		

Steps	Possible Points	First Attempt	Second Attempt
10. Discard the contaminated dressing, and gloves. Sanitize the hands once again, and put on sterile gloves to remove the sutures or staples.	10		
11. Cleanse the incision line.	5		
12. Grasp the first suture to be removed. Cut the suture at the skin level away from the suture line.	10		
13. Use the dressing forceps to lift the suture at the knot straight upward, away from the suture line, and out of the skin.	10		
14. Place each suture on the gauze square after being removed, and inspect and count the sutures on the gauze square after being removed. Inspect and count the sutures on the gauze square before discarding them. (Check to be sure the number of sutures applied and the number of sutures removed are the same.)	15		

To Remove Staples

Steps	Possible Points	First Attempt	Second Attempt
15. Carefully place the jaws of the staple remover under the staple to be removed.	10		
16. Firmly squeeze the staple remover handles until they are fully closed.	10		
17. Gently lift the staple remover upward to remove the staple from the incision line.	10		
18. Place the staple on a gauze square.	10		
19. Continue in this manner until all the staples have been removed.	5		
20. Inspect and count the staples on the gauze square before discarding.	10		

Cleansing and Dressing a Wound

Steps	Possible Points	First Attempt	Second Attempt
21. Cleanse the wound with an appropriate solution.	10		
22. Use the sterile gauze squares to absorb excess antiseptic.	10		
23. Apply a sterile dressing to cover and protect the wound and any remaining sutures.	10		
24. Once the wound is covered, remove your gloves and discard in the water-resistant waste container.	10		
25. Sanitize the hands before bandaging the dressing.	5		
26. Bandage the dressing.	10		
27. Use a spiral turn to apply the bandage to the suture site by anchoring the bandage with a circular turn. Then begin the spiral turns being sure to cover the previous turn by one third to one half of the distance. Be sure the turn does not stop on a pressure site.	20		
28. Check the patient's fingers and hand or toes and foot for adequate circulation.	10		
29. Assist the patient to a comfortable position.	5		
30. Instruct the patient when to return for removal of the remaining sutures if applicable.	10		
31. Disinfect the work area.	10		

Steps	Possible Points	First Attempt	Second Attempt
32. Remove gloves and sanitize the hands.	5		
33. Provide the patient with verbal and written wound care instructions.	10		
34. Document the procedure.	10		

Total Points Possible   300

Comments: Total Points Earned _____ Divided by _____ Total Possible Points = _____ % Score

Instructor's Signature _____

Student Name _____ Date _____

PROCEDURE 41-9: APPLY AND REMOVE ADHESIVE SKIN CLOSURES

TASK: Apply and remove a skin closure using a sterile technique.

CONDITIONS: Given the proper equipment and supplies, the student will apply and remove a skin closure using a sterile technique.

EQUIPMENT AND SUPPLIES
- Nonsterile disposable gloves
- Sterile cotton-tipped applicator
- Sterile gloves
- Adhesive skin closure strips
- Antiseptic solution
- Sterile 4 × 4-inch gauze squares
- Sterile dressing forceps
- Surgical tape
- Antiseptic swabs (povidone-iodine [Betadine])
- Tincture of benzoin
- Biohazardous waster container
- Patient's medical record

STANDARDS: Complete the procedure within _____ minutes and achieve a minimum score of _____ %.

Time began _____   Time ended _____

Steps	Possible Points	First Attempt	Second Attempt
1. Sanitize hands.	5		
2. Verify orders, and assemble equipment and supplies.	5		
3. Obtain the patient's medical record.	5		
4. Greet and identify the patient, and escort the patient to the examination room.	5		
5. Explain the procedure to the patient.	5		
6. Position the patient as required and inspect the wound.	5		
7. Position the Mayo stand so that it is within easy reach of the procedure site.	5		
8. Put on disposable gloves.	5		
9. Clean the wound thoroughly using an antiseptic solution and working from the center of the wound outward.	10		
10. Apply tincture of benzoin.	10		
11. Open the sterile adhesive strips.	5		
12. Apply sterile gloves.	5		
13. Verify that the skin surface is dry and position the first strip over the center of the wound.	10		
14. Continue applying adhesive strips from center outward, pulling the wound in the same direction with each strip applied.	10		
15. Apply a dry sterile dressing over the strips, as indicated by the physician.	5		

Steps	Possible Points	First Attempt	Second Attempt
16. Remove gloves and sanitize the hands.	5		
17. Provide the patient with verbal and written wound care instructions as ordered by the physician.	10		
18. Document the procedure.	10		
Removal of Skin Closures			
19. Sanitize hands.	5		
20. Verify orders and assemble equipment and supplies.	5		
21. Obtain the patient's medical record.	5		
22. Greet and identify the patient, and escort the patient to the examination room.	5		
23. Explain the procedure to the patient.	5		
24. Position the patient as required and remove the soiled dressing.	5		
25. Check the incision line.	5		
26. Place a 4 × 4-inch gauze square in close approximation with the wound. Apply clean gloves.	5		
27. Cleanse the site with antiseptic swab and apply a dry sterile dressing as indicated by the physician.	5		
28. Properly dispose of all contaminated supplies.	5		
29. Disinfect the work area.	5		
30. Remove gloves and sanitize hands.	5		
31. Provide the patient with verbal and written wound care instructions.	10		
32. Document the procedure.	10		

Total Points Possible   200

Comments: Total Points Earned _____ Divided by _____ Total Possible Points = _____ % Score

Instructor's Signature _____

CHAPTER QUIZ

Multiple Choice

Identify the letter of the choice that best completes the statement or answers the question.

1. Scissors, biopsy punches, and curettes are _____ instruments.
   A. clamping
   B. dissecting
   C. probing
   D. retracting

2. Scalpel blades range in size from _____.
   A. 5 to 10
   B. 10 to 15
   C. 10 to 25
   D. 10 to 35

3. _____ are two-pronged instruments used for grasping or holding body tissue.
   A. Forceps
   B. Curettes
   C. Retractors
   D. Scissors

4. _____ have delicate, straight blades for cutting through tissue.
   A. Bandage scissors
   B. Dissecting scissors
   C. Operating scissors
   D. Suture scissors

5. _____ does not show a break in the skin.
   A. Closed wound
   B. Open wound
   C. Deep wound
   D. Superficial wound

6. Local anesthetics produce unconsciousness.
   A. True
   B. False

7. _____ occurs when a large wound is not closely approximated and may heal from the base of the wound upward.
   A. Primary intention healing
   B. Secondary intention healing
   C. Tertiary intention healing
   D. None of the above

8. A _____ scalpel blade is used for incision and drainage.
   A. concave
   B. convex
   C. curved
   D. pointed

9. Probes are instruments used to feel inside a body cavity.
   A. True
   B. False

10. _____ drainage consists of serum.
    A. Purulent
    B. Sanguineous
    C. Serous
    D. Serosanguineous

11. Patients must return to the physician's office in approximately _____ days for a dressing change.
    A. 1 to 3
    B. 3 to 5
    C. 5 to 10
    D. 10 to 14

12. _____ is accomplished when a local anesthetic is injected into and around a set of nerves.
    A. Topical anesthesia
    B. Regional anesthesia
    C. General anesthesia
    D. Local anesthesia

13. _____ is a wound that does not extend beyond the subcutaneous layer.
    A. Open
    B. Superficial
    C. Closed
    D. Deep wound

14. The surgical scrub removes dead skin, dirt, and pathogenic microorganisms.
    A. True
    B. False

15. _____ may be used to close wounds.
    A. Band-Aids
    B. Staples
    C. Superglue
    D. All of the above

16. _____ are instruments with serrated rings at the tips used to hold gauze sponges.
    A. Hemostats
    B. Thumb forceps
    C. Sponge forceps
    D. Dressing forceps

17. _____ is used when nonsterile hands never touch the outside of the gown or glove.
    A. Aseptic technique
    B. Closed technique
    C. Open technique
    D. Sterile technique

18. _____ have a sharp, pointed, slender tip used to grasp fine objects.
    A. Hemostats
    B. Thumb forceps
    C. Splinter forceps
    D. Sponge forceps

19. Curettes are instruments used to hold back the edges of a wound.
    A. True
    B. False

20. Surgical asepsis is the highest level of protection for patients.
    A. True
    B. False

CHAPTER **FORTY-TWO**

Patient Education and Nutrition

VOCABULARY REVIEW

Matching

Match each term with the correct definition.

A. affective

B. anorexia

C. antioxidant

D. beriberi

E. bulimia

F. cellulose

G. cognitive

H. dermatitis

I. display panel

J. fad diet

K. glossitis

L. goiter

M. hydrogenated

N. major minerals

O. malabsorption

P. monounsaturated fats

Q. night blindness

R. osteomalacia

_____ 1. Minerals used by the body in small amounts

_____ 2. Chief part of a cell wall

_____ 3. Minerals used in significant amounts by the body

_____ 4. Type of learning based on motor skills to perform tasks

_____ 5. Type of learning based on feelings and emotions

_____ 6. Polyunsaturated fats are made solid

_____ 7. Vitamins not stored in the body

_____ 8. Panel on a label used for marketing purposes

_____ 9. Disease caused by a deficiency of niacin in the body

_____ 10. Condition caused by a lack of vitamin C in the diet

_____ 11. Condition caused by a deficiency of thiamine

_____ 12. Condition caused by a deficiency of vitamin A

_____ 13. Dietary fats that have been broken down into fatty acids and glycerol

S. pellagra

T. psychomotor

U. rickets

V. scurvy

W. synthesize

X. trace minerals

Y. triglycerides

Z. water-soluble vitamins

_____ 14. Diet that is structured to cause quick loss of weight

_____ 15. Inability of the digestive system to absorb required nutrients

_____ 16. Condition in children caused by vitamin D deficiency

_____ 17. Psychological fear of gaining weight; also lack of appetite

_____ 18. Inflammation of the tongue

_____ 19. Inflammation of the skin caused by irritation or riboflavin deficiency

_____ 20. To make or take in

_____ 21. Disorder characterized by compulsive overeating followed by self-induced vomiting or use of laxatives or diuretics

_____ 22. Abnormal bone softening caused by vitamin D deficiency

_____ 23. Type of learning based on what the patient already knows and has experienced

_____ 24. Enlarged thyroid

_____ 25. Substance that acts against oxidizing agents

_____ 26. Fats that are liquid at room temperature and help lower total cholesterol

THEORY RECALL

True/False

Indicate whether the sentence or statement is true or false.

_____ 1. The information on the food label is considered a legal document.

_____ 2. Foods that have been fortified with vitamins and minerals take the place of a well-balanced diet.

_____ 3. Sodium is found naturally in many foods.

_____ 4. Effective patient education is the key to helping patients understand the situation and the need for change.

_____ 5. It is okay for the medical assistant to tell the patient that he or she is not knowledgeable about the material being presented but that they will learn it together.

Multiple Choice

Identify the letter of the choice that best completes the statement or answers the question.

1. The food guide pyramid was developed by the _____.
   A. DHHS
   B. FDA
   C. RDA
   D. USDA

2. Honey is composed of _____% sugar.
   A. 10
   B. 25
   C. 50
   D. 75

3. _____ are organic substances that enhance the breakdown of proteins, carbohydrates, and fat.
   A. Carbohydrates
   B. Minerals
   C. Nutrients
   D. Vitamins

4. Complex carbohydrates supply the _____ with energy.
   A. heart and lungs
   B. muscles and brain
   C. brain and heart
   D. lungs and muscles

5. _____ is a type of learning.
   A. Affective
   B. Cognitive
   C. Psychomotor
   D. All of the above

6. RDAs are the nutritional guidelines that are published as the recommended dietary allowances whose name has been changed to read _____.
   A. recommended daily allowances
   B. daily allowances
   C. daily values
   D. has not been changed and still reads the same

7. _____ is an example of a fat-soluble vitamin.
   A. Vitamin B
   B. Vitamin C
   C. Vitamin K
   D. All of the above

8. _____ mg is the recommended intake of sodium per day.
   A. 1200
   B. 1500
   C. 2000
   D. 2400

9. _____ are liquid at room temperature and may help lower blood cholesterol.
   A. Saturated fats
   B. Monounsaturated fats
   C. Polyunsaturated fats
   D. Fatty acids

10. There are _____ amino acids in protein.
    A. 10
    B. 15
    C. 22
    D. 24

11. The recommended amount of water to ingest is _____ daily.
    A. 16 ounces
    B. 1 quart
    C. 2 quarts
    D. 3 quarts

12. _____ is(are) a group of substances composed of many amino acids linked together.
    A. Proteins
    B. Carbohydrates
    C. Cholesterol
    D. Minerals

13. High-protein diets are often used _____.
    A. before surgery
    B. when an infection is present
    C. with hypothermia
    D. all of the above

14. The daily allowance of saturated fats is _____ grams.
    A. 10
    B. 20
    C. 25
    D. 30

15. A diet low in saturated fats and cholesterol helps to maintain the blood cholesterol at levels below _____.
    A. 100
    B. 200
    C. 250
    D. 300

16. Fad diets can result in _____.
    A. revised eating habits
    B. slowed weight loss
    C. rapid weight loss
    D. long-term weight loss

17. Dietary fats break down into fatty acids and are passed into the blood to form _____.
    A. phospholipids
    B. enzymes
    C. hormones
    D. all of the above

18. The Mayo Clinic considers a person overweight when their body mass index is _____.
    A. 10 to 19.9
    B. 20 to 25.9
    C. 25 to 29.9
    D. 30 to 35.9

19. Which one of the following is not affected by proper nutrition?
    A. hair
    B. teeth
    C. reproduction
    D. all of the above are affected

20. _____ produces quick energy.
    A. Carbohydrates
    B. Protein
    C. Fatty acids
    D. Unsaturated fats

Sentence Completion

Complete each sentence or statement.

1. _____ learning is based on what a person already knows or has experienced.

2. _____ is the scientific study of how different food groups affect the body.

3. _____ vitamins are not stored in the body.

4. _____ are inorganic substances used in the formation of hard and soft body tissue.

5. _____ are usually solid at room temperature.

6. The primary function of _____ is to build and repair tissue and the formation of enzymes.

7. _____ is necessary for vitamin D and bile acid production.

8. _____ are liquid at room temperature and are thought to lower both HDL and LDL

   cholesterol levels.

9. _____ is important for elimination.

10. A person's _____ ability is concerned with the person's emotions and feelings.

Short Answers

1. List the two main panels of a food label and explain each.

   _____

   _____

   _____

   _____

   _____

   _____

2. List and explain the five tips for a balanced diet.

   _____

   _____

   _____

   _____

   _____

3. Explain three conditions a medical assistant should be looking for when doing an inventory of the patient's readiness to follow a new health plan.

   _____

   _____

   _____

CRITICAL THINKING

Select one of the four following diets and make a plan for three meals a day with a morning and afternoon snack diet for 7 days. Each diet should include a calorie count, fat count, carbohydrate count, and salt intake, regardless of which diet is selected.

1. A 1200-calorie diet   3. Low-carbohydrate diet

2. Low-fat diet   4. Low-sodium diet

INTERNET RESEARCH

Keywords: South Beach Diet, Atkins' Diet, Weight Watchers' Diet, Low-Fat Diet

Choose one e topic to research (South Beach Diet; Atkins' Diet; Weight Watchers' Diet; Low-fat diet) or pick a diet you are interested in learning more about. Write a one-page paper describing the advantages and disadvantages of the diet you selected to research. Cite your source. Be prepared to give a 2-minute oral presentation should your instructor assign you to do so.

WHAT WOULD YOU DO?

If you have accomplished the objectives in this chapter, you will be able to make better choices as a medical assistant. Take a look at this situation and decide what you would do.

Josephine, age 52, has just been diagnosed with type 2 diabetes mellitus related to obesity. Living in the home with Josephine are her mother, Susie, who is 80 years old; Josephine's daughter Jessie, who is 24 and pregnant; and Jessie's two very active children, ages 6 and 2. Susie has been diagnosed with a heart condition and must be on a soft diet that is low in cholesterol and sodium restricted.

Josephine's concern today is how she can maintain a diet acceptable for all the medical conditions in the household while being sure the other family members will eat what is prepared. She thinks the children need sugar, but her mother needs to watch her sugar and salt intake to remain in a stable condition and not gain weight. Susie also needs her meals to be soft and easily chewable because of her decreased intestinal motility. However, Jessie and her 2-year-old child both need a diet that allows the necessary fiber for adequate bowel activity.

If you were the medical assistant, how might you educate Josephine about nutrition and answer her questions?

1. **Why are learning styles important for the medical assistant to understand when teaching medical knowledge to the patient?**

   _____

   _____

   _____

2. **Why is it now so important for Josephine to read food labels? What information is found on these?**

   _____

   _____

   _____

   _____

   _____

   _____

3. Why is diet so important for Josephine to follow in the treatment of type 2 diabetes mellitus? Why does she need to know the glycemic index of foods?

_____

_____

_____

_____

_____

_____

4. What special requirements will be needed for Susie so that she maintains a low-cholesterol diet?

_____

_____

_____

_____

_____

_____

5. Jessie's children want to eat pizza and French fries like their friends. How will this affect the dietary changes of Josephine, Susie, and Jessie?

_____

_____

_____

_____

6. Because Jessie has elevated blood pressure and early signs of edema in the legs and feet, what type of diet would you expect her to maintain for the remainder of her pregnancy?

_____

_____

_____

_____

7. **What is found in a diabetic diet? A low-sodium diet?**

_____

_____

_____

_____

_____

_____

8. **What effect would low income have on this family?**

_____

_____

_____

_____

9. **What effect would culture have in planning this diet if the family were of Greek or Italian ethnicity?**

_____

_____

_____

_____

10. **Why is body mass index (BMI) a better guide for obesity than height-weight charts?**

_____

_____

_____

11. Why is it important that Josephine include a variety of foods in the diet for all members of the family?

_____

_____

_____

_____

_____

CHAPTER QUIZ

Multiple Choice

Identify the letter of the choice that best completes the statement or answers the question.

1. _____ are building blocks; byproducts of protein breakdown by enzymes.
   A. Amino acids
   B. Carbohydrates
   C. Major minerals
   D. Trans-fatty acids

2. _____ is learning based on what a person already knows or has experienced.
   A. Affective learning
   B. Cognitive learning
   C. Individual learning
   D. Psychomotor learning

3. Honey is _____% sugar.
   A. 20
   B. 40
   C. 60
   D. 75

4. _____ are chemical substances within food that are released and absorbed during the digestive process.
   A. Minerals
   B. Nutrients
   C. Vitamins
   D. Carbohydrates

5. _____ are in liquid form at room temperature and may help lower total blood cholesterol.
   A. Monounsaturated fats
   B. Polyunsaturated fats
   C. Trans-fatty acids
   D. None of the above

6. A medical assistant pretending to be knowledgeable about a subject is not acceptable.
   A. True
   B. False

7. The acceptable level of saturated fats daily is _____ grams.
   A. 10
   B. 15
   C. 20
   D. 25

8. An adult should consume a minimum of _____ of water a day.
   A. 16 ounces
   B. 32 ounces
   C. 1 quart
   D. 2 quarts

9. Sodium is found naturally in foods.
   A. True
   B. False

10. Cholesterol is necessary for vitamin _____ and bile production.
    A. A
    B. C
    C. D
    D. E

11. A patient undergoing chemotherapy for cancer must have a diet high in _____.
    A. carbohydrates
    B. fats
    C. vitamins
    D. all of the above

12. A body mass index of higher than _____ is considered to be obese.
    A. 20
    B. 30
    C. 40
    D. 50

13. _____ is a condition caused by the body's inability to absorb vitamin B12.
    A. Beriberi
    B. Night blindness
    C. Pellagra
    D. Pernicious anemia

14. The key to patient teaching is not to focus on how to make a patient do something but to create a situation in which the patient will want to do what is needed.
    A. True
    B. False

15. Vitamin _____ is a fat-soluble vitamin.
    A. B6
    B. B12
    C. C
    D. K

16. _____ are inorganic substances used in the formation of soft and hard tissues.
    A. Amino acids
    B. Carbohydrates
    C. Minerals
    D. Vitamins

17. _____ are the building blocks of fat that produce oil.
    A. Fatty acids
    B. Saturated fats
    C. Unsaturated fats
    D. None of the above

18. An infant should be fed between _____ times in a 24-hour period.
    A. 6 and 8
    B. 8 and 12
    C. 10 and 14
    D. 12 and 15

19. A food label is a legal document.
    A. True
    B. False

20. With a diagnosis of cancer, the patient should eat a _____ diet.
    A. full liquid diet
    B. high protein
    C. regular diet
    D. soft diet

CHAPTER **FORTY-THREE**

Basic First Aid and Medical Office Emergencies

VOCABULARY REVIEW

Matching

Match each term with the correct definition.

A. anaphylactic shock

B. automated external defibrillator

C. burn

D. cardiac arrest

E. cerebrovascular accident

F. defibrillation

G. direct pressure

H. epistaxis

I. fracture

J. full-thickness burn

K. Heimlich maneuver

L. hemorrhagic shock

M. hypothermia

N. insulin shock

O. Kussmaul breathing

P. metabolic shock

_____ 1. Severe infection with toxins that prevent blood vessels from constriction, causing blood to pool away from vital organs

_____ 2. Sudden cessation of breathing and heart activity

_____ 3. Not responding to stimuli

_____ 4. Break or crack in a bone caused by trauma or disease

_____ 5. Breathing pattern that begins with very deep, gasping respirations that become rapid and are associated with severe diabetic acidosis and come

_____ 6. Cerebrovascular accident; condition caused by narrowing cerebral vessels; hemorrhage into the brain; and formation of an embolus or thrombus resulting in a lack of blood supply to the brain

_____ 7. Form of hyperthermia caused by dehydration causing a loss of consciousness

_____ 8. Chronic brain disorder in which an individual has seizures

_____ 9. Severe allergic reaction caused by hypersensitivity to a substance

Q. neurogenic shock

R. "rules of nines"

S. seizure

T. splint

U. stoke

V. syncope

W. unconscious

X. septic shock

Y. heat stroke

Z. epilepsy

_____ 10. Methods of evaluating a surface area of a burn; the surface is divided into regions with percentage assigned

_____ 11. Fainting

_____ 12. Firm material used to immobilize above and below a fracture to prevent further damage

_____ 13. Electrical shock to the heart to maintain heart rhythm

_____ 14. Shock caused by inadequate blood supply to tissues as a result of trauma, burns, or internal bleeding

_____ 15. Machine that analyzes a patient's cardiac rhythm and delivers an electric shock if indicated

_____ 16. Loss of nerve control over the circulatory system causing decreased blood supply to an area

_____ 17. Burn that destroys the epidermis and dermis to include the nerve endings; third-degree burn

_____ 18. Decreased body temperature

_____ 19. Injury or destruction of tissue caused by excessive physical heat, chemicals, electricity, or radiation

_____ 20. Sudden involuntary muscle activity leading to a change in level of consciousness and behavior

_____ 21. Lack of oxygen to the brain caused by narrowing or ruptured cerebral vessels

_____ 22. Abdominal thrust used in an emergency to dislodge the cause of a blockage

_____ 23. Nosebleed

_____ 24. Type of shock caused by excessive loss of body fluids and metabolites

_____ 25. Pressure applied directly over a wound

_____ 26. State that occurs when the body has too much insulin and not enough glucose to use the insulin; severe hypoglycemia

THEORY RECALL

True/False

Indicate whether the sentence or statement is true or false.

_____ 1. When a patient is having an epileptic seizure, it is important to place something between the patient's teeth.

_____ 2. Indirect pressure is applied over the wound.

_____ 3. Insulin shock occurs when a patient has taken too much insulin in relation to the amount of food eaten, causing the available glucose to be depleted.

_____ 4. Abdominal thrust is an emergency procedure used to dislodge the cause of a blockage.

_____ 5. All chemical burns should be washed with water immediately.

Multiple Choice

Identify the letter of the choice that best completes the statement or answers the question.

1. _____ occurs when the brain does not receive enough oxygen.
   A. Cerebrovascular accident
   B. Heart attack
   C. Shock
   D. Fainting

2. Epilepsy seizures can be brought on by _____.
   A. low blood sugar
   B. high fever
   C. head trauma
   D. all of the above

3. Arterial blood is _____ color.
   A. bright red
   B. dark red
   C. pale red
   D. none of the above

4. _____ occurs when the body is subjected to excessive heat.
   A. Heat exhaustion
   B. Heat stroke
   C. Sunstroke
   D. Hypothermia

5. _____ is a fracture of a bone that does not break but bends the bone.
   A. Compound
   B. Greenstick
   C. Simple
   D. Open

6. _____ can lead to ketoacidosis.
   A. Infection
   B. Glucose overload
   C. Common cold
   D. All of the above

7. With infant CPR, the medical assistant needs to give _____ compressions, at a rate of 100 per minute, to _____ ventilation.
   A. 3:1
   B. 5:1
   C. 8:1
   D. 10:1

8. When a patient feels lightheaded, the medical assistant needs to _____.
   A. stand the patient up
   B. have the patient lower head to knee level
   C. help patient to lithotomy position
   D. place a warm compress on forehead

9. _____ occurs when one end of a bone is separated from its original position in a joint.
   A. Dislocation
   B. Fracture
   C. Sprain
   D. Strain

10. A patient who is having a CVA will complain of _____.
    A. lightheadedness
    B. warm tingly sensation
    C. sudden confusion
    D. difficulty concentrating

11. Epistaxis can be caused by _____.
    A. low altitude
    B. upper respiratory infection
    C. hypotension
    D. exercise

12. _____ is when the cardiac muscle can no longer pump blood throughout the body.
    A. Cardiogenic shock
    B. Hemorrhagic shock
    C. Insulin shock
    D. Septic shock

13. The body temperature of a person with heat exhaustion is _____.
    A. 100° to 102°
    B. 101° to 102°
    C. 102° to 103°
    D. 103° to 104°

14. With a sprain, the RICE treatment must begin within _____.
    A. 10 to 20 minutes
    B. 30 minutes
    C. 45 minutes
    D. 1 hour

15. Treatment for hypothermia requires the body part to be gradually warmed in water, which should not exceed _____ degrees.
    A. 99
    B. 100
    C. 105
    D. 108

Sentence Completion

Complete each sentence or statement.

1. _____ is the temporary care given to an injured or ill person until the victim can be

   provided complete emergency treatment.

2. _____ is a temporary loss of consciousness caused by an inadequate blood supply

   to the brain.

3. _____ is a progressive circulatory collapse of the body brought on by insufficient blood

   flow to all parts of the body.

4. _____ is the loss of blood from a ruptured, punctured, or cut blood vessel.

5. _____ occurs when the body is subjected to high temperatures and humidity for a long

   period of time.

6. A(n) _____ immobilizes an affected body part and can be made from any available firm

   material.

7. Respirations that become very deep and gasping and then become rapid is known

   as _____ breathing.

8. _____ is an injury to or destruction of body tissue caused by excessive physical heat.

Short Answers

1. Explain the symptoms of a heart attack.

_____

_____

_____

2. List the four steps in wound care.

_____

_____

_____

_____

3. Explain what the acronym RICE stands for.

_____

_____

_____

CRITICAL THINKING

You and a friend are out on a lunch-time jog when she starts complaining of shortness of breath. You both write it off as being out of shape and continue. Once back at the office, you notice your friend's lips are bluish in color and her skin tone is gray. You ask her if she is feels okay. She states she is sweaty and her chest feels a little heavy. What would you do next? Explain what the friend's statement tells you.

INTERNET RESEARCH

Keyword: Poisons

Choose one of the following topics to research: Inhaled poisons—Ingested poisons. Give examples and remedies. Cite your source. Be prepared to give a 2-minute oral presentation should your instructor assign you to do so.

WHAT WOULD YOU DO?

If you have accomplished the objectives in this chapter, you will be able to make better choices as a medical assistant. Take a look at this situation and decide what you would do.

Mariah has type 1 diabetes mellitus and takes insulin on a regular basis. Dr. Naguchi is aware that Mariah does not follow her diet as she should and that her exercise habits are not consistent, so her diabetes is often not stable.

Mariah lives in the southern United States, where it is currently 100° F outside and very humid. Earlier today, Mariah was in the garden gathering vegetables. Later she started canning the vegetables. Her house has minimal air-conditioning. In her haste to complete what needed to be done in the garden, Mariah did not eat her lunch as she should have, although she took her entire dose of insulin.

During the afternoon Mariah began to feel weak, experiencing dizziness and sweating, and her skin felt cool and clammy. Don, her husband, drove her the three blocks to Dr. Naguchi's office because she started complaining of chest pain and difficulty breathing. As soon as she arrives, Mariah appears to faint and falls, injuring her left ankle. As the medical assistant, Janis is the first health care professional to see what is happening to Mariah. After seeing Mariah, Dr. Naguchi orders an x-ray of her ankle to see whether she has a sprain, strain, or fracture.

If you were in Janis's place, would you know what to do in this situation?

1. **What are the external factors that could have caused the symptoms that Mariah showed?**

2. **How should Janis handle this problem when several persons are in the waiting room with Don and Mariah?**

3. **What questions should Janis immediately ask Don?**

4. **What recent activities could have contributed to Mariah's problems?**

_____

_____

_____

_____

_____

5. **If Mariah fainted and you were the medical assistant, what would you do for her immediately while someone was notifying the physician?**

_____

_____

_____

_____

_____

6. **Knowing that Mariah has diabetes, what might you think happened, and what would you expect Dr. Naguchi to order for her?**

_____

_____

_____

_____

_____

7. **Why would you be suspicious of hyperthermia? What should Janis do for these symptoms?**

_____

_____

_____

_____

_____

_____

8. **What symptoms does Mariah have that might indicate a heart attack?**

_____

_____

_____

_____

_____

9. **How do a sprain, strain, and fracture differ, and how is each treated? What treatment is common to all three conditions?**

_____

_____

_____

_____

_____

_____

_____

_____

APPLICATION OF SKILLS

1. Perform Procedure 43-1: Perform the Heimlich Maneuver

2. Perform Procedure 43-2: Open an Airway

3. Perform Procedure 43-3: Perform Rescue Breathing

4. Perform Procedure 43-4: Perform One-Person Adult CPR

5. Perform Procedure 43-5: Perform Two-Person Adult CPR

6. Perform Procedure 43-6: Perform One-Person Infant CPR

Student Name _____ Date _____

PROCEDURE 43-1: PERFORM THE HEIMLICH MANEUVER

TASK: Remove airway obstruction.

CONDITIONS: Given the proper equipment and supplies, the student will demonstrate the Heimlich maneuver to remove airway obstruction to an adult.

EQUIPMENT AND SUPPLIES
* Nonsterile disposable gloves (optional for practice)
* Pocket ventilation mask (optional for practice)
* Adult-sized CPR mannequin (approved for FBAO practice)

STANDARDS: Complete the procedure within _____ minutes and achieve a minimum score of _____%.

Time began _____   Time ended _____

Steps	Possible Points	First Attempt	Second Attempt
1. Assess the victim.	5		
2. Ask, "Are you choking?" If affirmative response, ask, "Can you speak?" If unable to speak, reassure victim that you are going to help.	10		
3. Position yourself behind the victim with feet slightly apart.	5		
4. Wraps arms around the body just above waist with the fist and thumb against the abdomen, above umbilicus, and below sternum.	5		
5. Grasp your fist with your other hand and place the thumb of that fist toward the victim.	5		
6. Firmly press your fist into the victim's abdomen with a quick inward and upward thrust.	5		
7. Repeat thrusts until the obstruction is removed or until the victim becomes unconscious.	5		
8. If the victim becomes unconscious or unresponsive, immediately activate the emergency response system.	5		
9. Apply gloves if available (optional during practice), and open the victim's mouth to perform a finger sweep.	15		
10. Begin ventilation by opening the victim's airway using the head-tilt, chin-lift or jaw thrust. Use a protective barrier.	10		
11. Provide the victim with two slow breaths. If ventilation is unsuccessful, reposition the head and try again.	10		
12. Position yourself for abdominal thrusts by moving toward the victim's feet and straddling the victim across the thighs.	10		
13. Position the heel of one hand above the navel but below the xiphoid process. Place the other hand on top of the first hand. Lift fingers off the victim's abdomen.	15		

Steps	Possible Points	First Attempt	Second Attempt
14. Administer five abdominal thrusts.	10		
15. Return to the victim's head, reposition the head, and perform a finger sweep.	5		
16. If the obstruction has not released, repeat steps 10 and 11 until EMS personnel arrive or the obstruction is expelled.	5		
17. If the obstruction is expelled, monitor the victim's breathing and circulation. If the victim has a pulse but is not breathing, perform rescue breathing. If the victim is not breathing and has no pulse, initiate CPR.	15		
18. Remain with the victim until he or she has stabilized or EMS personnel assume responsibility for the victim.	10		

Total Points Possible   150

Comments: Total Points Earned _____ Divided by _____ Total Possible Points = _____ % Score

Instructor's Signature _____

Student Name _____ Date _____

PROCEDURE 43-2: OPEN AN AIRWAY

TASK: Open the airway of an unresponsive victim using head-tilt, chin-lift or jaw thrust maneuver.
CONDITIONS: Given the proper equipment and supplies, the student will demonstrate opening an airway
to restore breathing to an adult.

EQUIPMENT AND SUPPLIES
• Nonsterile disposable gloves (optional for practice)
• Adult-sized CPR mannequin (approved for FBAO practice)

STANDARDS: Complete the procedure within _____ minutes and achieve a minimum score of _____%.

Time began _____   **Time ended** _____

Steps	Possible Points	First Attempt	Second Attempt
1. Assess the environment for safety issues.	5		
Head-Tilt, Chin-Lift Maneuver			
2. Tilt the head.	5		
3. Apply gentle pressure to the forehead while lifting the chin upward until the teeth are touching but the mouth is not completely closed.	5		
4. Look, listen, and feel for air movement. If there is no air movement, proceed with rescue breathing.	5		
Jaw Thrust Maneuver			
5. Position yourself above the victim's head.	5		
6. Place both thumbs on the victim's cheekbones, and place the index and middle fingers on both sides of the lower jaw where it angles toward the ear.	5		
7. While using the cheekbones to stabilize the head, lift the jaw upward, without tilting the head or flexing the cervical spine.	10		
8. Look, listen, and feel for air movement. If there is no air movement, proceed with rescue breathing.	10		
Total Points Possible	50		

Comments: Total Points Earned _____ Divided by _____ Total Possible Points = _____ % Score

Instructor's Signature _____

Student Name _____ **Date** _____

PROCEDURE 43-3: PERFORM RESCUE BREATHING

TASK: Perform rescue breathing.
CONDITIONS: Given the proper equipment and supplies, the student will demonstrate rescue breathing.

EQUIPMENT AND SUPPLIES
• Nonsterile disposable gloves (optional for practice)
• Pocket ventilation mask (optional for practice)
• Adult-sized CPR mannequin (approved for FBAO practice)

STANDARDS: Complete the procedure within _____ minutes and achieve a minimum score of _____%.

Time began _____   **Time ended** _____

Steps	Possible Points	First Attempt	Second Attempt
1. Assess the environment for safety issues.	5		
2. Establish responsiveness. Tap the victim on the shoulder and shout, "Are you OK?" Wait for a response. If no response, proceed with rescue breathing.	15		
3. Look, listen, and feel for breathing. Assess for 5 seconds.	10		
4. Open the airway with the head-tilt, chin-lift or jaw thrust maneuver.	10		
5. Once the need for rescue breathing has been established, alert EMS.	10		
6. Seal your mouth or mask completely around the victim's mouth while pinching the nose and maintaining the airway. Deliver two slow breaths while observing for chest to rise out of the corner of your eye. Each breath should take 1.5 to 2 seconds to deliver.	20		
7. Assess for circulation. If pulse is present, administer one breath every 5 seconds for an adult and one breath every 3 seconds for an infant or child until the victim begins to breathe adequately.	15		
8. If breathing does not resume, continue with steps 3 and 4 until EMS arrives and assumes responsibility.	15		

Total Points Possible   100

Comments: Total Points Earned _____ Divided by _____ Total Possible Points = _____ % Score

Instructor's Signature _____

Student Name _____ Date _____

PROCEDURE 43-4: PERFORM ONE-PERSON ADULT CPR

TASK: Perform one-person CPR on an adult.
CONDITIONS: Given the proper equipment and supplies, the student will demonstrate the proper procedure to perform one-person adult CPR.

EQUIPMENT AND SUPPLIES
- Nonsterile disposable gloves (optional for practice)
- Pocket ventilation mask (optional for practice)
- Adult-sized CPR mannequin

STANDARDS: Complete the procedure within _____ minutes and achieve a minimum score of _____%.

Time began _____   Time ended _____

Steps	Possible Points	First Attempt	Second Attempt
1. Assess the environment for safety issues.	5		
2. Establish responsiveness. Tap the victim on the shoulder and shout, "Are you OK?" Wait for a response. If no response, proceed with rescue breathing.	15		
3. Look, listen, and feel for breathing. Assess for 5 seconds.	10		
4. Open the airway with the head-tilt, chin-lift or jaw thrust maneuver.	5		
5. Once the need for rescue breathing has been established, alert EMS.	10		
6. Seal your mouth or mask completely around the victim's mouth while pinching the nose and maintaining the airway.	5		
7. Deliver two smooth breaths while observing for chest rise out of the corner of your eye. Each breath should take 1.5 to 2 seconds to deliver.	15		
8. Assess for circulation. Check the carotid pulse for at least 5 seconds. If no pulse, place index and middle fingers of the dominant hand along the margins of the ribs, and then slide up the breastbone. Place the heel of the dominant hand at the base of the breastbone and place the heel of the other hand directly over the hand on the sternum; interlock fingers.	15		
9. Perform four cycles of 15 compressions to every 2 ventilations by rocking from the hip and compressing the sternum 1½ to 2 inches at a rate of 80 to 100 per minute. Count out loud " and 2 and 3 and 4 and so on."	15		

Steps	Possible Points	First Attempt	Second Attempt
10. Maintain correct body position with arms straight and shoulders, elbows, and the heels of your hands in alignment directly over the victim's sternum.	15		
11. Recheck the pulse after every four cycles.	15		
12. Continue CPR until the victim stabilized or EMS personnel arrive and assume responsibility.	10		
13. If pulse and breathing return, place person in the rescue position.	15		

Total Points Possible   150

Comments: Total Points Earned _____ Divided by _____ Total Possible Points = _____ % Score

Instructor's Signature _____

Student Name _____ Date _____

PROCEDURE 43-5: PERFORM TWO-PERSON ADULT CPR

TASK: Perform two-person adult CPR.
CONDITIONS: Given the proper equipment and supplies, the student will demonstrate competency performing two-person CPR on an adult.

EQUIPMENT AND SUPPLIES
- Nonsterile disposable gloves (optional for practice)
- Pocket ventilation mask (optional for practice)
- Adult-sized CPR mannequin

STANDARDS: Complete the procedure within _____ minutes and achieve a minimum score of _____%.

Time began _____   Time ended _____

Steps	Possible Points	First Attempt	Second Attempt
1. Assess the environment for safety issues.	5		
2. Establish responsiveness. Tap the victim on the shoulder and shout, "Are you OK?" Wait for a response. If no response, proceed with rescue breathing.	15		
3. Look, listen, and feel for breathing. Assess for 5 seconds.	10		
4. Open the airway with the head-tilt, chin-lift or jaw thrust maneuver.	5		
5. Once the need for rescue breathing has been established, alert EMS.	10		
6. Seal your mouth or mask completely around the victim's mouth while pinching the nose and maintaining the airway.	5		
7. Deliver two smooth breaths while observing for chest rise out of the corner of your eye. Each breath should take 1.5 to 2 seconds to deliver.	10		
8. Assess for circulation. Check the carotid pulse for at least 5 seconds. If no pulse, place index and middle fingers of the dominant hand along the margins of the ribs, and then slide up the breastbone. Place the heel of the dominant hand at the base of the breastbone and place the heel of the other hand directly over the hand on the sternum; interlock fingers.	15		
9. The person performing compression performs the compressions at a rate of 5 compressions to 1 ventilation.	15		
10. Maintain correct body position with arms straight and shoulders, elbows, and the heels of your hands in alignment directly over the victim's sternum.	15		
11. The carotid pulse is checked after the first minute and every few minutes thereafter.	10		

Steps	Possible Points	First Attempt	Second Attempt
12. The positions may be changed to prevent exhaustion of the providers. To do so, the person performing ventilation delivers a breath as usual and then moves into position to do compressions and the second person moves in to perform ventilation.	15		
13. Continue with CPR until the victim stabilizes or EMS personnel arrive and assume responsibility.	5		
14. If pulse and breathing return, place person in rescue position.	15		

Total Points Possible   150

Comments: Total Points Earned _____ Divided by _____ Total Possible Points = _____ % Score

Instructor's Signature _____

Student Name _____ **Date** _____

PROCEDURE 43-6: PERFORM ONE-PERSON INFANT CPR

TASK: Perform one-person infant CPR.
CONDITIONS: Given the proper equipment and supplies, the student will demonstrate competency
in performing CPR to an infant.

EQUIPMENT AND SUPPLIES
- Nonsterile disposable gloves (optional for practice)
- Pocket ventilation mask (optional for practice)
- Infant-sized CPR mannequin

STANDARDS: Complete the procedure within _____ minutes and achieve a minimum score of _____%.

Time began _____ **Time ended** _____

Steps	Possible Points	First Attempt	Second Attempt
1. Establish unresponsiveness.	5		
2. Gently shake or click the sole of the foot. If unresponsive, position the infant for CPR.	10		
3. Look, listen, and feel for breathing.	5		
4. Check for an open airway using the head-tilt, chin-lift maneuver.	5		
5. If the infant is not breathing, maintain head position, make a seal over the infant's mouth and nose, and give two breaths. Observe chest rise and fall. If the chest does not rise, reposition the infant and reopen the airway. Attempt rescue breathing again. If the chest still does not rise and there is no air exchange, suspect a blocked airway. Open the airway by performing 2 back blows, 2 finger abdominal thrusts; repeat this step until airway is open.	15		
6. Give two slow breaths.	10		
7. Assess circulation by palpating the brachial artery.	10		
8. If no pulse, perform compressions by placing middle and ring fingers in the midline and one finger below the nipple line. Depress the lower sternum 1/2 to 1 inch at a rate of 100 compressions per minute. After each 5 compressions, give one breath.	15		
9. Maintain correct body position while performing chest compressions.	5		
10. Perform CPR for 1 minute and check pulse.	10		
11. Activate EMS.	15		
12. Continue with chest compressions and breaths. Recheck the pulse very minute.	5		

Steps	Possible Points	First Attempt	Second Attempt
13. Continue with CPR until the victim stabilizes or EMS arrives and assumes responsibility.	10		
14. Place in recovery position on left side if pulse and breathing return.	5		

Total Points Possible   125

Comments: Total Points Earned _____ Divided by _____ Total Possible Points = _____ % Score

Instructor's Signature _____

CHAPTER QUIZ:

Multiple Choice:

Identify the letter of the choice that best completes the statement or answers the question.

1. _____ can lead to ketoacidosis.
    A. Infection
    B. Common cold
    C. Glucose overload
    D. All of the above

2. With vein damage, the color of the external bleeding will be _____.
    A. bright red
    B. light red
    C. dark red
    D. pale red

3. _____ shock is when there is a loss of nerve control over the circulatory system, causing decreased blood supply to an area.
    A. Insulin
    B. Metabolic
    C. Neurogenic
    D. Psychogenic

4. Patients who are being seen for heat exhaustion will have a core temperature of _____ degrees.
    A. 99 to 101
    B. 101 to 102
    C. 102 to 103
    D. 103 to 104

5. When performing adult CPR, the first thing that must happen is _____.
    A. to start compressions
    B. to call 911
    C. to rescue breath
    D. to call for help

6. A sprain is a full or partial tear of a ligament.
    A. True
    B. False

7. _____ is a form of hyperthermia marked with pale, cool, and clammy skin.
    A. Shock
    B. Heat exhaustion
    C. Heat stroke
    D. None of the above

8. _____ burn is a burn that destroys the epidermis and dermis, including the nerve endings.
    A. Full-thickness
    B. First-degree
    C. Second-degree
    D. Minor

9. Heimlich maneuver should be done only on conscious patients with an airway obstruction.
   A. True
   B. False

10. A child must be older than _____ years to feel for the carotid pulse as a part of CPR.
    A. 1
    B. 3
    C. 5
    D. 7

11. When one end of bone is separated from its original position in a joint, it is called _____.
    A. dislocation
    B. fracture
    C. strain
    D. sprain

12. When warming an area due to frostbite, the warming solutions should be no warmer than _____ degrees.
    a. 105
    b. 120
    c. 125
    d. 130

13. A(n) _____ fracture pierces through the skin.
    A. closed
    B. open
    C. greenstick
    D. compound

14. Treatment for a sprain should begin within _____ minutes.
    A. 10 to 20
    B. 15 to 30
    C. 20 to 40
    D. 30 to 45

15. When a patient has an epileptic seizure, it is important to remember not to place anything between the patients's teeth as it could become an airway obstruction.
    A. True
    B. False

CHAPTER FORTY-FOUR

Beginning Your Job Search

VOCABULARY REVIEW

Matching

Match each term with the correct definition.

A. chronological resume

B. cover letter

C. employment agencies

D. functional resume

E. heading

F. job application

G. job interview

H. networking

I. objective

J. placement service

K. references

L. resume

_____ 1. Agencies that assist job seekers in finding employment

_____ 2. Type of resume that lists education and job experience from most recent to earliest

_____ 3. Document that provides an employer with the work history and personal information about a potential employee

_____ 4. Form that, when completed, provides information about the person applying for employment

_____ 5. Part of a resume that states the career goal(s) of the person looking for employment

_____ 6. Agencies that charge a fee to an individual for finding employment or to an employer for finding an employee

_____ 7. Verbal, face-to-face interaction that allows the employer to form an impression about the job applicant

_____ 8. Resume section that includes the demographics about the applicant

_____ 9. List of people who can vouch for the job seeker's characteristics and work habits; can be provided to a potential employer on request

_____ 10. Job tool that serves to introduce an applicant to the person in charge of screening resumes for employment opportunities

_____ 11. Interacting with people met through various professional, education, and social activities to assist in job search

_____ 12. Type of resume that relates the person's skills to the type of employment sought

THEORY RECALL

True/False

Indicate whether the sentence or statement is true or false.

_____ 1. The classifieds can only list medical assistants in the medical section of the "Help Wanted" section of the newspaper.

_____ 2. All schools have a placement service to help students find jobs.

_____ 3. Networking is only for professional office personnel.

_____ 4. Greet your interviewer with direct eye contact.

_____ 5. A resume needs to pique a potential employer's interest.

Multiple Choice

Identify the letter of the choice that best completes the statement or answers the question.

1. Answer all questions at an interview _____.
   A. honestly
   B. with what you think they want to hear
   C. with one-word answers
   D. none of the above

2. When writing your cover letter, it is okay to _____.
   A. rely on the computer to correct spelling
   B. not correct errors because the employer will not notice
   C. have two people proofread it
   D. ask the receptionist at the interview to proof it

3. The objective section of a resume should be reflective of _____.
   A. the demographic information of the applicant
   B. the career goal of the applicant
   C. the educational history of the applicant
   D. references available to the applicant

4. Ads will describe _____ of the position.
   A. duties
   B. hours
   C. pay scale
   D. location

5. The medical assistant who practices patient-centered professionalism means being _____.
   A. diligent
   B. responsible
   C. honest
   D. all of the above

6. The medical assistant should be _____ when an interview does not result in a job offer.
   A. disappointed
   B. angry
   C. encouraged to improve
   D. all of the above

7. A follow-up note/thank-you note should be sent to the interviewer following an interview _____.
   A. always
   B. only if you think it went well
   C. does not matter if you do or do not
   D. only when you think it went badly

8. The impression that will be remembered by the interviewer is _____.
   A. the first 10 seconds of the interview
   B. the follow-up
   C. when the applicant is leaving the interview
   D. the interaction during the interview

9. Your _____ is a major part of your overall image.
   A. communication style
   B. attire
   C. hairstyle
   D. none of the above

10. When interviewing over the telephone, make sure you have _____.
    A. a second person listening on another line
    B. a pen and paper
    C. soft music playing in the background
    D. used a cellphone so it cannot be traced

11. The medical assistant will need to revise his or her cover letter _____.
    A. once a year
    B. only when changing jobs
    C. for each job interview
    D. never if you have a well-written cover letter

12. A cover letter should be _____.
    A. accurate
    B. brief
    C. concise
    D. all of the above

13. When developing your resume, it is a good practice to _____.
    A. inform your reference names that you are interviewing and that they may be called
    B. ask for permission to include a potential references name on your resume
    C. not include references on your resume; it is not required and you need to provide them only if you are hired
    D. all of the above are correct

14. A private employment agency _____.
    A. does not charge a placement fee
    B. charges only the client a placement fee
    C. charges only the employer a placement fee
    D. can charge the employer and/or the potential employee

15. Larger facilities will list employment opportunities _____.
    A. with an employment agency only
    B. only in the newspaper
    C. on a telephone hotline
    D. only within the company

Sentence Completion

Complete each sentence or statement.

1. _____ is interacting with contacts or people you have met through various professional, educational, and social activities.

2. A(n) _____ accompanies a resume and basically introduces the medical assistant to the person in charge of screening job applicants.

3. _____ argue about salary when you think it is too low.

4. A(n) _____ should be a win-win situation for both the employer and applicant.

5. _____ is a type of resume that relates the person's skill to the type of employment sought.

6. _____ is(are) a list of people who can vouch for the job seeker's character and work habits.

7. _____ is a form that, when completed, provides information about the person applying for employment.

8. The _____ is the part of a resume that states the career goals of the person looking for employment.

Short Answers

1. List the five information sections of a resume.

_____

_____

_____

_____

_____

2. List the four ways to contact an employer.

_____

_____

_____

_____

3. List the seven traits that a job interviewer will remember about an applicant.

_____

_____

_____

_____

_____

_____

_____

CRITICAL THINKING

You are a newly graduated medical assistant and are very excited to be entering the medical workforce. After doing a job search on a medical Website, you find the job of your dreams. You have a resume from last summer that is not updated to reflect your most recent accomplishments. Even so, you decide it is better to get your resume there quickly; instead of taking the time to rewrite it you decide to Fax it to the potential employer.

Describe your thoughts on this approach and support your answer.

INTERNET RESEARCH

Keyword: Current Resume Styles

Choose one of the following topics to research: Reverse Chronological Resume; Functional Resumes. Cite your source. Be prepared to give a 2-minute oral presentation should your instructor assign you to do so.

WHAT WOULD YOU DO?

If you have accomplished the objectives in this chapter, you will be able to make better choices as a medical assistant. Take a look at this situation and decide what you would do.

Dora has recently completed a medical assisting program and will be looking for new employment as a medical assistant in an ambulatory care setting. As she begins her search, she goes to the school placement office to see if the counselor knows of any jobs in the area. The counselor, Ms. Smith, states that she is unaware of any openings at present but will keep Dora in mind should someone call.

Next, Dora turns to the newspaper ads. She writes her resume and cover letter quickly because she is excited about a position she saw advertised in the classifieds. She is typically good at writing, so she does not bother to ask a friend to proofread her resume and cover letter this time. (After all, it would only slow her down.) She is in such a hurry to apply for the job in the newspaper that she does not proofread or spell-check her materials. As a result, several words are misspelled, and the information that is supposed to be in chronological order is not.

Despite the errors on Dora's resume and cover letter, she obtains an interview with a potential employer. When she arrives, she is surprised that the employer expects her to complete an application before the interview. After completing the application, she answers the employer's interview questions and asks a few of her own. Overall, she has a good feeling about this interview.

After the interview, Dora returns home and waits to hear from the potential employer, taking no further action and hoping that she has been chosen for the job.

Do you think Dora would be hired for this job? What would you have done differently?

1. **What are the advantages of using a newspaper ad?**

   _____

   _____

   _____

2. **With whom would you network when seeking employment in your area?**

   _____

   _____

   _____

3. **If you were the employer, how would you feel about a resume that had misspelled words? Would you still consider hiring this person?**

_____

_____

_____

_____

4. **Who should proofread a resume? Why?**

_____

_____

_____

5. **Why is the order of work experience on a resume important?**

_____

_____

_____

_____

6. **If an ad requests that an applicant apply "in person" and you send a Fax or e-mail, do you think the employer would consider your application? Explain your answer.**

_____

_____

_____

_____

_____

7. **Why is a cover letter so important?**

_____

_____

_____

_____

8. Why do you think that an employer may ask applicants to complete an application at the interview? What do you need to do to make a good impression on the application?

_____

_____

_____

_____

_____

9. Why is a thank-you letter after an interview important?

_____

_____

_____

_____

10. Do you think you would have been chosen for the job if you had made the above mistakes? Explain your answer.

_____

_____

_____

_____

_____

APPLICATION OF SKILLS

1. Write a cover letter.

2. Write a resume.

3. Write a reference sheet.

4. Write a thank-you card.

CHAPTER QUIZ

Multiple Choice

Identify the letter of the choice that best completes the statement or answers the question.

1. A chronological resume is a type of resume that lists education and job experience from most recent to earliest.
   A. True
   B. False

2. _____ is a job tool that serves to introduce an applicant to the person in charge of screening resumes for employment opportunities.
   A. Cover letter
   B. Job application
   C. Resume
   D. Interview

3. _____ is a document given to the interviewer to provide him or her with an applicant's work history and personal information.
   A. Job application
   B. Cover letter
   C. Resume
   D. Reference sheet

4. An ad may describe the potential employee's _____, duties, and desired characteristics.
   A. hours
   B. qualifications
   C. pay scale
   D. location

5. Public employment agencies _____.
   A. charge a fee to the applicant who is looking for a job
   B. charge a fee to the employer who is hiring
   C. offer free placement service
   D. none of the above

6. Networking is interacting with people you have met through various professional, educational, and social activities.
   A. True
   B. False

7. The cover letter should be _____.
   A. updated every year
   B. updated for each job applied for
   C. updated only when changing jobs
   D. it is not necessary to update

8. When a telephone interview is done, the applicant should _____.
   A. have music in the background
   B. use a cell phone only
   C. have a pen and paper available
   D. none of the above

9. Typical information asked on a job application might be _____.
    A. age of children
    B. Social Security number
    C. references
    D. next of kin

10. The applicant should answer questions _____.
    A. with what you think the employer wants to hear
    B. completely
    C. with one-word answers
    D. with excitement

11. The cover letter is what the employer most wants to read.
    A. True
    B. False

12. When using a person as a reference, the applicant should _____.
    A. ask permission before putting them on the list
    B. tell them you are using them
    C. there is no need to tell them about it
    D. none of the above

13. When the applicant is not offered a job, he or she should _____.
    A. be angry
    B. learn from the experience
    C. be disappointed
    D. be happy

14. To send a follow-up note is strictly the applicant's decision.
    A. True
    B. False

15. When greeting your interviewer, the applicant should _____.
    A. have a firm handshake
    B. not look them in the eyes
    C. lead the conversation
    D. have dressed flashy